PRENATAL DIAGNOSIS AND SCREENING FOR DOWN SYNDROME

Edited by **Subrata Dey**

Prenatal Diagnosis and Screening for Down Syndrome
Edited by Subrata Dey

Published by InTech
Janeza Trdine 9, 51000 Rijeka, Croatia

Publishing Process Manager Romina Krebel

Technical Editor Teodora Smiljanic

Cover Designer InTech Design Team

Additional hard copies can be obtained from orders@intechopen.com

Prenatal Diagnosis and Screening for Down Syndrome, Edited by Subrata Dey
p. cm.
ISBN 978-953-307-355-2

For EU product safety concerns:
IN TECH d.o.o., Prolaz Marije Krucifikse Kozulić 3, 51000 Rijeka, Croatia,
info@intechopen.com or visit our website at intechopen.com.

Meet the editor

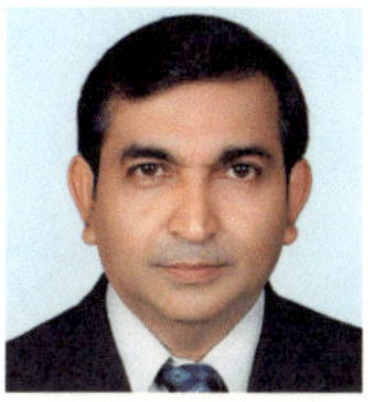

Subrata Dey was born in India and grew up in the state of Assam. He received his Ph.D. from the University of Kalyani, West Bengal. He joined the faculty of West Bengal University of Technology as Professor of Biotechnology in 2005. In 2006 he became the Director of the School of Biotechnology and Biological Sciences. His laboratory has long been involved in research on Genetics of Down syndrome & other congenital disorders, Genetics of Alzheimer's disease, radiation induced genomic instability, radioprotection by antioxidants & stem cell biology. He has been teaching courses in Genetics, Molecular Biology, Evolution & Developmental Biology for more than thirty years. Prof. Dey received golden jubilee award of excellence from Presidency College (Presidency University), Kolkata, in recognition of his contributions to undergraduate and post graduate teaching. He is also the founder Director of the Centre for Genetic Counselling. Prof. Dey is the author of many scientific papers resulting from research funded by University Grants Commission, Council of Scientific & Industrial Research, Inter-University Accelerator Centre, National Tea Research Foundation & Department of Biotechnology.

Contents

Preface

This book features up-to-date, well referenced research and review articles on Down syndrome. It provides a concise yet comprehensive source of current information on behaviour and learning, orthopaedic features, congenital heart disease and acute lymphoblastic leukemia in individuals with Down syndrome. Development of multimedia softwares and artificial intelligence techniques plays an important role in the learning process of Down syndrome. Attention has been focussed on the present status of research on prenatal diagnosis of Down syndrome with the subsequent option of termination of pregnancy. Down syndrome has been and continues to be a central focus of prenatal testing technology due to its high frequency of live births.

Over the last three decades, prenatal screening for Down syndrome and other chromosomal abnormalities has become a routine practice during antenatal care. Prenatal diagnosis of Down syndrome has changed from second to first trimester because of the higher detection rate and earlier diagnosis. While it is never easy for a couple to decide to pursue prenatal diagnosis, because of the possibility of subsequently having to consider termination of pregnancy, this is an option which is chosen by many couples at high risk of having a child with a serious hereditary disorder. Moreover, the ethical issues surrounding prenatal diagnosis and selective termination of pregnancy are both complex and emotive. Prenatal diagnosis can be carried out by both invasive and non invasive methods. The most common indication for prenatal diagnosis for Down syndrome is advanced maternal age.

This book will be useful not only for research workers and medical practitioners, but will also be an important reference for the management of Down syndrome.

This book consists of four sections. All sections include chapters on recent advances in Down syndrome research.

Section I describes the behaviour and learning aspects of Down syndrome. People with intellectual disability require education to help them resist abuse. Individuals with Down syndrome can live full, productive and quality lives with help from modern medicine, multimedia technology and lifetime educational/support programs.

Section II deals with dental and orthopaedic features of a child with Down syndrome. Dental problems are very common in Down syndrome with an incidence about five times greater than that of normal child. Skeletal development has also been assessed in individuals with Down syndrome.

Section III describes the incidence of Acute lymphoblastic leukemia in Down syndrome child. Compared to children without this syndrome, there is ten to twenty fold higher risk of developing acute leukemia in Down syndrome.

Section IV presents both invasive and noninvasive methods of prenatal diagnosis. Recent advances in the detection of cell free fetal DNA in maternal circulation, Down syndrome screening after assisted reproduction techniques have been reviewed.

All the Articles are very interesting and provide an up-to-date knowledge on recent progress in the area of prenatal diagnosis in Down syndrome.

Acknowledgements

The editor wants to acknowledge the superb assistance of staff members and management of Intech Publisher. In particular, Ms. Romina Krebel for her co-ordination and editorial assistance. We are also grateful to all contributing authors and scientists who made this book possible by providing valuable research and review articles.

Subrata Dey
Salt Lake City,
Kolkata

Part 1

Behavior and Learning

1

Imitation as an Element of Social Interaction of Children with Down Syndrome at School

Patrícia Páfaro Gomes Anhão, Luzia Iara Pfeifer
and Jair Lício Ferreira Santos
*Ribeirão Preto Medical School, University of São Paulo
Brazil*

1. Introduction

Because of the development of new health practices, mainly those related to prevention and early diagnosis, life expectancy of people with Down Syndrome (DS) in developed countries increased from 12 years in 1940 (Penrose, 1949) to 60 years nowadays (Bittles, 2004; Glasson, 2002). Different kinds of treatment and therapies, especially early stimulation, have contributed to the development and social performance of persons with DS (Moreira, 2000), so that she/he can experience new situations such as inclusion in regular schools.

Diagnosing trisomy is not significant in the prognosis or determines strong more or less pronounced physical aspects. It does not establish higher or lower intellectual effectiveness, either. There is a consensus in the scientific community that there are no different levels of DS and that the developmental differences occur because of individual characteristics that stem from genetic inheritance, stimulation, education, environment, and clinical problems, which are all inter-related (Silva & Kleinhans, 2006).

Children with DS can have difficulties adapting socially because of the delay in mental and motor development. Thus, family support and motivation are needed to help the development of stronger autonomy when performing daily life activities (Glat, 1995). Because the family can help those children to, or prevent them from integrating in life contexts, it is extremely important to educate and advise the family from diagnosis on in order to make them aware that the child will go through all stages inherent to development, which imply different needs, including professional help involving objectives and strategies that will consider not only the level of impairments, motor and language changes but also the child's potential and skills to perform daily tasks and live in different community settings (Glat, 1995).

Although children with DS present lower functional performance when compared to children with typical development, that difference does not remain consistent throughout their development because the child with DS, little by little, develops mobility skills that are gradually incorporated to his/her daily repertoire, affecting his/her independent performance in several daily activities (Mancini et al., 2003).

In DS, sequential auditory memory problems somehow block attention and make it difficult to stay focused as long as necessary, which shows those subjects' difficulty storing sequential information. Physical tiredness itself and brain synaptic communication prevents information from flowing properly, which is understood as lack or loss of attention

(Troncoso & Cerro, 1999). That shows the importance of imitation and the presence of a role model for an individual with DS, when his/her attention fails, as pointed out by the authors, he/she can, by imitating the model, find ways of regaining the content missed because of the lack of attention.

2. The role of school in social interaction

Throughout the history involving disabled people there has been a world wide concern regarding their integration into society and, as with any ordinary citizen, their civic life starts in school, thus, it is only fair that those people be included in these socio-educational settings.

School is a very rich environment for the development of social skills, and it is noticeable that children from well-structured school settings tend to be more sociable, show more developed social interaction, play more advanced games with their peers, and exhibit more solid knowledge of social rules (Bonome-Pontoglio & Marturano, 2010).

The objective of child education is to make the child develop a positive image of him/herself, be more and more independent, trust his/her abilities and perceive his/her limitations; to find out and know his/her body little by little, his/her potentials and limitations by taking care of his/her health and well-being; to establish affective and exchanging bonds with adults and other children, strengthen self-esteem and expand possibilities of communication and social interaction gradually; to establish and expand social relations by learning how to articulate his/her interests and points of view, respect differences and develop aid and cooperation actions; to observe and explore the environment out of curiosity and feel as part of it, as an agent that will be dependent on and transform the environment, valuing attitudes which contribute to its preservation; play, express emotions, feelings, thoughts, desires and needs; use different languages (body, musical, artistic, verbal and written languages) for different intentions and communication situations, in a way to understand and be understood, express ideas, feelings, needs, desires and progress in the process of meaning construction, enriching his/her expression skills; learn about some cultural manifestations, showing interest, respect and participation and value diversity (Brazil, 1998).

Entering school is the child's first contact with the world outside the family environment. It is a big step as well as a challenge to those who participate in that new stage. To understand child development it is necessary to observe him/her not only as an individual but also in his/her social relations. It is important to observe the way the child expresses him/herself in a group in order to understand him/her. The school can help the development of his/her individual identity and favor his/her future social relationships in a determinant way through relationships with the others.

A disabled child's inclusion in regular schools is getting more and more common and the way it happens is closely related to local culture and policies (Luiz, 2009), that is the reason why it may happen in many different ways in cities, regions and countries (Buckley & Bird, 1998).

Inclusion foresees school integration in a radical, complete and systematic way in which all students should be in regular school classrooms. There is a proposal of a way of organizing the educational system which considers the need of all students and it is designed according to those needs in inclusive schools. Therefore, it involves not only the disabled students but also all those who have any kind of learning difficulties. The inclusive view eliminates the subdivision of special and regular school systems. According to that view, the school should address differences without discriminating, without working separately with some students and without establishing specific rules to plan, learn and evaluate. For the proponents of school inclusion it is mandatory that the educational establishments eliminate architectural barriers and employ teaching practices appropriate to the students' differences in general, providing alternatives which contemplates diversity besides the teaching resources and special equipment that can meet all educational needs of the students with deficiencies or not but without discriminations (Mantoan, 2003).

According to Buchley and Bird (1998), there is evidence that inclusive schools have been seen as the best schools for all kinds of children, and those that are prepared to receive children with special needs and have changed the teaching system, have improved education for all children. In such inclusion process not only the children with special needs experience positive aspects, but also all children who start living with diversity become more prepared as human beings for adversities and differences in life. In this case, the society will be responsible for the inclusion of all people who present some kind of difference, in other words, the society must adapt, accept and live together with all its elements, regardless of their abilities or their difficulties.

According to Vieira and Denari (2005), for school inclusion to take place, besides school structural, ideological and professional transformations, it is essential to consider the social and objective aspects of the process. Misinformation and lack of daily contact among people with typical development and people with special educational needs, can contribute to the build up of prejudice and difficulties in social interactions. That is the reason why it is necessary to boost direct contact and access to information and encourage thinking about diversity from an early childhood.

The objective of pre-school is to facilitate learning of basic concepts, provide socialization and development of skills of autonomy in self-care activities. Thus, when parents and teachers include a DS child in pre-school, they expect that they can, mainly, develop their comprehension of rules for social living, acquire autonomy to perform self-care activities such as eating and hygiene (Ferraz, Araujo & Carreiro, 2010) and become literate (Rubim, 2009).

Although DS children exhibit lower social interaction than their peers with typical development, when they are included in pre-school, they accelerate their language development, decrease their aggressive behavior and learn social rules (Monteiro, 1997).

Nowadays it is widely accepted that neurobiological functioning and environmental experience are reciprocally influenced (Cichetti & Toth, 2009) and advances in neuroscience have contributed to the understanding of a young child's development in his/her interaction with the environment (Bonome-Pontoglio & Marturano, 2010).

Living together in an environment which promotes a variety of stimuli and different possibilities of discoveries will allow the individuals' brain reorganization and plasticity (Silva & Kleinhans, 2006). It is undeniable that adults strongly influence a child's life in relation to cognitive and social development, however, children can also learn from their peers (Flynn & Whiten, 2010). Thus, schools become a very important place for learning.

Social interaction is one of the most important tasks of a child's initial development because it is characterized by the expansion and improvement of one's social behaviors repertoire and, simultaneously, by a gradual understanding of values and rules which govern life in society (Del Prette & Del Prette, 2005).

Studies have shown that the inclusion of disabled children is beneficial and promotes gains not only in terms of academic achievement but also in terms of skills related to speech and social behavior (Buckley & Bird, 1998; Buckey, Bird, Sacks & Archer, 2006).

By making an association between the process of social interaction and school inclusion of DS children it is possible to consider that when they enter school, interpersonal relationship with their school mates offers wider range of role models and demands for the acquisition of new social skills. Social performance and quality of relationships at school are based on behavioral resources previously acquired by the children in their family environment. Considering recent inclusion policies, it is possible to understand that interpersonal development (especially problem solving skills, self-control and pro-social behavior) is an essential component of that process. Such stance is consistent with those adopted by several researchers who promote the improvement of relationships among peers as one of the main objectives of inclusion: motivation of acts of comprehension and understanding of differences on the part of peers and teachers (Del Prette; Del Prette, 2005).

Several authors mention that children with regular development prefer to imitate adult behavior in order to meet a specific goal (Huang, Heyes & Charman, 2006; McGuigan, Whiten, Flynn & Horner, 2007; Whiten, Flynn, Brown & Lee, 2006). Children do that because they want to get socially involved and show that they are similar to the others around them (Nielson, 2006; Nielsen & Carpenter, 2008).

Imitation, as any other cognitive processes, is not innate, it changes due to the subjects' actions on the objects in the environment, firstly it is an extension of the action, that is, movements where the child can see her/himself doing the action and it evolves to a moment when the action becomes internalized and the child acquires the possibility of imitating events even in the absence of role models (Piaget, 1964/1978).

In child development, imitation presents two different but complementary functions, one of them is the cognitive function that makes learning about world events possible, and the other is an interpersonal one, which allows sharing experiences with the others (Uzgiris, 1981). Imitation occurs primarily because the child needs to understand the others' intention in communicating, that is, he/she is going to imitate whatever she/he thinks that his/her peer wants to be imitated, thus "feeding" social interaction (Nielsen & Hudry, 2010). As can be seen, imitation is a very important characteristic of the construction of social skills.

There has been increasing evidence that children with DS are strongly likely to copy the others (Wright, Lewis & Collis, 2006; Anhão et al., 2010). Children with DS are very observant and they use imitation as an instrument for creating social skills.

In an observational, non experimental study conducted by Anhão et al. (2010) with three to six-year-old children with DS from the regular educational system, it was possible to observe that, among several observed characteristics of social interaction, when compared to their peers with regular development, only two kinds of skills presented statistically significant results: "makes first contact" and "imitates (an) other child/children".

3. Contacting others

The typical development group had higher number of "makes first contact" behaviors. Such behavior indicator tried to investigate how often the study subjects (with Down Syndrome and regular development) started social interaction, that is whether she/he tried to make contact with another child, suggested games, started a dialogue with another child, or invited a peer to play by touching (Anhão, 2009).

Those results suggest that children with typical development, the study subjects, found it easier to start social contact. Angélico (2004) classified that kind of behavior as social communication skills in his study about the social repertoire of teenagers with DS. The same author verified that in the situations studied most of the subjects with DS had a deficit of responses for assertive coping in their behavioral repertoire.

According to Soresi and Nota (2000), many studies have shown that people with mental retardation have poor interaction with the others. The same authors, through a meta-analysis of different studies, claimed that DS school children and those with developmental disorders (moderate or severe) poorly adapt to school demands and, in general, experience difficulties achieving reasonable levels of school performance. They especially have difficulties in two wide classes of behaviors which are fundamental for school adaptation: relationship with peers and relationship with teachers. The latter is related to the ability of meeting the teachers' requests within school settings and the former is related to the ability of participating in group dynamics, facing negotiation skills and start positive relationships with schoolmates. Those difficulties decrease the quality and number of social experiences, which potentially results in serious negative effects on their abilities to adapt to adult life and on their social integration. That ability must be stimulated by the school environment for a complete development of life aspects, both in DS children and in children with typical development. Thus, inclusion is founded on the human and socio-cultural dimension which tries to enhance forms of positive interaction, possibilities and support for difficulties, and meeting needs, all of which is done by listening to students, parents, and school community.

Among other aspects, children with DS have been shown to present a deficit in social assertive abilities, those that depend on a stronger initiative and to develop better passive social skills, meaning those in which the influence of the environment is determinant (Anhão et al., 2010).

The set of abilities that allows children to understand, make references and consider their own and the others' state of mind and compare them, participating socially based on that comprehension is known as the theory of mind (Alves et al., 2007). The theory of mind is an area that investigates pre-school children's ability to understand their own and the others' state of mind and, thus, predicts their actions or behavior (Astington & Gopnik, 1988, 1991; Dias, 1993; Feldman, 1992; Lourenço, 1992; Siegel & Beattie, 1991; Wellman, 1991). Research on the theory of mind by Baron-Cohen and colleagues (Baron-Cohen, 1991 and Baron-Cohen, Leslie & Frith, 1985) with autistic and DS children were very important for the development of the innatist perspective. Leslie (1987) argues that the sheer absence of ability for popular psychology in autistic and DS children would support the opinion that those children have an innate neurological deficit.

A child, from a very early age, has the ability to regulate shared attention (Baron-Cohen, 1991). According to Fodor (1992) human beings are born with a social module which allows them to acquire the popular psychology typical of the culture they belong to. To that author, the theory of mind is related to the innate capacity of elaborating theories, that capacity would involve an intellectual process aiming to infer a group of beliefs guided by certain rules, which is another group of beliefs.

4. Imitating the others

Anhão et al. (2010) found out that a group of DS children presented greater "imitates (an) other child/children" behavior in comparison with their peers with typical development. That social ability referred to moments when the child observed his/her peers performing some kind of action (during a pedagogical activity or a game) and reproduced it in his/her own way. "Imitates the teacher" behavior, which referred to moments when the child (with

DS and with typical development) observed the teacher's action, his/her way to gesture or speak, and reproduced it in his/her own way, did not show significant differences in frequency between DS children and those with typical development (Anhão et al., 2010).

These data may suggest that DS children are more likely to imitate other children's behavior, and not to seek a performance "model" among teachers. Comparing the latter observed in this study it was possible to notice that this difference does not mean that the teacher does not have an important role in the process of social interaction and inclusion, but rather that children in that age require more interaction with others who have the same interests as their own, thus they imitate their peers. Such results show the importance of school settings in inclusion as a positive aspect in the process of social and academic development since that setting influences a stronger contact with DS children as well as with other children with typical development in the same age, which does not happen in protected settings of special learning or even in therapeutical settings. School inclusion has proved to be really effective providing models of social performances which are effective for DS children, helping them to create social symbols which are determinant for the development of social aspects (Anhão et al., 2010).

Rosin-Pinola (2006) believes that interpersonal development of students with some disabilities can be seen as an adjuvant in the process of integration and inclusion of those in regular school, as it increases the number of demands for communication with peers and a better use of social conditions of development and learning.

Social skills are learned and the demands for their performance vary according to the stage in which the subject is as a result of environmental contingencies to which he/she is exposed to (Angélico, 2004). Thus, a pre-school child does not have the same social abilities as one from elementary school, and the abilities of a teenager would exhibits are not the same as the ones expected in an adult or an elderly (Soresi & Nota, 2000).

The results by Anhão et al. (2010) show the importance of providing children with special educational needs with an inclusive education system as soon as possible, as Stainback and Stainback (1999) have noted.

As mentioned before, imitation of others is widely recognized as a fundamental behavior for the learning process in the first years of life because it supports the development of relationships others and it is the basis of social learning (Hurley & Chater, 2005). Although children with DS are considered good imitators, the study by Vanyuchelen, Feys and De Weerdt (2011) pointed that that behavior seems be more associated to age than to some specificity of the syndrome.

As several important authors talk about imitation in children with regular development, it makes sense to bring such observations to the world of children with DS.

Therefore, it is necessary to understand how DS children's behavior occurs in the school setting as opposed to imitation actions in their peers with typical development, which contributes to their social interaction and learning. Thus, it is important to understand how imitation happens according to different authors.

5. Imitative action

Wallon (1979) presents the situation by focusing on two different ways of determining imitation. The first one says that imitation is an action which reproduces a model, but that implies admitting acting previous to it. He believes that imitation stems from postural activity and distinguishes spontaneous imitation from intelligent imitation. The role model does not impose him/herself as something external to the subject and although it has originated as a perception it seems to be intimate and impels him/her to an imitative action which complements and reestablishes a psychomotor agreement. The second one, imitation is different from the model: the subject decides to imitate or not something felt as external. The change from one to another is, however, a slow and complex process. Intelligent imitation tends to establish dissociation between what is noticed, desired or imagined and what is done. That opposition provides an acting plane. Acting would be, according to him, the result of the replication of reality, in other words, a development from the sensitive, concrete plane into a similar one, formed by images, symbols and ideas.

The similarity between imitation and acting leads us to think about the influence or participation of imitation during acting too. It is clear that both processes develop to different planes: one in the motor plane and the other in the plane images and symbols. But the strength of the analogy is due to the fact that both processes have a problem in common: turning an intimate formula, a result of a condensation of impressions and several experiences, into successive terms, that must be localized in time (Pedrosa, 1994).

Studies by Nadel (1986) and Nadei and Baudonnière (1981) show some kinds of imitative behavior among children, and they state that the main basis of social relationships among three-year-old children is an immediate imitation. Echerman, Davis and Didow (1989) showed that in children who are around 2 years old, interacting with peers who are not familiar, a new behavioral organization appears: the child repeatedly imitates the others' games creating social games which seem to be constructions of the moment and not a reestablishment of the script previously rehearsed with familiar peers.

Eckerman and Stein (1990) compared 24-month-old children interacting in dyads with and adult during a game. For eight children, the adult reacted as if following a program, imitating the child's movements during the game, for the other eight, the adult reacted to the same game material but in a different way, not related to the child's actions, this procedure is similar to the way the partner of a child reacts when they are below 24 months old, according to some previous observations. The authors mentioned above assumed that imitative actions, which occurs more often at around 24 months is one of the elements which contribute to a new form of behavioral organization identified in peer children of that age: imitation motivates imitation and leads to the generation of social games in dyads. The results of the experiment described, conducted with child-adult dyads, point to the authors' assumption and they emphasize the need of continuing with the studies with children interacting in natural situations.

Nadei et al. (1989) believe that imitation among young children, who still do not command a verbal linguistic code, makes up a transitory system of socially sustained exchange and has a fundamental role in communication among peers.

According to Winnicott (1996), cognitive, social and intellectual development depends mainly on the relationship of the child and the transition object, which is the peak of a good individual development and the game of imitating relatives, teachers and friends start from that. Therefore, imitation games contribute to growth and health and lead to group relationships.

Imitation is based on the perception-action mechanism which combines the visual kinematic characteristics of an action perceived with the motor kinematic characteristics of the action itself (Prinz, 2002). That visual-motor skill starts much earlier than the development of language for the children, which is very clear in children with typical development soon after the birth (Meltzoff & Moore, 1977) as well as in DS children (Heimann, Ullstadius & Swerlander, 1998; Heimann & Illstadius, 1999).

When a child imitates another person there is a discharge on the mirror neurons (Gallese, 2007). Those neurons are brain cells which fire when a subject copies an action or simply observes someone performing some actions (Rizzolatti, 2006). The activation of these neurons helps children to understand other actions and, therefore, they play an important role in learning, how children learn about the world, how they act and how they play (Stagnitti, 2009).

6. Imitation in school routine

In school routine imitation is many times understood negatively because it limits creativity and neutralizes students' free expression, as in the sentence "he who copies, does not create", and in the discussion about the relation between copy and re-reading of works of art. Thus, imitation is doing the same as somebody else in a mechanic way and does not represent the subject's cognitive potential (Pimentel, 2000). Here, however, imitation is being considered not as a copy but as a reproduction of an action after an observation the way that the observer understood and learned the mentioned action, in an attempt to feed social interaction.

According to Fernandes (2005), it is through imitation that children in general recreate and not just make a copy of the world they live in. He also states that imitation is inherent to the learning process, changing according to historical and cultural determinations, not in a mythical or mechanics way, but as a determinant factor for acquisition of knowledge and future development of the students. Imitation is an intellectual activity when the individual acts under others' influence, however, he/she grasps knowledge according to his/her development level.

Teaching imitation skills is, many times, the first step of interventions with children with intellectual disabilities (Vanyuchelen & Vochten, 2011), DS children can be included here.

In psychological studies, imitation is studied through different theories. According to the genetic theory, imitation follows the level of development, forming structures of inner symbolic representation that evidence intelligence and is a copy of images which have been interiorized (Piaget, 1978).

In the behaviorist conception, imitation is the objective and mechanic copy of what is around and it is able to modify an individual's behavior and make up his/her own habits. Thus, the child learns by modeling and observing (France, 2998).

Vygotski states that imitation is a dynamic process which contributes to learning and makes it easier, demystifying the mechanic or restricted aspect attributed to it (Gasparin, 2002). Vygotski, however, does not rule out the possibility that there are times when imitation becomes simply mechanic. However, he tries to expand that restricted sense to a wider one in which imitation is the basis on which acquisition of human knowledge and development occurs. That premise counts if imitation is observed as an intentional and intellectual human activity. Thus, a dialectical unit is formed between mechanical imitation and intellectual one (Fernandes, 2005).

Vygotski (2001), in a social historical view, believes that a proximal development zone is more important for intellectual development and improvement than the actual level of development because it confirms the thesis that a child who is helped can do more than when he/she does that alone. He adds that it is only possible to imitate what is in the area of intellectual potential, in other words, to imitate it is necessary to have some possibilities to go beyond what is already known. Development derived from collaboration via imitation is the capacity to transform what children can already do into what he/she still cannot do, providing a basis for learning and subsequent development.

When it is said that a child imitates, it does not mean that she/he looks at another person and imitates him/her like a mirror, it indicates that a future action can present characteristics of the way the other does things. Such aspect is subjectively implied in daily relationships in a classroom. Thus, learning through imitation means that the child performs better when he/she learns together with other people (Fernandes, 2005).

7. DS children imitation in school routine

Fernandes (2005) points that when the human being imitates, he/she does it according to cultural references that he/she has as basis and establishes new associations and combinations according to his/her interests and needs. The individual never simply copies the other, he/she makes a connection between imitation and creation.

Memory has an important role in the development of the human being's intelligence and learning. Children with DS hardly ever forget what they learn well. Those children's visual memory develops faster than the auditory one because of the bigger amount of stimuli, thus, they acquire good sensory memory, recognizing and searching for stimuli. Progressive learning facilitates the development of the sequential auditory, visual, tactile and kinesthetic memory (Escamilla, 1998). Once again the hypothesis that imitating a model could help individuals with DS develop better memory aspects comes up.

Troncoso and Florez (1997) believe that DS individuals do not have difficulties performing old activities using common knowledge even if they are long, but they have problems when it is necessary to develop new conducts which request programmed organization, in other words, a new sequence of actions.

Learning requires responses which can be motor, verbal or graphic. A DS child's response is poor because of the limitations that they can possibly have. However, the possibility of expanding and determining certain responses will depend on environmental support. The more a demanding environment is offered, one that promotes autonomy and offers different possibilities of discoveries of their potential, the better DS child's development will be. By recognizing the characteristics of the phenotype of people with DS, it is better to focus on proposed activities in areas of greater potential to be developed. Thus, an individual who notices that he/she can perform such tasks successfully will be more satisfied and motivated to face more challenging tasks. Education needs patience, dedication and consistency, and above all, professionals' and parents' love and affection. Everyone has abilities and difficulties, it is necessary to know them and learn how to deal with them (Silva & Kleinhans, 2006).

Ciciliato et al. (2010) compared a group of children with DS and a group of children with typical development, 12 to 36 months old, to characterize the development of symbolic abilities present in those two groups. Among the results, it was possible to confirm the hypothesis of the delay in symbolic abilities for the group of DS children. But sonic and gestural imitation was not statistically different between the two groups. Children with DS in this study explored objects repeatedly through few actions and, using sensory motor activities with no organization of objects and imitating words and visible gestures of their own.

Making first contact as proposed by children with regular development shows that they are open to new experiences and interactions in general, they try to make social contact by themselves. Imitating their classmates for DS children shows that they look for new ways of acting and performing in their settings. DS children have a deficit of assertive social abilities, in other words, of those that depend on a stronger initiative and develop better passive social abilities, meaning those where the role of the environment is determinant (Anhão, 2009).

8. Final considerations

The development of social interaction of DS children occurs in fairly similar ways to that of their peers with typical development, differing only in rhythm and in the way DS children try to sustain that relationship. Thus, it is important that some practical educational changes are made in order to achieve real inclusion of those students in regular educational setting, turning them into actions that will be beneficial for the maturity and growth of children with typical and non typical development.

Establishing contact with the other and imitating another child's behavior are important aspects for the development and establishment of abilities and social interactions, so, it is important to mention school environment as a facilitator that will promote a stronger contact of DS child with other children in the same age group, helping the development of social abilities of those children.

Therefore, it is possible to highlight the importance of the inclusion of DS children in the regular educational system, favoring living with educators and peers, helping their acquisition of social abilities and necessary behaviors in society.

This way, it is possible to see that the results show the importance of providing children with special educational needs with an inclusive educational system as early as possible as Stainback and Stainback (1999) have noted. All children with any kind of difficulty, regardless of physical, cognitive or emotional conditions, are children who have the same basic needs of affection, attention and protection, and the same desires and feelings as any other children. They are able to live together, interact, exchange, learn, play and be happy, although, sometimes in a different way. That different way of being and acting is what makes them unique and special. They must be seen not as a failure, but as people with different potential, with some difficulties that, many times become challenges from which we can learn and grow, as people and professionals who try to help their neighbor. With inclusion, we can make students with special educational needs be exposed to positive forms of communication and interaction, of assistance and of different social exchanges, to challenging learning conditions where they are required to think, solve problems, express feelings, desires and take initiatives.

9. References

Angélico, A. P. Estudo descrivo do repertório de habilidades sociais de indivíduos com Síndrome de Down. 2004. ___126f. Dissertação de Mestrado, Universidade Federal de São Carlos. São Carlos, SP. 2004.

Anhao, P. P. G.; Pfeifer, L. I.; Santos, J. L. Interação social de crianças com Síndrome de Down na educação infantil. *Rev. bras. educ. espec.*, Marília, v. 16, n. 1, abr. 2010.

Batista, M. W.; Enumo, S. R. F. Inclusão escolar e deficiência mental: análise da interação social entre companheiros. *Estud. psicol. (Natal)*, Natal, v. 9, n. 1, 2004. Disponível em:

<http://www.scielo.br/scielo.php?script=sci_arttext&pid=S1413 294X2004000100012&lng=pt&nrm=iso>. Acesso em: 23 Ago 2008. doi: 10.1590/ S1413-294X2004000100012

Bittles, A. H.; Glasson, E. J. Clinical, social and ethical implications of changing life expectancy in Down syndrome. *Dev Med Child Neurol.* 2004; 46:282–6.

Bonome-Pontoglio, C. F.; Marturano, E. M. Brincando na creche:atividades com crianças pequenas. *Estudos de Psicologia* (Campinas), v.27 (3), p.365-373, jul-set., 2010.

BRASIL. Ministério da Educação e do Desporto. Secretaria de Educação Fundamental. Referencial curricular nacional para a educação infantil / Ministério da Educação e do Desporto, Secretaria de Educação Fundamental. – Brasília: MEC/SEF, 1998. 3v.: Il Disponível em: http://portal.mec.gov.br/seb/arquivos/pdf/rcnei_vol1.pdf

Buckley, S.; Bird, G.; Sacks, B.; Archer, T. A comparison of mainstream and special education for teenagers with Down syndrome: implications for parents and teachers. *Downs Syndr Res Pract*, Inglaterra, v. 9, n. 3, p. 54-67, 2006.

Buckley, S.; Bird, G. Including children with Down Syndrome. *Down Syndrome News & Update*. Vol. 1, No. 1, PP 5-13, 1998.

Cavalcanti, A.; Galvão, C. Terapia Ocupacional: fundamentação & prática. Rio de Janeiro, Ed. Guanabara Koogan, 2007.

Cicchetti, D., & Toth, S. L. (2009). The past achievements and future promises of developmental psychopathology: the coming of age of a discipline. *Journal of Child Psychology & Psychiatry, 50*(1/2), 16-25.

Ciciliato, M. N.; Zilotti, D. C.; Mandrá, P.P. Caracterização das habilidades simbólicas de crianças com síndrome de down. *Rev. Soc. Bras. Fonoaudiol.* 2010; 15(3): 408-14.

Del Prette, Z.A.P.; Del Prette, A. Psicologia das habilidades sociais na infância: teoria e prática. Petrópolis, Rio de Janeiro, Editora Vozes, 2005.

Escamilla, S. G. *El niño con Síndrome del Down*. México: Diana, 1998.

Eckerman, C. O.; Davis, C.C: e Didow, S. M. (1989). Toddler's emerging ways of achieving social coordinations with a peer. *Child Development*, 60, 440-453.

Eckerman, C. O. e Stein, M. R. (1990). How imitation begets imitation and toddler's generation of games. *Developmental Psychology*, 26(3), 370-378.

Fernades, V. L. P. A imitação no processo de ensino e aprendizagem em arte. Dissertação de mestrado da Universidade Federal do Mato Grosso do Sul. 2005.

Ferraz, C. R. A.; Araujo, M. V. ; CARREIRO, L. R. R.. Inclusão de crianças com Síndrome de Down e paralisia cerebral no ensino fundamental I: comparação dos relatos de mães e professores. *Rev. bras. educ. espec.* [online]. 2010, vol.16, n.3, pp. 397-414. ISSN 1413-6538.

Flynn E.; Whiten A. Studying children's social learning experimentally "in the wild" Whiten *Learning & Behavior 2010, 38 (3), 284-296 doi:10.3758/LB.38.3.284*

França, A. C.; Santos, J. R.; Rei, V. A. F. Um estudo preliminar sobre aprendizagem por modelação com sujeitos Rattus Novergicus. 1998. Disponível em: <http://www.nead.unama.br /revista/lato/pdf/lato41a8.pdf >. Acesso em: 17 out. 2003.

Flórez, B. J.; Troncoso, V. M. (Eds.). *Síndrome de Down y educacíon*. 3. reimp. Barcelona: Masson - Salvat Medicina y Santander, 1997.

Gallese, V. Before and below 'theory of mind': embodied simulation and the neural correlates of social cognition *Phil. Trans. R. Soc. B* 2007 362, 659-669

Gasparin, J. L. Uma didática para a Pedagogia histórico-crítica. Campinas: Autores Associados, 2002. Comênio ou da arte de ensinar tudo a todos. Campinas, SP: Papirus, 1994. (Coleção Magistério, Formação e Trabalho Pedagógico).

Huang, C., Heyes, C., & Charman, T. (2006). Preschoolers behavioural reenactment of 'failed attempts': The roles of intention-reading, emulation and mimicry. *Cognitive Development*, 21, 36–45.

Jou, G. I.; Sperb, T. M.. Teoria da Mente: diferentes abordagens. Psicol. Reflex. Crit., Porto Alegre, v.12, n.2, 1999. Disponívelem <http://www.scielo.br/scielo.php?script=sci_arttext&pid=S0102-79721999000200004&lng=pt&nrm=iso>. Acessos em 02 mar. 2011. doi: 10.1590/S0102-79721999000200004.

Luiz, F. M. R. Experiência de famílias de crianças com Síndrome de Down no processo de inclusão na rede regular de ensino. Dissertação de mestrado da Escola de Enfermagem de Ribeirão Preto da Universidade de São Paulo. 2009.

Mancini, M. C. et al. Comparação do desempenho funcional de crianças portadoras de síndrome de Down e crianças com desenvolvimento normal aos 2 e 5 anos de idade. *Arq. Neuro-Psiquiatr.*, São Paulo, v. 61, n. 2B, Junho 2003.

Mantoan, M.T.E. Inclusão escolar: O que é? Por quê? Como fazer? São Paulo: Moderna, 2003. - (Coleção Cotidiano Escolar)

Mcguigan, N., Whiten, A., Flynn, E., & Horner, V. (2007). Imitation of causally opaque versus causally transparent tool use by 3- and 5-year-old children. *Cognitive Development*, 22, 353-364.

Monte, F. R. F.; Santos, I. B. Saberes e práticas da inclusão. Brasília: MEC, SEESP, 2004.

Moreira, L. M. A.; El-Hani, CH. N.; Gusmão, F. A. F. A síndrome de Down e sua patogênese: considerações sobre o determinismo genético. *Rev. Bras. Psiquiatr.*, v. 22, n. 2, p. 96-99, 2000.

Moeller, I. Diferentes e Especiais. *Rev. Viver Mente e Cérebro*, n. 156, p. 26-31, Jan, 2006.

Nadel, J. (1986) Imitation et Communication entre Jeunes Enfants. Paris: Presses Universitaires de France.

Nadel, J.; Baudonnière, P. (1981) Imitação, modo preponderante de intercâmbio entre pares durante o terceiro ano de vida. *Cadernos de Pesquisa*, 39, 26-31.

Nadel, J.; Fontaine, A. (1989) Communicating by imitation: a developmental and comparative approach to transitory social competence. In, B. H. Schneider et al. Social Competence in Developmental Perspective. Kluwer Academic Publishers

Nielsen, M. (2006). Copying actions and copying outcomes: Social learning through the second year. Developmental Psychology, 42, 555–565.

Nielsen, M., & Carpenter, M. (2008). Reflecting on imitation in autism: Introduction to the special issue. Journal of Experimental Child Psychology, 101, 165–169.

Nielsen, Mark AND Hudry, Kristelle(2010) 'Over-imitation in children with autism and Down syndrome', Australian Journal of Psychology, 62: 2, 67 — 74, First published on: 25 March 2009 (iFirst). DOI: 10.1080/00049530902758613URL: http://dx.doi.org/10.1080/00049530902758613

Oliveira, LA, Oliveira, DC. O desenvolvimento de crianças com Síndrome de Down: um estudo de caso (Dissertação de Mestrado). Rio de Janeiro (RJ): Universidade do Estado do Rio de Janeiro; 2001. Disponível em Anais do 4º Congresso Brasileiro de Educação Especial, 2010.

Pedrosa, M. I. A imitação como um processo de construção de significados compartilhados. Temas psicol., v. 2, n.2, Ribeirão Preto, ago. 1994.

Penrose, L. S. The incidence of Mongolism in the general population. J Ment. Sci. 1949; 95:685–8.

Piaget, J. (1978). *A formação do símbolo na criança*. Rio de Janeiro: Zahar.(Texto original publicado em 1964)

Pimentel, V. & Szpigel, M. - "Cópia ou releitura? como não levar gato por lebre" In Pátio Revista Pedagógica, nº 14, Porto Alegre, 2000, pp.61-65

Rizzolatti, G., Fogassi, L., & Gallese, V. (2006). Espelhos na mente. *Scientific American, 55*, 44-51.

Rosin-Pinola, A. R. Avaliação de professores sobre o repertório social e acadêmico de alunos com deficiência mental incluídos no ensino regular. 2006. ___94F. Dissertação de Mestrado (apresentada ao Programa de Pós-graduação em Educação Especial) Universidade Federal de São Carlos - SP, 2006.

Rubim, D. L. M. Pais de alunos com Síndrome de Down: significados atribuídos à inclusão escolar e expectativa de escolarização. 2009. Dissertação (Mestrado) - Universidade Presbiteriana Mackenzie, São Paulo.

Salisbury, C. L.; Galucci, C.; Palombaro, M.M. & Peck, C. A. Strategies that promote social relations among elementary students with and without severe disabilities in inclusive schools. Exceptional Children, v. 65, n. 2, p. 125-197, 1995.

Silva, M. F. M. C.; Kleinhans, A. C. S. Processos cognitivos e plasticidade cerebral na Síndrome de Down. Rev. Bras. Ed. Esp., Marília, jan-abr. 2006, v. 12, n. 1, p. 123-138.

Stagnitti, K. (2009). Children and pretend play. In K. Stagnitti and R. Cooper (Eds.) *Play as Therapy: Assessment and therapeutic interventions.* (pp.59-69). London: Jessica Kingsley Publishers.

Stainback, S.; Stainback, W. Inclusão: um guia para educadores. Trad. Magda França Lopes. Porto Alegre: Artes Médicas Sul, 1999.

Soresi, S.; Nota, L. A social skill training for persons with Down Syndrome. European Psychologist, v. 5, n. 1, p. 33-43, 2000.

Schwartzman, J. S. *Síndrome de Down*. São Paulo: Mackenzie, 1999.

Teixeira, F. C.; Kubo, O. M. Características das interações entre alunos com Síndrome de Down e seus colegas de turma no sistema regular de ensino. Rev. bras. educ. espec., Marília, v. 14, n. 1, abr. 2008. Disponível em <http://www.scielo.br/scielo.php?script=sci_arttext&pid=S14136538200800010000 7&lng=pt&nrm=iso>. Acesso em 31 maio 2009.

Troncoso, V. M.; Cerro, M. M. *Síndrome de Down:* lectura y escritura. Barcelona: Masson, 1999.

Uzgiris, I. (1981). Two functions of imitation during infancy. *International Journal of Behavioural Development*, 4, 1–12.

Vanvuchelen, M.; Feys, H.; De Weerdt, W. Is the good-imitator-poor-talker profile syndrome-specific in Down syndrome?: Evidence from standardised imitation and language measures. *Research in Developmental Disabilities*, v. 32, p. 148–157 (2011).

Vanvuchelen, M., Vochten, C. How much change is true change? The smallest detectable difference of the Preschool Imitation and Praxis Scale (PIPS) in preschoolers with intellectual disabilities of heterogeneous aetiology *Research in Developmental Disabilities* 32 (1), pp. 180-187

Vieira, C. M.; Denari, F. E. O acesso a informações sobre deficiência mental como veículo de transformação de concepções infantis. Universidade Federal de São Carlos. Transcrito para publicação. Livro de Programas e Resumos do II Congresso Brasileiro de Educação Especial e II Encontro da Associação Brasileira de Pesquisadores em Educação Especial, (p.227). São Carlos, SP, 03 de novembro de 2005.

Vygotsky, L. S.; Luria, A. R.; Leontiev, A. N. Linguagem, desenvolvimento e aprendizagem. 1 ed., São Paulo, Icone: Editora da USP, 1988.

Vigotski, L. S. Psicologia concreta do homem. Educação e Sociedade, Campinas, n.71, p. 23-43, jul. 2000.

Vygotsky, L. S. *A formação social da mente:* o desenvolvimento dos processos psicológicos superiores. 6. ed. São Paulo: Martins Fontes, 1998.

Wallon, H. (1979) Do Acto ao Pensamento: Ensaio de Psicologia Comparada. Lisboa: Moraes.

Winnicott(1996)Pensando sobre crianças. Trad. de Maria Adriana Veríssimo Veronese. Porto Alegre, Artes Médicas, 1997. W21 - Thinking About Children, eds. R.Shepherd/J.Johns/H.T.Robinson. London, Karnac Books.

Whiten, A., Flynn, E., Brown, K., & Lee, T. (2006). Imitation of hierarchical action structure by young children. *Developmental Science*, 9, 574-582

Wright, I., Lewis, V., & Collis, G. M. (2006). Imitation and representational development in young children with Down syndrome. *British Journal of Developmental Psychology*, 24, 429-450.

2

Adaptive and Behavioral Development in Children with Down Syndrome at School Age with Special Emphasis on Attention Deficit Hyperactivity Disorder (ADHD)

Asher Ornoy[1], Tanya Rihtman[2] and Shula Parush[2]
[1]*Israel Canada Institute for Medical Research, Hebrew University Hadassah Medical School and Israeli Ministry of Health, Jerusalem*
[2]*School of Occupational Therapy, Hebrew University Hadassah Medical School, Jerusalem, Israel*

1. Introduction

Down syndrome (DS) is the most common chromosomal anomaly occurring in live births (Capone et al, 2004; Menkes & Falk, 2005) and it has been described as a syndrome-complex of genetic origin with protean neurobiological consequences, and several characteristic neurodevelopmental and neuropsychological manifestations. Down syndrome is also considered to be the most common single cause of mild, moderate and severe mental retardation (MR) with over half of individuals with DS attaining an IQ of between 50 and 25 by the end of the first decade of life (Bittles & Glasson, 2004; Capone, 2004; Hanson, 2003; Menkes & Falk, 2005; Roubertoux & Kerdelhue, 2006; Van Cleve & Cohen, 2006; Vicari, 2006). Individuals with Down syndrome experience a reduced life expectancy, but within the DS population, life expectancy is increasing.

Clinically, individuals with Down syndrome have typical physical and anatomical characteristics (Van Cleve &, Cohen, 2006). An issue of major medical importance is the participation and function on the health of individuals, communities and society. A holistic approach is now vital when assessing the individual, from body functions and IQ to learning abilities, attentional skills, daily activities and participation defined by the ICF as 'the execution of a task or action' with involvement in a life situation (WHO, 2001). Despite these shifts, there is limited investigation into the activity performance, participation, learning and behavior of children with DS, as measured by their adaptive functioning.

The cognitive limitations of individuals with Down syndrome have an important influence on the level of functioning attained and a significant correlation between IQ and all areas of function has been noted. Relatively preserved visual-spatial and visual-motor skills are often noted, yet the influence of these skills on the activity performance of the child with DS is unclear (Fiddler, et al 2005; Vicari 2006; Vicari & Carlesimo 2006).

The few existing studies investigating the holistic functional profile of children with DS have tended to be qualitative and investigated adult populations, even though all these children will display some form of intellectual disability requiring functional intervention. Few studies have measured specific skills appropriate to the wide range of abilities presented by children with Down syndrome or reported attainment levels for children in different age groups (Turner & Alborz 2003). There remains, therefore, a dearth of investigation into the functioning and participation of children with DS based on age-appropriate, socially acceptable activities. Up-to-date information is needed to guide parents and professionals with regard to reasonable expectations.

Attention deficit hyperactivity disorder (ADHD), characterized by symptoms of inattention, with or without impulsivity and hyperactivity, (Barkley, 1997; Biederman & Faraone, 2005 DSM - fourth edition, 2000; Furman 2005) is estimated to affect between 6-12% of typically developing school age children worldwide (Biederman & Faraone, 2005). In typically developing populations, ADHD is more commonly diagnosed amongst boys than girls; (Bauermeister et al., 2007; Biederman et al., 2005; Biederman & Faraone, 2005; Furman, 2005; Stefanatos & Baron, 2007). In clinical samples, boys are six to ten times more likely to be referred and three to four times more likely to be diagnosed with ADHD (Biederman et al., 2005; Stefanatos & Baron, 2007) while in non-referred samples, gender differences have been reported to be in the range of 1:1 to 1:3 (Biederman et al., 2005; Stefanatos & Baron, 2007).

Children with Down syndrome, due to their intellectual disabilities may have an increased risk for ADHD behaviors over and above that associated with their developmental delays, (Hastings et al, 2005) and clinically, attention function and hyperactive behaviors are commonly reported to be problem areas for children with DS (Brown et al., 2003). However, an investigation into the literature reveals a lack of information regarding the frequency and characteristics of these deficits in this population at different ages, (Määttä, et al, 2006) as well as no data on possible gender differences in these deficits. Children with DS are not exempt from having a dual-diagnosis with ADHD (Capone et al, 2006) and, indeed, the risk of "diagnostic overshadowing" (Reiss et al, 1982) is apparent in this population. Since attention deficits are not inherently incorporated into the phenotype of individuals with MR, (Burack et al, 2001) it is important to investigate the frequency and types of attention deficits/hyperactivity amongst children with DS.

As it is now essential to adopt a holistic approach when assessing the individual especially the mentally retarded, ADHD being a commonly reported deficit can not be overlooked when assessing children with DS. Accurate information regarding the frequency of a dual-diagnosis such as ADHD amongst children with DS is important since the symptoms of this diagnosis are not inextricably linked with the cognitive impairment characteristic of DS and as such could potentially be treated under a medical model (Capone et al., 2006). The alleviation of attention deficit behaviors has the potential of improving the effectiveness of intervention for children with DS and, as a result, lead to improved function and quality of life.

Despite the limited information available, (Brown et al., 2003; Hastings et al., 2005) it was hypothesized that children with DS would show attention deficit/hyperactive behaviors at a higher frequency than that noted in typically developing populations, and that these deficits would be more common amongst older children. In addition, (based on the fact that it was a non-referred sample), it was hypothesized that no gender differences in the frequency of these deficits would be found. Finally, it was assumed that the severity of attention deficit/hyperactive behaviors would be correlated with the child's adaptive behavior and IQ.

In our study we assessed the developmental profile of 60 children with Down syndrome between the ages of 6 and 16 years who had received a holistic early intervention program from birth until their entry into an appropriate educational framework. A focus was placed on investigating the frequency of attention deficit/hyperactive behaviors amongst these children and to assess whether it differs between sexes and whether it changes across age groups. The influence of the severity of attention deficit/hyperactive behaviors on adaptive behavior and their correlation with the child's intelligence quotient (IQ) was investigated The relationship between body function variables and participation as well as the performance of specific school-related activities was also studied.

2. Method

2.1 Sample

This study included 60 Hebrew-speaking children (33 males, 27 females) with Down syndrome, all of whom were treated at the Jerusalem Institute for Child and Family Development of the Israel Ministry of Health from birth until their entry into an appropriate special educational framework between the ages of 3 and 4 years. The children were between the ages of 5 years 10 months and 15 years 8 months (mean 9y 3mo; SD 28.8mo) at the time of testing. No child was receiving treatment at the Institute at the time of the study. The children were divided into the following three similarly sized age groups: youngest (*n*=20; 12 males, eight females; mean age 6y 11mo, SD 7.1mo; range 5y 10mo–7y 8mo); middle (*n*=21; nine males, 12 females; mean age 9y, SD 9.9mo; range 7y 9mo–10y) and oldest (*n*=19; 12 males seven females; mean age 12y 2mo, SD 20.3mo; range 10y 2mo– 15y 8mo). These age groups were selected since it seems feasible to expect greater differences between groups of children between the ages of 6–8 (younger pre-teens) and 8–10 (older pre-teens) as compared to teenagers.

2.2 Instruments

Psycho-social intake questionnaire

A non-standardized measure developed by the Jerusalem Institute for Child and Family Development for internal use, completed by caregiver interview. This questionnaire provided demographic information including gender, age and whether the child received medication for attention deficits (methylphenidate) at the time of testing or in the past.

ADHD Rating scale for parents and teachers (Pelham et al, 1992)

Parents and teachers both completed the Parent-Teacher ADHD Rating Scale based on the DSM-III-R criteria (American Psychiatric Association, 1987) as described by Pelham et al. (1992). The questionnaire includes 14 items, for which the informant responds on a scale of 0-3, resulting in a maximum score of 42. For each informant (parent and teacher) the total score was calculated, with higher scores indicating greater difficulties. A cut-off score above 15 was used to suggest attention deficit and hyperactive behavior with scores of 21 and above suggestive of more pronounced difficulties.

Vineland Adaptive Behavior Scales, interview edition (VABS) (Sparrow, et al, 1984)

A 577-item norm-referenced and standardized parent/caregiver interview measuring personal and social skills and intended for use in populations from birth to 18 11/12 years. Standard scores are measured (in normative populations, M=100 and SD=15). Reliability has been demonstrated using internal consistency (split half means for Domains .91 to .95; for Adaptive Behavior Composite .97). In the current study, composite scores were attained for three domains (communication skills, daily living skills and socialization skills).

Stanford-Binet Intelligence Scale, fourth edition (SBIS)(Thorndike, et al, 1986)

A reliable and valid measure developed to test cognitive ability in individuals from 2 years-23 years, administered by a psychologist, provided an IQ score. In normative populations, the general score has a mean of 100 and SD of 16 while subtests have a mean of 50 and a SD of 8. The Brief IQ including the verbal reasoning, abstract/visual reasoning, quantitative reasoning and short-term memory scales were used in the current study.

2.3 Procedure

This study was performed as part of a larger study (Rihtman et al., 2009) and was approved by the ethics committee of the School of Occupational Therapy, Hebrew University Hadassah Medical School, Jerusalem. Letters were sent to the parents of all the children born with Down syndrome in the Jerusalem vicinity between 1988-1998 who were treated with a standard intervention protocol at the Jerusalem Institute for Child and Family Development of the Israel Ministry of Health (N=119). Eight children had passed away, 30 children were not traced and 21 declined to participate, leaving the study group with 60 children. Parents signed a consent form and all participants were invited to the Institute for a testing session. A written summary was sent to the parents of each participant.

2.4 Statistical analysis

A Type 1 error rate of 0.05 was used for all analyses. Statistical Package for Social Sciences 13 (SPSS 13) for Windows was used for all calculations. Descriptive statistics were used to reveal the frequency of attention deficit/hyperactive behaviors. One-way ANOVA's were performed to assess age-group differences and independent sample t-tests were performed to assess gender differences on parent and teacher reports of attention deficit/hyperactive behaviors. Chi square tests were used to assess age group and gender differences on medication for attention deficit/hyperactive behaviors. Independent sample t-tests were performed to assess parent and teacher report ADHD Rating Scale score group differences in adaptive behavior. Pearson coefficient correlations were calculated to assess the correlations between parent and teacher ADHD Rating Scale scores and adaptive behaviors. One-way MANOVA's were employed to assess ADHD Rating Scale score group differences and the Stanford Binet subscales. Effect sizes were ascertained by means of Eta squared, which reflects the proportion of the total variance attributed to or accounted for by an effect, with 0.01 reflecting a small effect size, 0.06 reflecting a medium effect size and 0.14 reflecting a large effect size (Cohen 1988; Hays 1994).

3. Results

3.1 Frequency of attention deficit/hyperactive behaviors

Reports of attention deficit/hyperactive behaviors were initially considered in individual settings (home or school). Based on parent report on the ADHD Rating Scale (Figure 1), for the total group, 28.8% attained scores of 16 and above, indicative of deficits, with 11.9% attaining scores of 21 and above, indicative of more pronounced deficits. Amongst boys, 34.4% attained scores of 16 and above, while 15.6% attained scores of 21 and above.

Amongst girls, 22.2% attained scores of 16 and above, while 7.4% attained scores of 21 and above.

Based on teacher's report on the ADHD Rating Scale (Figure 1), for the total group, 25.6% attained scores of 16 and above, with 9.3% attaining scores of 21 and above. Amongst boys, 32.0% attained scores of 16 and above, while 8.0% attained scores of 21 and above. Amongst girls, 16.7% attained scores of 16 and above, while 11.1% attained scores of 21 and above.

When the frequencies of attention deficit/hyperactive behaviors were considered based on parent and teacher reports combined (Figure 1), within the total group, 11.9% attained scores of 16 and above in two settings, with 4.8% attaining scores of 21 and above in both settings. Amongst boys, 12.5% attained scores of 16 and above in two settings, with none attaining scores of 21 and above. Amongst girls, none attained scores of 16 and above in two settings, but 10.5% attained scores of 21 and above.

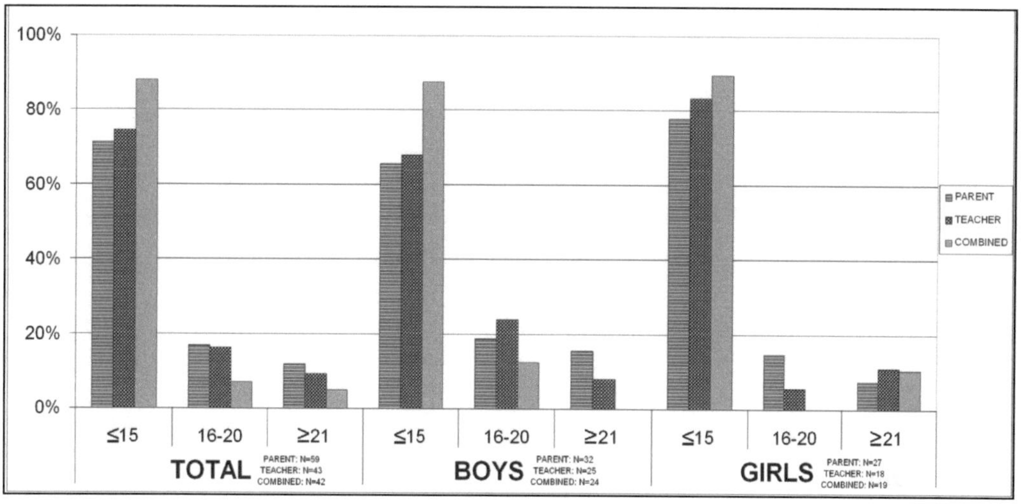

Fig. 1. ADHD Rating Scale Parent, Teacher and Combined Reports: Frequencies of attention deficit/hyperactive behaviors based on parent report, teacher report and parent and teacher report combined.

The frequencies of whether the child had never been medicated for attention deficit/hyperactive behaviors, had been medicated in the past or was medicated at the time of the study, by gender, are presented in Table 1 In order to shed light on the frequency of children with Down syndrome who had ever had behaviors warranting medication for attention deficit/hyperactive behaviors, both the children who had been medicated in the past and those who were medicated at the time of the study (past/present) were included. Of the total study population, 11.7% had been medicated for attention deficit/hyperactive behaviors at some time (present/past). Amongst the boys, 15.2% had received medication at some time, as opposed to 7.4% of the girls.

The frequency of medication use was also considered based on the severity of reported attention deficit/hyperactive behaviors for the total study sample. Based on parent report, 9.52% of children with ADHD Rating Scale scores of 15 and below, were medicated at some time (past/present), while this was true for 30% of those who attained scores between 16 and 20; none of the children with scores of 21 and above were medicated (past/present). Of those children who attained ADHD Rating Scale scores of 15 and below based on teacher report, 12.5% were medicated or had been medicated at some time, while 14.3% of those who attained score between 16 and 20 were medicated (past/present). Again, none of the children with scores of 21 and above were medicated or had been medicated in the past (Table 1).

		Boys N=33	Girls N=27	Total N=60	Parent (N=59)	Teacher (N=43)
Never Medicated		28 (84.8%)	25 (92.6%)	53 (88.3%)	-	-
Medicated in Past		2 (6.1%)	1 (3.7%)	3 (5.0%)	-	-
Medicated at Time of Study		3 (9.1%)	1 (3.7%)	4 (6.7%)	-	-
Total Medicated at Some Time		5 (15.2%)	2 (7.4%)	7 (11.7%)	-	-
ADHD Rating Scale Score Group	≤15	-	-	-	N=42 Medicated*=4 (9.5%)	N=32 Medicated*=4 (12.5%)
	16-20	-	-	-	N=10 Medicated*=3 (30%)	N=7 Medicated*=1 (14.3%)
	≥21	-	-	-	N=7 Medicated*=0 (0%)	N=4 Medicated*=0 (0%)

*At the time of the study or in the past

Table 1. Frequencies of medication use for attention deficit/hyperactive behaviors, by gender, and by severity of these behaviors based on parent and teacher report

ANOVA's performed to investigate age group differences in parent report total ADHD Rating Scale score (Table 2) revealed no group differences, however significant differences between age groups on the teacher's report of total ADHD Rating Scale score were found, with a large effect size ($F(2,41)=3.84$, $p=0.030$, $\eta^2=0.16$). A Scheffe post-hoc analysis was performed to assess this result; the oldest group had a significantly higher score on the ADHD Rating Scale teacher report (M=13.63; SD=7.70) than the youngest group (M=6.79; SD=4.17; $p=0.030$) but the middle group had an intermediate score (M=10.89; SD=8.87) that did not differ significantly from the oldest or youngest groups. There were no significant gender differences on the ADHD rating scales between boys and girls.

To analyze age-group differences in the need for medication for attention deficit/hyperactive behaviors, only those children who were medicated at the time of the study were included in the analysis (Table 1) as the inclusion of those who had been medicated in the past may have skewed the results. A chi^2 test performed to assess age group differences in whether the child received medication for attention deficit/hyperactivity behaviors at the time of the study revealed no group differences (χ^2[2, N=60]=0.43, p=0.81, not significant).

Independent sample t-tests performed to assess gender differences on parent report total ADHD Rating Scale score and teacher report total ADHD Rating Scale score, revealed no significant differences (Table 2). No gender differences in whether the child received medication for attention deficit/hyperactivity behaviors at the time of the study were revealed using a chi² test (χ^2[1, N=60]=0.69, p=0.40, not significant).

	Youngest M(SD)	Middle M(SD)	Oldest M(SD)	Boys Total Score M(SD)	Girls Total Score M (SD)	t	df	p
Parent report	n=20 12.50(5.02)	n=18 13.67(8.62)	n=21 13.90(6.80)	14.22(5.03)	12.33(8.45)	1.06	57	0.29(NS)
Teacher report	n=15 7.47(4.81)	n=9 10.89(8.87)	n=19 13.63(7.70)	11.44(6.99)	10.17(8.21)	0.55	41	0.59(NS)

Table 2. Average parent and teacher ADHD Rating Scale score by age group and independent sample t-tests to assess gender differences based on parent report and teacher report total ADHD Rating Scale score

3.2 ADHD Rating scale score group differences in measures of adaptive behavior

The results of independent sample t-tests performed to assess the differences between parent report ADHD Rating Scale score groups (15 and below; 16 and above) on the sub-scores of the three Vineland Adaptive Behavior Scale (VABS) domains (communication skills, daily living skills and socialization skills) are presented in Table 3. A significant difference with a medium effect size was found on the daily living skills standard score (t[57]=2.03; p=0.047) and a significant difference with a medium-to-large effect size was found on the communication skills standard score (t[56]=2.58; p=0.013)..

Independent sample t-tests performed to assess the differences between teacher report ADHD Rating Scale score groups (15 and below; 16 and above) on the sub-scores of the three VABS domains (communication skills, daily living skills and socialization skills) revealed no group differences (Table 3). Due to the discrepancy between parent and teacher report in terms of adaptive behavior, we applied Pearson Coefficient correlations between the parent and teacher ADHD Rating Scale total scores. Results yielded only moderate significant correlations (r=0.46; p=<0.01).

3.3 Correlations between parent and teacher ADHD rating scale scores and adaptive behaviors

Pearson Coefficient correlations between the VABS and parent report total ADHD Rating Scale score revealed significant moderate correlations for the communication skills standard score (r=-0.38) and the daily living skills standard score (r=-0.37) but not for the socialization skills standard score. Pearson Coefficient correlations between the VABS and teacher report total ADHD Rating Scale score revealed no significant correlations (Table 3).

Measure	Informant	Group	Mean(SD)	t-test	η^2	r	CI
Communication Skills Standard Score	Parent	≤15	54.02(11.64)	t[56]=2.58 p=0.013*	0.11	-0.38 p=0.003*	[-0.58]-[-0.13]
		≥16	45.53(10.81)				
	Teacher	≤15	53.19(11.00)	t[40]=0.46 p=0.65	N/A	-0.24 p=0.131	[-0.50]-[0.07]
		≥16	51.10(16.47)				
Daily Living Skills Standard Score	Parent	≤15	50.38(14.64)	t[57]=2.03 p=0.047*	0.07	-0.37 p=0.004*	[-0.57]-[-0.13]
		≥16	41.71(15.50)				
	Teacher	≤15	51.06(15.14)	t[41]=1.09 p=0.28	N/A	-0.25 p=0.107	[-0.51]-[0.06]
		≥16	44.91(18.80)				
Socialization Skills Standard Score	Parent	≤15	56.74(15.15)	t[52]=0.54 p=0.474	N/A	-0.21 p=0.124	[-0.45]-[-0.06]
		≥16	53.81(8.76)				
	Teacher	≤15	56.14(12.44)	t[37]=-0.53 p=0.60	N/A	-0.04 p=0.822	[-0.35]-[0.28]
		≥16	59.00(20.91)				

*Statistically significant, P<,0.05; CI confidence interval

Table 3. Independent sample t-tests between ADHD Rating Scale score groups (parent and teacher; 15 and below; 16 and above) and subscales of the Vineland Adaptive Behavior Scales and Pearson Coefficient correlations between total ADHD Rating Scale scores (parent and teacher) and the standard scores of the Vineland Adaptive Behavior Scales:

3.4 IQ differences based on parent and teacher ADHD rating scale score groups

The cognitive profile of the study sample has been previously reported (Rihtman et al., 2009). In the current study, the IQ scores were compared between children identified as having attention deficit/hyperactive behaviors and those without. One-way MANOVA's were employed to assess ADHD Rating Scale score group differences (≤15; ≥16) in the four Stanford Binet subscales. Based on parent report, no significant group differences were found (Wilk's Λ=0.91, F(4,50)=1.29, p=0.28, NS). Likewise, no significant group differences were found based on teacher report (Wilk's Λ=0.88, F(4,36)=1.26, p=0.30, NS).

4. Discussion

A high rate of Attention Deficit Disorder (ADHD) was previously observed by us in several groups of children; among the offspring of mothers with pregestational diabetes (Ornoy et al, 1998), among children born to mothers with gestational diabetes (Ornoy et al, 1999), as well as among offspring of heroin dependent mothers (Ornoy et al, 2001). These and other studies emphasize the importance of environmental factors to which the developing embryo and fetus were exposed in the etiology of ADHD. This is in addition to the well known genetic etiology of ADHD (Biederman et al., 2005; Biederman & Faraone, 2005; Furman, 2005). In the present study we were interested to assess the possible impact of DS, where trisomy 21 induces changes in many different genes, on the rate of ADHD, using accepted assessment measures.

In our previous study (Rithman et al, 2009) on the same group of children, we did not find any age related decline in the IQ scores of the children with DS. There was a significant correlation between IQ and different neurodevelpomental and adaptational measures (visual-motor integration and adaptive behavior) supporting previous findings implying that the IQ of children with Down syndrome is related to their success at implementing functional components and participating in specific activities. There was an age-related body function improvements and correlations between specific body functions and participation.. We also found sex differences on the short-term memory and motor function, with females performing better than males. However, functional sex differences on the specific VABS measures of copying, handwriting and free writing were not found. It was therefore of interest to see whether the occurrence of inattention is related to the IQ or to gender differences.

As stated above, the goals of the current study were to investigate the frequency of attention deficit/hyperactive behaviors amongst children with Down syndrome between the ages of 6 and 16, to assess age-group and gender differences in these behaviors and to analyze the relationship between the severity of these deficits and adaptive behavior and IQ. The findings have the potential of being both clinically significant as well as opening avenues for further investigation of the attentional function of children with DS.

The investigation into the frequency of attention deficit/hyperactive behaviors in this population in different settings revealed that it may be prudent to consider these behaviors from a number of perspectives. While current diagnostic criteria require deficits in two settings to warrant a diagnosis of attention deficit hyperactivity disorder (ADHD) (American Psychiatric Association, 2000), the results from the investigation of these behaviors at home and at school, as well as an analysis of combined parent and teacher reports, suggest that amongst children with DS, these behaviors should be considered from both angles. When the reports of the parent or teacher ADHD Rating Scale were considered individually, the frequency of attention deficit/hyperactive behaviors amongst children with DS appeared to be more common than that found in typically developing populations. When behavioral reports from both the child's home and educational environments were considered (as required to warrant a diagnosis of ADHD), reported deficits in the total study group were similar to that found in typically "normal" developing populations (~12%), with a similar frequency noted amongst children who had been medicated for these deficits at some time.

It may be feasible to assume that children with DS with more severe attention deficit/hyperactive behaviors reveal these deficits in both the home and educational environments and are those children whose deficits are pronounced enough to warrant medical intervention. Moreover, it should be considered that two of those children medicated for attention deficit/hyperactive behaviors at the time of the study had parent

ADHD Rating Scale scores below 15 and three had teacher ADHD Rating Scale scores below 15. Thus, even though these children were not included within the group of children demonstrating attention deficit/hyperactive behaviors, it is feasible to assume that they were medicated due to these behaviors and the medication was responsible for the lower scores on the ADHD Rating Scale; thus, the frequency of attention deficit/hyperactive behaviors is even higher than reported. This finding implies that, based on current diagnostic criteria, ADHD is apparently more prevalent amongst children with DS than amongst typically developing children (Biederman & Faraone, 2005).

However, the diagnostic potential of individual parent or teacher report in this population should not be overlooked. Our findings of inconsistencies between parent and teacher reports reinforce the need to consider not only whether or not the child with DS has a diagnosis of ADHD according to diagnostic criteria, but also whether the attention deficit/hyperactive behaviors may be expressed differently in different environments amongst non-referred samples in this population. The findings of reported deficits in individual environments are important to consider amongst this population, particularly when considering our findings of correlations between attentional function and adaptive behavior. Indeed, in a genetic study, Gizer et al., (2008) recently found that, while the combination of mother and teacher reports yielded the strongest association for hyperactive-impulsive symptoms, teacher reports alone were sufficient for identifying inattentive symptoms. This finding of a discrepancy on a genetic level reinforces the point that attention deficit/hyperactive behaviors can not be overlooked in individual settings, since there may be key differences in how parents and teachers rate attention deficit/hyperactive behaviors. Moreover, varying manifestations of this disorder (for example, hyperactive as opposed to inattentive symptoms) may be identified based on reports of different deficits in diverse environments, since different environments place different demands on children. As this deficit has an important impact on adaptive functioning amongst children with DS, this warrants consideration even if there are reports of deficits in one setting alone.

In the current study, when reports of deficits in only one environment (school or home) were considered, it appeared that the frequency of these deficits may be more common (~27%) than that found in typically developing populations.. While this may not conform to a diagnosis of ADHD, this frequency warrants consideration, since these deficits appear to impact on the functioning of these children in important areas. Deficits in only one setting may reflect a less severe form of ADHD or an environment-specific form of ADHD which may be similar in its severity to non-referred samples. However, these frequencies suggest that more than a quarter of children with DS will show some form of attention deficit/hyperactive behaviors in at least one setting.

The findings of relatively high percentages of medication use within the groups of children with scores below 15 on the ADHD Rating Scale, based on both parent and teacher report, and the lack of medication use within the groups of children scoring 21 and above on the ADHD Rating Scale may not be altogether surprising. It is likely that many of the medicated children attained lower scores due to their medication use, while those who attained extreme high scores did so since they were not medicated. Moreover, it is important to bear in mind that the use of medication for attention deficit/hyperactive behaviors is also dependent on parental opinion and preferences, the age of diagnosis of attention deficit/hyperactive behaviors and the opinions of the treating physician regarding the use of these medications in young children. Thus, those children with severe manifestations of attention deficit/hyperactive behaviors may be un-medicated due to parental preference and not due to a lack of need.

No age-group differences in the attentional profile of the cohort were found based on parent report, yet differences were found based on teacher's report, potentially due to different demands of the different environments which shift with age. The finding of age-group differences based on teacher report is particularly noteworthy, and may shed light on a potentially shifting attentional profile within the educational environment amongst children with DS with age, due to increased academic demands. While no age differences were noted between the youngest (younger pre-teen) and middle (older pre-teen) which is intermediate in its scores between the three groups, or middle and oldest (teenage) groups, the oldest group differed significantly from the youngest group and may suggest that attention deficit/hyperactive behaviors increase gradually as children with DS become teenagers.

Since this was a non-referred sample, the investigation into gender differences seems to be of particular importance. The findings appear to conform to the opinion regarding non-referred samples of typically developing children that gender differences are not as pronounced as in clinical samples. When both settings (i.e. parental and teacher's ADHD Rating Scale) were considered, the frequency of deficits was indeed in the realm of 1:1 (12.5%:10.5%; boys to girls respectively). While the differences did not reach significance, it should be noted that boys appeared to be medicated more than girls (15.2% and 7.4% respectively), potentially due to the clinical manifestations of their difficulties. Likewise, when only one setting (home/school) was considered, boys appeared to have higher frequencies of reported difficulties (~33%) as opposed to girls (16.7% [teacher] -22.2% [home]) yet, again, these differences did not reach statistical significance. Once again, this reinforces the need to consider reports of attention deficit/hyperactive behaviors in both the education and home environment of the child with DS.

The investigation of adaptive functioning in light of attention deficit/hyperactive behaviors amongst children with DS sheds light on a vital area of investigation for this population. It may not be surprising that no differences were found between children above and below the cutoff point for attention deficit/hyperactive behaviors on the socialization domain of the Vineland Adaptive Behavior Scales (VABS) in either the teacher or parent report as this is known to be an inherent area of strength for individuals with DS (Fidler et al 2006) and may therefore be less influenced by attention deficit/hyperactive behaviors. However, the finding of an association between attention deficit/hyperactive behaviors based on parent report and adaptive behaviors in the realms of daily living and communication skills, with greater impairments in attentional function leading to greater adaptive behavior impairments, has immense clinical significance. It would appear that skills in these realms are more based on learning and acquired behaviors and abilities than those required for successful social functioning which is a strength of this population, regardless of the lack of an association between IQ scores and attentional function in the current study since learning and attention are associated at every level of cognitive functioning. If this were the case, since intact attentional functioning is a major component of learning, (Posner et al, 2008) this association between impairments in attention and these elements of adaptive behavior is not surprising. It is, however, important to note as this association particularly reinforces the need to consider possible treatment of attention deficit/hyperactive behaviors in this population, even if these deficits are apparent only in one setting, since learning occurs both within the school environment and outside of it.

The lack of an association between adaptive behavior and attention deficit/hyperactive behaviors based on teacher report also raises a number of points to consider. This finding may reflect an important principle of current health paradigms, (World Health Organization, 2001) namely, that deficits in participation in different settings may not always result from deficits in body functions and structures. As such, a child with attention deficit/hyperactive behaviors in the classroom may not necessarily have participation deficits in their overall school functioning. An alternative explanation may be that, since the VABS was completed by parents while the ADHD Rating Scale was completed by teachers, the lack of an association between the VABS and the teachers ADHD Rating Scale may be due to informant differences. Indeed, only a moderate correlation between the parent and teacher report ADHD Rating Scale was found. In addition to the lack of congruence between parents and teachers with regard to the adaptive behavior of children with DS, Crystal et al (2001) stress that varying informant sources can produce significantly different descriptions of attention deficit/hyperactive behaviors. Different aspects of adaptive behavior may be stressed in different environments, and what may be considered to be adaptive behavior at home may not necessarily be perceived as such at school. It therefore seems prudent for future studies investigating the attention deficit/hyperactive profile of children with DS to assess adaptive behavior based on educator report as well.

In our previous study on the same population we assessed the functional and behavioral profile of these 60 children with Down syndrome. There were sex differences on the short-term memory as well as motor function, with females performing better than males. It is not clear whether the developmental continuum differs between males and females, and our findings begin to shed light on such differences.

We also found previously an association between IQ and measures of visual-motor integration and adaptive behavior. This supports previous findings implying that the IQ of children with DS is related to their success at implementing functional components and participating in specific activities. This result is also important when considering reports that functional attainments earned in childhood seem to be maintained into adulthood in this population (Brown et al, 1990). Adults with Down syndrome who are the most accomplished in terms of independence in daily living and maintaining paid employment are those who participated in structured school experiences aimed at teaching them specific skills. Yet reports of an IQ plateau or decrease beginning in early adulthood are common (wang, 1996).

Children with Down syndrome who show improved performance on structured tests may be those with greater motivational levels and thus predisposed to greater adaptive functioning by virtue of having a greater tendency toward experience and learning. Alternatively, more successful adaptive functioning may occur in children with the physical foundation of better functional components. It is possible that these children are then the ones who are better able to participate successfully in functional activities. If this is true, it would lend empirical support for intervention that is directed at improving functional components while using these functions to create a bridge with actual participation in age-appropriate activities.

A number of limitations are evident in the present study. Foremost, the study sample was small and was not compared to a typically developing population. An interesting idea for further investigation would be to compare the adaptive functioning of children with ADHD with and without DS. In addition, the use of the Parent-Teacher ADHD Rating Scale only provides limited information and future studies would benefit from using more extensive ADHD testing. Furthermore, the age group division could have been more homogenous with larger groups. Finally, the correlations performed in this study can not necessarily be considered to reveal a causal relationship between ADHD and adaptive behavior or IQ. While the findings begin to shed light on this area, further research should apply interventional studies which may provide a clearer picture regarding causal relationships between attention deficit/hyperactive behaviors and adaptive functioning of children with DS.

An additional limitation of the study is the wide age range of the oldest group, as a result of the attempt to include all teenagers within the same group and to examine differences between younger (6–8y) and older (8–10y) pre-adolescent school-aged children. However, future studies should ensure improved homogeneity of age groups and should also attempt to attain objective measures of handwriting performance. Finally, this study applied a cross-sectional study design that limits the interpretation of the developmental continuum of the child with Down syndrome. Further research should seek to apply longitudinal study designs.

5. Conclusions

Changing international health measures and intervention in children with developmental disorders also focuses in treating children with Down syndrome, with increased emphasis being placed on participation and on the acquisition of specific, functional skills and functional independence, all being vital element of their quality of life. Moreover, the fact that there is a high rate of ADHD among children with Down syndrome forces us to pay attention to that possibility in each child with trisomy 21 as proper medical or other treatment may help the child with Down syndrome to get better help.

Our findings of continuous improvement in function with age, if such intervention has been provided, is further evidence supporting the need for pediatric DS intervention to encourage improved body functions while emphasizing the acquisition of functional skills that enable enhanced participation in age-appropriate activities. In addition, this study raises doubts as to whether or not children with DS do indeed reach a functional plateau and offers the possibility of changing our perception with regard to the functional and educational potential of children with trisomy 21.

6. References

American Psychiatric Association. (1987). *Diagnostic and statistical manual of mental disorders* (3rd ed., Rev.). Washington, DC:

American Psychiatric Association. (2000). *Diagnostic and statistical manual of mental disorders* (4th ed., Text Revision). Washington, DC:

Barkley, RA. (1997). Behavioral inhibition, sustained attention, and executive functions: Constructing a unifying theory of ADHD. *Psychological Bulletin*, 221.,65-94.

Bauermeister, JJ, Shrout PE, Cha´vez, L, Rubio-Stipec, M, Ramı´rez, R, Padilla, L& Canino, G. (2007). ADHD and gender: Are risks and sequela of ADHD the same for boys and girls? *Journal of Child Psychology and Psychiatry*, 48, 831–839.

Biederman, J & Faraone SV. (2005). Attention deficit hyperactivity disorder. *Lancet,366,* 237-248.

Biederman J., Kwon A., Aleardi M., Chouinard V, Marino T., Cole, H.&, Faraone SV. (2005). Absence of gender effects on attention deficit hyperactivity disorder: Findings in non referred subjects. *American Journal of Psychiatry, 162,* 1083–1089.

Bittles, A H, & Glasson, E J. (2004). Clinical, social and ethical implications of changing life expectancy in Down syndrome. *Developmental Medicine & Child Neurology, 46,* 282-286.

Brown FR, Greer MK, Aylward EH, Hunt HH. (1990). Intellectual and adaptive functioning in individuals

with Down syndrome in relation to age and environmental placement. *Pediatrics* 85, 450–452.

Brown, JH, Johnson MH, Paterson, SJ, Gilmore, R, Longhi, E, & Karmiloff-Smith A. (2003). Spatial representation and attention in toddlers with Williams syndrome and Down syndrome. *Neuropsychologia, 41,* 1037–1046.

Burack J A,, Evans, DW, Klaiman, C & Iarocci, G. (2001). The mysterious myth of attention deficits and other defect stories: Contemporary issues in the developmental approach to mental retardation. *International Review of Research in Mental Retardation, 24,* 299-320.

Capone, G, Goyal, P, Ares, W & Lannigan, E. (2006). Neurobehavioral disorders in children, adolescents, and young adults with Down syndrome. *American Journal of Medical Genetics, Part C, 142C,* 158–172.

Carr J (2003). Patterns of aging in 30–35-year olds with Down's syndrome. *J Appl Res Intellect* 16, 29–40.

Cohen, J. (1988). *Statistical power analysis for the behavioral sciences (2nd ed.).* Hillsdale, NJ: Erlbaum.

Crystal, DS, Ostrander, R, Chen, RS, & August, GJ. (2001). Multimethod assessment of psychopathology among DSM-IV subtypes of children with attention-deficit/ hyperactivity disorder: Self-, parent, and teacher Reports. *Journal of Abnormal Child Psychology, 29,* 189–205.

Fidler, D J., Hepburn, S, & Rogers, S. (2006). Early learning and adaptive behavior in toddlers with Down syndrome: Evidence for an emerging behavioral phenotype? *Down's Syndrome, Research and Practice, 9,* 37-44.

Furman, L. (2005). What is attention-deficit hyperactivity disorder (ADHD)? *Journal of Child Neurology, 20,* 994–1002.

Gizer, IR, Waldman ID, Abramowitz A, Barr CL, Feng Y, Wigg KG, Misener VL, & Rowe DC. (2008). Relations between multi-informant assessments of ADHD symptoms, DAT1, and DRD4. *Journal of Abnormal Psychology, 117,* 869–880.

Hanson MJ. (2003). Twenty-five years after early intervention: A follow-up of children with Down syndrome and their families. *Infants and Young Children, 16,* 354-365.

Hastings RP, Beck A., Daley, D & Hill C. (2005). Symptoms of ADHD and their correlates in children with intellectual disabilities. *Research in Developmental Disabilities, 26,* 456–468.

Hays WL.(1994). Statistics. 5th edn. Belmont, CA: Wadsworth.

Määttä, T, Tervo-Määttä, T, Taanila, A, Kaski, M, & Iivanainen, M. (2006). Mental health, behaviour and intellectual abilities of people with Down syndrome. *Down's Syndrome, Research and Practice, 11*, 37-43.

Menkes, JH, & Falk,RE. (2005). Chromosomal anomalies and continuous-gene syndromes. In J. H. Menkes, H. B. Sarnat, & B. L. Maria (Eds.), *Child Neurology, 7th Ed.* (pp. 227-257). Philadelphia, PA: Lippincott Williams and Wilkins.

Ornoy, A, Ratzon, N, Greenbaum, C, Peretz E, Soriano D & Dulitzky M. (1998). Neurobehavior of children born to diabetic mothers a early school age. *Arch Dis Chil* 79, F94-F99.

Ornoy, A. Wolf, A., Ratzon, N., Greenbaum, C & Dulitzky, M. (1999). neurodevelopmental impact of diabetic alterations on early school-age children born to mothers with Gestational Diabetes. *Arch. Dis. Child*, 81, F10-F14.

Ornoy A, Segal J, Bar-Hamburger R & Greenbaum, C. (2001). The developmental outcome of school age children born to heroin- dependent mothers: Importance of environmental factors. *Dev. Med. Child. Neurol.* 43, 668-675.

Pelham, W.E, Gangy, E M, Greenslade, KE, & Milich, R. (1992). Teacher ratings of DSM-III-R symptoms for the disruptive behavior disorders. *Journal of the American Academy of Child and Adolescent Psychiatry, 31*, 210-218.

Posner, MI, Rothbart, MK, & Rosario Rueda, M. (2008). Brain mechanisms and learning of high-level skills. In A. M. Battro, K. W. Fischer, & P. J. Léna (Eds.), *The educated brain: Essays in neuroeducation.* Cambridge, UK: Cambridge University Press pp. 151-165.

Reiss, S., Levitan, G. W., & Szyskzo, J. (1982). Emotional disturbances and mental retardation: Diagnostic overshadowing. *American Journal of Mental Deficienty, 86*, 567-574.

Rihtman, T., Tekuzener, E., Parush, S., Tenenbaum, A., Bachrach, S.J., & Ornoy, A. (2009). Are the cognitive functions of children with Down syndrome related to their participation? *Developmental Medicine & Child Neurology, 52*, 72-78.

Roubertoux P& Kerdelhue B (2006). Trisomy 21: from chromosomes to mental retardation. *Behav Genet*; 36, 346–54.

Sparrow, SS, Balla, DA & Cicchetti DV. (1984). *Vineland Adaptive Behavior Scales interview edition: Expanded form manual.* Minnesota, MO: American Guidance Service.

Stefanatos, GA, & Baron, IS. (2007). Attention-deficit/hyperactivity disorder: A neuropsychological perspective towards DSM-V. *Neuropsychology Review, 17*, 5-38.

Thorndike, RL, Hagen, EP, & Sattler, J. M. (1986). *The Stanford Binet Intelligence Scale, Fourth Edition: Guide for administering and scoring*. Chicago, IL: Riverside Publishing.

Turner, S & Alborz, A. Academic attainments of children with Down's syndrome: a longitudinal study. *Br J Educ Psychol* 2003; 73: 563–83.

Van Cleve, SN & Cohen WI. (2006). Part I: Clinical practice guidelines for children with Down syndrome from birth to 12 years. *Journal of Pediatric Health Care, 20*(1), 47-54.

Vicari, S. (2006). Motor development and neuropsychological patterns in persons with Down syndrome. *Behavior Genetics, 36*, 355-364.

Vicari S & Carlesimo GA (2006). Short-term memory deficits are not uniform in Down and Williams syndromes. *Neuropsychol Rev* 2006; 16: 87–94.

Wang PP. (1996). A neuropsychological profile of Down syndrome: cognitive skills and brain morphology. *Ment Retard Dev Disabil Res Rev* 2, 102–108

World Health Organization. (2001). *International Classification of Functioning, Disability and Health.* Geneva:

3

Motor Behavior in Down Syndrome: Atypical Sensoriomotor Control

Regiane Luz Carvalho[1] and Délcia Adami Vasconcelos[2]
[1]*Centro Universitário de São João da Boa Vista-FAE. São João da Boa Vista*
[2]*Puc Minas Gerais*
Brasil

1. Introduction

In addition to the phenotype characteristics, the Down syndrome is accompanied by multi-system pathological conditions. These conditions involve delays in basic motor skills, motor impairments and abnormalities in postural and gait control. A large body of literature has documented delays in basic motor skills, such as walking, reaching and grasping, in children with Down syndrome. Also their movements are slower and more variable. There has been debate in the literature over the real cause of atypical motor behaviors observed in individuals with DS. Possible explanations are related to cognitive limitations, biomechanical deficits, neurological disorder, abnormal sensorimotor integration, compromised somatosensory system or adaptive choice. In this chapter, we will first discuss similarities in the control of movement, posture and balance between nonhandicapped individuals and those with DS, and then consider differences. Second, we will review the evidence that relates to whether individuals with DS have specific sensoriomotor deficits. Finally we will explore possible explanations for the cause of atypical postural behaviors observed in individuals with DS.

2. General characteristics of individuals with Down syndrome

Down syndrome (DS) is a chromosomal anomaly that leaves the individual affected with an additional chromosome (the21th). The syndrome is associated with approximately 1/800 live births and is one of the leading causes of intelectual disabilities. Intelectual disability of some degree is invariably presente in individuals with DS, but, unusual for any major chromosomal disorder, levels of impairment vary greatly acroos individuals. Most of those with DS fall within the moderate to severe range of disability, but some show levels of cognitive abilities that are bordeline normal while others experience profound mental retardation (Roizen, 2002).
In addition to the phenotype characteristics, the Down syndrome (DS) is accompanied by multi-system pathological conditions. The individual with DS faces numerous movement control challenges. These challenges involve delays in basic motor skills, motor impairments and abnormalities in postural and gait control.
The literature has documented delays in basic motor skills, such as walking, reaching and grasping, in children with Down syndrome (Palisano et al., 2001). The complexity of this

developmental pattern is also exhibited in what is described as differences in the structure of cognitive and sensoriomotor functioning. That is, children with DS have been found to exhibit particular difficulties in certain areas (e.g., linguistic skills; visual scanning; ability to attend, to discriminate and encode complex stimuli) compared with their overall level of mental function.

One of the most established findings is that children with DS are slower at both initiating and executing goal-directed movements compared to typically developing peers (Savelsbergh, et al., 2000). They also exhibit greater movement time advantages as the accuracy demands of the movement goal are increased (Hodges, et al., 1995). Commonly reported sensorimotor deficits exhibited by children with DS also include perceptual-motor slowness (Elliott & Bunn, 2004), limb control problems and decreased motor proficiency (Wuang, Lin, & Su, 2009). Also the motor items that required aspects of strength and balance (such as standing and walking) developed more slowly than other motor behaviors.

In summary, researchers have found the normal sequencing of motor development in infants with DS, although the pattern of development is slower and the variability higher (Van Dujin et al., 2010). Much of this developmental delay continues to be attributed to isolated factors such as low muscle tone. Ulrich et al., (1997) explain this delay by perception difficulty of postural responses, which undermines the sense of movement and its consequences. Uyanik et al., (2003) suggest the sensory integration dysfunction as a result of limited sensory experience.

Besides the development delay it is generally accepted that motor impairments are inevitably present, to greater or lesser extents, in individuals with DS. Their movements are slower and more variable. Evidences of slowness and lack of smoothness has been observed even in simple elbow-flexion movements (Almeida, et al., 1997), as well as in multijoint pointing tasks (Aruin & Almeida, 1997). As point out by Anson (1992) in a review of DS and reaction time, differences in simple reaction time have varied from 25% to greater than 300%. This slowness in reaction time can have two consequences. First, in all movements made in response to an external stimulus, the initiation of the movement is likely to be delayed and can therefore give the impression of slowness even if the actual movement itself is reasonably quick. Second, when individuals with DS are asked to perform sequences of movements, if each movement in the sequence is treated as a separate movement the sequence will be performed extremely slowly because of the increased reaction time to program each component movement.

3. Postural control

Also individuals with DS are characterized by instable postural control. They are unable to respond rapidly to changes in the environment (Haley1986). Typically they take longer to initiate and complete a motor task and have difficulty maintaining equilibrium (Galli et al. 2007; Vuillerme et al. 2001). Ulrich et al., (2004) compared levels of stiffness and forcing in preadolescents with and without DS, analyzing gait patterns on a treadmill at different speeds and showing the same adaptation mechanism: all participants increased their stiffness and forcing. The difference between the two groups is explained by the authors in terms of diferente goals: people with DS actuated the adaptation as a compensatory strategy, in order to maintain stability and to overcome the ligament laxity and hypotonia that characterize DS, while the control group's aim was to optimize metabolic efficiency. Kubo and Ulrich (2006) compared toddlers with DS, to control group and observed that individuals with DS showed wider step widths but not a larger ML displacement. The authors explained this finding speculating that the increase in step width contributes to ML stability by creating a wider base of support, but toddlers with DS cannot allow their nascent walking system to rock from side to side more than minimally, without losing control.

Although maintaining a bipedal position may appear to be simple, it requires integration of information arriving at the central nervous system (CNS) through the proprioceptive organs and senses, especially vision and the vestibular apparatus of the inner ear. In recent years, study of the behavior of the center of pressure (CoP) has emerged as a way of indirectly understanding the neuromuscular control of equilibrium. The CoP is the point location of the vertical ground reaction force vector. It represents a weighted average of all the pressures over the surface of the area in contact with the ground.

The analysis of the time and frequency domains of CoP data obtained from subjects on a strength platform has been used on several occasions to analyze healthy populations, as well as populations diagnosed with a pathology. Some studies on

the equilibrium of individuals with DS performed using this method conclude that this population shows deficient motor control compared to individuals without DS. Adults with DS show significantly higher postural sway velocity than control subjects during a resting stance (Galli et al. 2007; Rigold et al 2011) and adopt different patterns of anticipatory postural adjustments (Aruin & Almeida 1997). Specifically they react using a generalized pattern of co-activation.

3.1 Co-contraction

The simultaneous activation of agonist and antagonist (co-contraction) muscles has also been described during quiet conditions (Gomes & Barela 2007), gait (Smith et al. 2007, Rigoldi et al. 2010) and balancing on seesaw (Carvalho & Almeida 2009). The seesaw has been used to study CNS response to external forces because it demands more from the control system and requires an essential change in mode of utilization of incoming proprioceptive information. According to (Ivanenko et al. 1997) healthy subjects primarily use proprioceptive cues for motion perception and postural control when they are supported by a stable surface. For these authors, vestibular information is used to determine the state of the support surface, and, if the support surface is unstable, vestibular information is used to aid balance control. In a previous study we observed that neurologically normal individuals adopted an alternated EMG pattern between agonist and antagonist bursts of ankle muscles and scaled their postural response with the increment of the seesaw`s degree of instability (Almeida et al. 2006). Specifically they kept balance by alternating the activation of tibialis anterior and the gastrocnemius medialis muscles. The activation of the gastrocnemius started before the ankle moved from dorsal into plantar flexion and remained until the time the ankle shifted again into dorsal flexion. The activation of the tibialis anterior started before the ankle shifted into dorsal flexion, and remained active until the ankle shifted again into plantar flexion (Figure 1). On the other hand, the individual with DS kept balance by a continuous and simultaneous activation of TA and GM muscles, despite the direction of the ankle movement being into dorsal or plantar flexion (Figure 1). They were able to keep their balance on the seesaw without falling but they did so by using a pattern of muscle activity characterized by a co-activation of the agonist and antagonist muscles while control group did so by using an alternated muscles pattern. Also, contrary to control group the individuals with DS were not able to graduate the displacement magnitude of ankle joint with seesaw instability. The question is: why did they adopt unusual strategies to keep their balance on the seesaw?

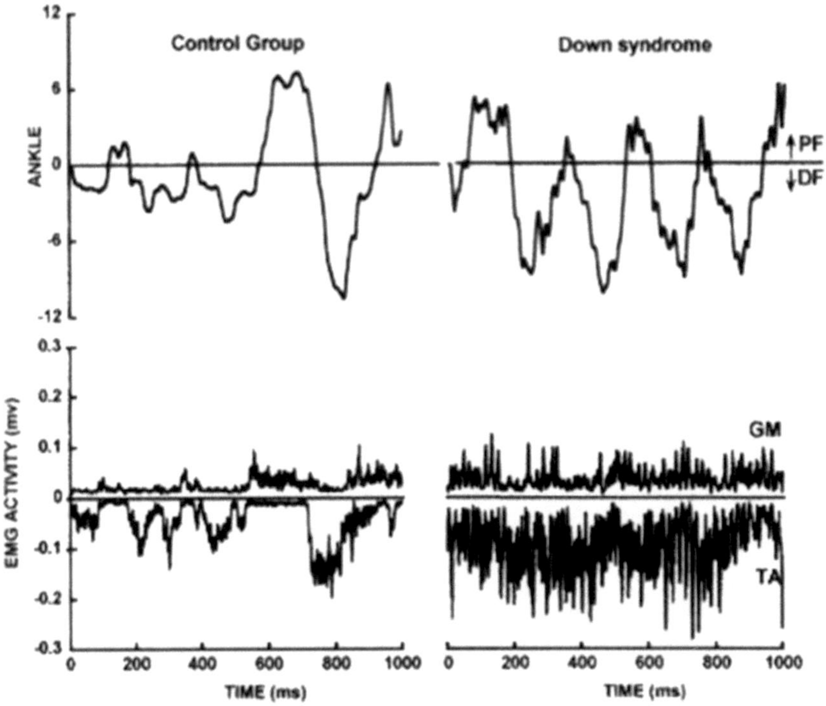

Fig. 1. Balance on a seesaw. Left panel are for control group subject and right for subject with DS. Positive values are for plantar flexion (PF) and gastrocnemius medialis (GM) activity and negative values for dorsal flexion (DF) and tibialis anterior activity.(Carvalho & Almeida 2009)

4. Explanations of atypical postural behaviors

There has been debate in the literature over the real cause of atypical postural behaviors observed in individuals with DS. Possible explanations are related to cognitive limitations (Latash & Anson 1996), neurological disorder (Moldrich et al. 2007), abnormal sensorimotor integration (Vuillerme et al. 2001), compromised somatosensory system (Brandt 1995) biomechanical deficits (Cioni et al. 1994) such difference in bone density, hypoplasia of cartilage, ligaments properties changes. These changes may affect the ability to generate joint torque and strength in isokinetic contractions. For Shields & Dodd (2004) the muscle weakness can also influence the ability to perform daily tasks such as equilibrium.

4.1 Neurological disorders

The brains of individuals with DS are smaller and lighter than those of normal individuals and exhibit a lower neuronal density; they also show synaptic irregularities due to the reduction of neurotransmitters and anomalies in myelination processes.

Favour to idea of neurological disorders are the studies investigating cerebral development have indicated that although persons with Down syndrome depend on their right hemisphere for speech perception, their left hemisphere appears to play the executive role in speech production (Maraj et al., 2002). Of relevance to the motor behaviour domain, left hemisphere specialisation for speech production is associated with a general lateralised proficiency for specifying the magnitude and timing of muscular force. That is, persons with Down syndrome appear to perceive speech with their right cerebral hemisphere, but depend on their left cerebral hemisphere for the organisation and control of movement thus, exhibiting atypical patterns of brain organisation.

In the motor domain, relating to visual and verbal-motor development, persons with Down syndrome have demonstrated relative proficiency on skills involving the visual demonstration of movement (Maraj et al., 2002). Several studies have shown that adults with Down syndrome exhibit more errors performing single manual oral gestures to a verbal command (e.g., "place your finger on your nose") than following the visual demonstration of a task. Elliott, Gray and Weeks (1991) proposed that the functional isolation of the speech perception (right hemisphere) and movement production (left hemisphere) systems has led to a breakdown in communication between these systems, adversely affecting tasks that require verbal-motor behaviour. This proposal had been previously formalised into a model of cerebral specialisation.

Subsequent research based on this model has indicated that individuals with Down syndrome experience difficulties in performing motor tasks based on verbal instruction. The model has been used in accounting for the information processing difficulties on the basis of verbal instruction. Further, there is some evidence to suggest that persons with Down syndrome may consolidate visual information such that positive transfer is seen when they are switched from a visual to verbal mode of learning. Although much work has been done on simple upper limb movements, real progress toward influencing broader health and education practices demands that we assess gross motor skills. Gross motor skills are an important component of many physical activities. Moreover, the acquisition of these types of motor skills can facilitate many other activities of daily living.

4.2 Adaptive choice

Other explanations are adaptive choice used in unexpected situations to enhance security and stability (Latash & Anson 1996). For these authors, while the movements produced by those with DS appear clumsy, they can be viewed as adaptive reactions due to changed priorities within the central nervous system. The central nervous system is able to generate solutions to provide movement outcomes accept to itself such as a wrong co-contraction pattern of pre-programed response to increase the stability. On the other hand, wrong reciprocal contraction pattern would increase the effects of perturbation. Interesting fact is that with the extensive practice of simple movements, these individuals are able to adopt a tri-phasic pattern of contraction, favoring the idea that the co-contraction is a choice made by the nervous system in view of its flexibility and adaptability. Although it is a mechanically sub-optimal choice, co-contraction offers more security and reflects insecurity of postural system to generate universal postural reactions. On the other hand, the high levels of co-contraction described above does not match with the characterization of lower tone and low ability to generate force of teenagers with SD. Exists therefore an inconsistency between the clinical evaluation of tone in this population and the abovementioned findings remain the relationship between hypotonia and co-contraction little understood. For Webber et al., (2004) and Vuillerme et al., (2001) evaluation of tone about passive conditions can provide limited information about the strategies used by SNC.

Among the explanations for the postural deficits found in individuals with DS, the favored explanatory hypothesis is that of a compromised sensorimotor system (Carvalho & Almeida 2009). Moreover, children with DS often exhibit significant perceptual problems. Auditory problems, often in association with ophthalmologic disorders such as cataracts, strabismus, nystagmus, visual and tactual impairments have been reported. However sometimes the apparent visual-perceptual problems in children with DS are actually due to deficits in the ability to physically perform the required task. Only a small proportion of children with DS were able to perform successfully on tactual and kinesthetic discrimination tasks (e.g., to discriminate among objects by texture, size, and weight while blindfolded), although the inclusion of visual input improved tactual performance in these children. In sum, children with DS show both motor and perceptual impairments that may influence the development and learning of various fundamental and complex actions. These influences have been widely reported over the years, but unfortunately not many findings have addressed the functional coupling of information and movement such as coupling of information and postural control.

4.3 Sensory contribution to postural control

One of the most widely used experimental approaches for understanding the sensory contribution to postural control is the manipulation of sensory information during postural disturbance. Galvanic vestibular stimulation (GVS) can induce postural reactions that are useful in determining the influence of vestibular function on balance (Fitzpatrick & Day, 2004). The vibration of muscle tendons is commonly used to determine the relative role of muscle proprioception in human posture control (Ruget, Blouin, Teasdale & Mouchnino, 2008). A number of studies have demonstrated that tendon vibrations, which almost selectively activate the primary endings of muscle spindles and elicits a discharge in the fast-conducting large-diameter Ia afferent fibers, can induce postural and orientation imbalance (Kavounoudias, Gilhodes & Roll, 1999). In order to better understand the sensory contribution to postural adjustments, we analyzed the effect of bipolar galvanic stimulation (GVS) and the vibration of Aquilles tendon on the pattern of muscle activity and joint displacements of individuals with DS.

Experiencing GVS, individuals with DS lacked the ability to maintain balance. The lack of balance under the effect of GVS cannot be explained by a change in muscle strategy as the pattern of co-activation was not changed by GVS. The DS individuals were more sensitive than control subjects to GVS (Carvalho & Almeida 2011). If somatosensory loss due to chronic neuropathy (Brandt 1995) or vibration (Carvalho & Almeida 2009) increases the reliance on vestibular information for control of postural orientation and individuals with DS also increases the reliance on vestibular information (shown by increased responses to GVS), we would suggest that individuals with DS have somatosensory deficits, and because of this, they were not able to compensate for a deficit of vestibular information with somatosensory feedback. Consistent with these findings are the results with vibration. The vibration was more detrimental to the balance performance of control group compared with group with DS. One possible reason is that vibration disrupted the somatosensory information of control group but not in individuals with DS already disrupted by some deficit. It is possible that their proprioceptive deficit may prevent them from detecting the vibration effects. Previous studies showed that postural sway in subjects with somatosensory loss was significantly larger than normal on a firm surface but not on the sway-referenced surfaced, suggesting that sway-referencing disrupts somatosensory information for postural control already disrupted by neuropathy (Horak et al 2002).

Our findings support the hypothesis of somatosensory deficits defended by such authors as Cole, Abbs & Turner (1988) showing that individuals with DS failed to modulate the grip force when were asked to lift one object with different surfaces and Brandt & Rosen (1995) showing low amplitudes for sensory nerve action potential following stimulation of the thumbs suggesting impaired peripherical somatosensory functions. Other possible explanation is a delay in central processing the afferent and efferent information at the cerebellum level because the cerebellum weight has been reported to be lower (Bellugi et al., 1990).

Despite the importance of knowledge of sensory changes, biomechanical and neurobiology for understanding motor deficits, characteristics such as environmental context, experience and practice have great influence over these deficits. The positive effects of the practice have been demonstrated. Repeated room mobile exposure of babies (illusory) led to a more coherent and stable coupling between visual information and the body oscillation (Polastri e Barela, 2005). Reduced stiffness over the trials during maintenance of static posture signaled the ability of adults to vary its stiffness with practice (Webber et al., 2004). Similarly Smith et al., (2007) observed the reduction of muscle stiffness values in tweens with SD after treadmill training, although the kinematic patterns adopted before and training have deferred of the control group patterns. According Tudela et al., (2011) the intervention should be started up to the 3rd month so that the infant can have adequate stimulus in different postures. If stimulation is started earlier, it can be a way of minimizing long periods necessary to improve a skill in the motor development required by the infants with Down syndrome, and thus facilitate motor acquisitions, mainly antigravitational postures.

Overall, the motor control studies in individuals with DS indicate deficits in postural control mechanisms. The acquisition of this control is delayed and postural mechanism seems to be organized in order to maximize stability, adapting them to the slowness and poverty of the responses to environment changes. The functional consequence of this principle is the reduction of speed and coordination of movements that become clumsy. Although restricted in laboratory conditions to practice has influenced positively the postural control. We believe that this practice should be focus in the function and not in the correction of compensatory adjustments since the SNC can adopt numerous motor patterns to realize motor tasks successfully (normal variability).

5. Conclusions

The Down syndrome is a multimodal disability affecting several systems therefore it is very difficult to pinpoint specific organic dysfunction for motor problems in these individuals. However, taking into consideration the lack of balance under the effect of GVS together with the fact that somatosensory loss increases the reliance on vestibular information, we could suggest that the balance difficulties observed in DS individuals during GVS can reflect deficits in the proprioceptive system.

6. References

Almeida GL, Corcos DM, Latash ML. Practice and transfer effects during fast single-joint elbow movements in individuals with Down syndrome. *Physical Therapy* 1994; 74(11): 1000-1016.

Aruin AS, Almeida GL. A. coactivation strategy in anticipatory postural adjustments in person with Down Syndrome. *Motor Control* 1997; 1: 178-191.

Brandt BR, Rosen I, Impaired Peripheral Somatosensory Function in children with Down syndrome. *Neuropediatrics* 1995; 26: 310-312.

Bellugi U, Jernigan TL, Anomalous brain morphology on magnetic resonance images in Williams syndrome and Down syndrome. *Arch Neurol.* 1990 May;47(5):529-33

Carvalho RL, Almeida GL. The effect of galvanic vestibular stimulation on postural response of Down syndrome individuals on the seesaw. *Res Dev Disabil.* 2011 Mar 17.

Carvalho R.L., Almeida G.L. (2009) Assessment of postural adjustments in persons with intellectual disability during balance on the seesaw. *J Intellect Disabil Res.* 53(4), 389-95.

Cole K.J., Abbs J.H., Turner G.S. (1988) Deficits in the production of grip force in Down syndrome. *Developmental Medicine and Child Neurology* 30, 752-758.

Elliott, D., & Bunn, L. (2004). Motor disorders in children with intellectual disabilities. In D. Dewey & D. E. Tupper (Eds.), Developmental motor disorders: A neuropsychological perspective (pp. 142–). New York: Guilford Publications.

Elliott, D., Gray, S. & Weeks, D. J. (1991). Verbal cueing and motor skill acquisition for adults with Down syndrome. *Adapted Physical Activity Quarterly*, 8, 210-220.

Fitzpatrick R.C., Day B.L. (2004) Probing the human vestibular system with galvanic stimulation. *J Appl Physiol* 96, 2301-2316.

Galli M., Rigoldi C., Mainardi L., Tenore N., Onorati P., Albertini G. (2007) Postural control in patients with Down syndrome. *Disabil Rehabil.* 9, 1-5.

Gomes MM, Barela JA. Postural control in down syndrome: the use of somatosensory and visual information to attenuate body sway. *Motor Control* 2007; 11(3): 224-34.

Haley S.M. (1986) Postural reactions in infants with Down syndrome: Relationship to motor milestone development and age. *Physical Therapy* 66, 17-22.

Hodges, N. J., Cunningham, S. J., Lyons, J., Kerr, T. L., & Elliott, D. (1995). Visual feedback processing and goal-directed movement in adults with Down syndrome. *Adapted Physical Activity Quarterly*, 12, 176–186.

Horak FB, Dickstein R, Peterka RJ. Diabetic neuropathy and surface sway-referencing disrupt somatosensory information for postural stability in stance. *Somatosens Mot Res.* 2002;19(4):316-26.

Kavounoudias A, Gilhodes JC, Roll R, Roll JP. From balance regulation to body orientation: two goals for muscle proprioceptive information processing? *Exp Brain Res.* 1999 Jan;124(1):80-8.

Kubo, M., & Ulrich, B. D. (2006). Early stage of walking: Development of control in mediolateral and anteroposterior directions. *Journal of Motor Behavior*, 38(3),229–237.

Maraj, B.K.V., Robertson, S.D., Welsh, T.N., Weeks, D.J., Chua, R.C., Heath, M., Roy, E.A., Simon, D.A., Weinberg, H.A. & Elliott, D. (2002). Verbal-motor behaviour in persons with Down syndrome. In M. Cuskelly, A. Jobling & S. Buckley (Eds) Down Syndrome Across the Lifespan. Pp. 175-193. London, England: Whurr Publishers Ltd

Latash ML, Anson JG. What are normal movements in atypical populations? *Behavioral and Brain Sciences* 1996; 19: 55-68.

Moldrich R.X., Dauphinot L., Laffaire J., Rossier J., Potier M.C. (2007) Down syndrome gene dosage imbalance on cerebellum development. *Prog Neurobiol* 82(2), 87-94.

Palisano RJ, Walter SD, Russell DJ, Rosenbaum PL, Gémus M, Galuppi BE, Cunningham L. Gross motor function of children with down syndrome: creation of motor growth curves. *Arch Phys Med Rehabil* 2001; 82(4): 494-500.

Polastri PF, Barela JA. Perception-action coupling in infants with Down syndrome: Effects of experience and practice. *Adapted Physical Activity Quarterly* 2005; 22: 39-56.

Rigoldi, C, Galli M, Mainardi L, Crivellini M, Albertini G. Postural control in children, teenagers and adults with Down syndrome *Research in Developmental Disabilities* 32 (2011) 170–175

Roizen, N. (2002). Down syndrome. In M. L. Batshaw (Ed.), Children with disabilities (5th ed.). Baltimore, ML: Paul H. Brookes.

Ruget H, Blouin J, Teasdale N, Mouchnino L. Can prepared anticipatory postural adjustments be updated by proprioception? *Neuroscience.* 2008 Aug 26;155(3):640-8. Epub 2008 Jun 17.

Savelsbergh, G., van der Kamp, J., Ledebt, A., & Planinsek, T. (2000). Information coupling in children with Down syndrome. In D. J. Weeks, R. Chua, & D. Elliott (Eds.), Perceptual-motor behavior in Down syndrome (pp. 251–275). Champaign, IL: Human Kinetics.

Smith BA, Kubo M, Black DP, Holt KG, Ulrich BD. Effect of practice on a novel task-walking on a treadmill: preadolescents with and without Down syndrome. *Phys Ther* 2007; 87(6): 766-77.

Shields N, Dodd KA, systematic review on the effects of exercise programms designed to improve strength for people with Down syndrome. *Phys Therapy Reviews* 2004; 9: 109-115

Tudella,E.,etal. Description of the motor development of 3–12month old infants with Down syndrome: The influence of the postural body position. *Research in Developmental Disabilities* (2011), doi:10.1016/ j.ridd.2011.01.046

Ulrich BD, Ulrich DA, Chapman DD. Sensitivity of infants with and without Down syndrome to produce treadmill steps. *Phy Ther* 1997; 75: 14-23.

Ulrich, B. D., Haehl, V., Buzzi, U. H., Kubo, M., & Holt, K. G. (2004). Modelling dynamic resource utilization in populations with unique constraints: Preadolescents with and without Down syndrome. Human Movement Science, 23(2), 133–156.

Uyanik M, Bumin G, Kayihan H. Comparison of different therapy approaches in children with Down syndrome. *Pediatrics International* 2003; 45: 68-73.

Van Dujin Van Braeckel K, Butcher PR, Geuze RH Difference rather than delay in development of elementary visuomotor processes in children born preterm without cerebral palsy: a quasi-longitudinal study.*Neuropsychology.* 2010 Jan;24(1):90-100.

Vuillerme N, Marin L, Debu B. Assessment of Static Postural Control in teenagers with Down syndrome. *Adapted Physical activity Quarterly* 2001; 18: 417-431.

Webber, A Babul V, Edwards R. Stiffness and postural stability in adults with Down syndrome. *Exp Brain research* 2004; 155: 450-458..

Wuang, Y. P., Lin, Y. H., & Su, C. Y. (2009). Pasch analysis of the Bruininks–Oseretsy test of motor proficiency-second edition in intellectual disabilities. *Research in Developmental Disabilities*, 30, 1132–1144.

Part 2

Dentistry and Skeletal Features

4

Skeletal Age of Down Syndrome Individuals

Mari Eli Leonelli de Moraes and Luiz Cesar de Moraes
São Paulo State University - UNESP, School of Dentistry of São José dos Campos
Brazil

1. Introduction

Down syndrome (DS) is a genetic disorder caused by the presence of all or part of an extra 21st chromosome and the most likely cause is non-disjunction occurring during gametogenesis (meiosis). It was first described in 1866 by a British physician named John Langdon Down and it is also known as trisomy 21 and trisomy G. This syndrome is the most common congenital mental disability and affects individuals independent of social status or ethnic group. (Jensen et al., 1973; Coe et al., 1999; Oliveira, 2001) The incidence of Down syndrome ranges between 1 in 600 and 1 in 350 live births. (Mustacchi & Rozoni 1990, Moraes 2007c) There are around 184.000 people with DS in Brazil and over 5.8 million people in the world.

The DS involves a set of signs that characterize a delay in the pre-natal and post-natal development, mental and general alterations with stature values observed to be generally below the normal standards. Regarding mental aspects, the average of intelligence quotient (IQ) in DS individuals are around 36.5. (Coelho & Loevy, 1982; Mustacchi & Rozone, 1990; Rey, 1991; Hayes & Batshaw, 1993; Moraes, 2002; Schwartzman, 2003; Barata & Branco, 2010) The general alterations involved slanting eyes, almond-shape, plica palpebronasalis (epicanthus), strabismus, myopia; flattening of the nose bridge, small, short nose with broad nasal bridge, pug nose; lop with flat or absent helix of the ears, auricles with a low implantation; wide and short neck with abundant skin; wide hands and short fingers; clinodactyly; brachydactyly; muscular hypotony and atlanto-axial instability (Ali 2006; Moraes, 2007c). They also can present dove-like chest, small genitalia, alterations of motor coordination, obesity, short stature (Cohen & Winer, 1965) thyroid diseases. Individuals with DS are more susceptible to leukemia and other types of malignant than the population at large. (Hill et al., 2003)

The systemic alterations with special dental significance in DS patients are congenital cardiopathy, pneumonia, allergy, bronchitis, tonsillitis, convulsion and blood dyscrasia. (Mariano et al., 1999; Pilcher, 1998; Ribeiro et al., 2003) The degree of systemic problems varies from individual to individual. (Jara 1993) Some people may have all the alterations, while others may have only a few of the problems. (Nadel, 2003; Mustacchi & Rozone, 1990)

The facial features of DS individuals include brachycephaly (condition where the head is disproportionately wide), hypotonic facial muscles, with a flat profile, normodivergent vertical pattern, lip incompetence, an ogival and deep hard palate, (Higa & Vargas-Machuca, 2004), and Class II malocclusion (Cohen & Winer, 1965). It is possible to observe

brachycephaly; small and underdeveloped maxilla; a fissured tongue with papillary hypertrophy and macroglossia, with an incidence of 11-60%. Labial fissures and angular cheilitis are some other common findings. (Aguiar et al., 2002)
The teeth of these patients present complete mineralization, but with a great variation in the eruption pattern, although it maintains a certain similarity in the sequence and symmetry. (Pilcher, 1998) It has been reported (Alpöz & Eronat, 1997) that these individuals usually have late eruption of the deciduous and permanent teeth, although Jara et al. did not find any differences on the sequence of eruption in DS people. Delay was also found in the mineralization chronology development of the canines and second molars. (Santos, 2004)
It is a universal finding in the literature that they have high prevalence of periodontal diseases and low prevalence of caries (Castilho & Marta, 2010). The higher prevalence of periodontal disease is probably related to the impaired host-response rather than to specific periodontal pathogens. (Reuland & Bosma, 2001; Cavalcante, 2009) The low caries prevalence seems to be due to immune protection caused by the elevated salivary *S.mutans* specific IgA concentrations. (Lee et al., 2004, Murakami et al., 2008)
Dental anomalies are very common, both in the primary and permanent teeth and in the patients with DS, dental anomalies occur with an incidence five times greater than in the normal population (Ingalls & Butler, 1953; Kumasaka et al., 1997). The most common dental associated with DS are variations in tooth number and morphology. (Seagriff-Curtin et al., 2006) Tooth eruption may be delayed, may occur in an unusual order and can be 2 to 3 years behind a child's normal eruption pattern. Over-retained primary teeth are also common. (Moraes, 2004) In the primary dentition, the most commonly absent teeth are lateral incisors, while in the permanent dentition, third molars, second premolars and lateral incisors, in this sequence, are the most frequently missing teeth. (Thompson 1976) Desai, 1997, described the oral anomalies that may require medical consultation, but also emphasized that these patients are routinely managed in an office setting to treat cases of microdontia, hipoplasia, partial anodontia, taurodontism and others manifestations. According to Moraes et al., 2007c, there was a high incidence of different types of dental anomalies, such as taurodontism (50%), anodontia (50%), conic teeth (8.3%) and impacted teeth (5.9%) and in most cases, the same individual presented more than one dental anomaly.
It is noteworthy that the variations of the development parameter in relation to the skeletal and dental age were deemed normal. (Moraes et al., 1998; Moraes et al. 2007a, 2007b) The variation degree was evaluated in order to assess how different the skeletal age was difference in DS individuals when compared with non DS group.
Only a few researchers have assessed the skeletal development of individuals with DS. Pozsonyi et al. (1964) and Sannomiya et al. (1998) observed a delay of skeletal development at the earlier years in relation to individuals without DS. They also observed that the process of skeletal maturation of individuals with DS was completed at around 15 years of chronological age.
The aim of this research was evaluate skeletal age of DS individuals in order to verify if they are delayed or advanced when compared with control group of non DS individuals.

2. Material and methods

This research was authorized by the Local Ethical Committee under the protocol no. 050/2005-PH/CEP.

Seventy-five hand and wrist films of DS individuals from the archive of the Discipline of Radiology at the School of Dentistry - São Paulo State University (UNESP) - São José dos Campos -SP, Brazil, were initially evaluated. The final study population comprised 40 hand and wrist radiographs of individuals with DS (19 males, 21 females). They had to fulfill the following inclusion criteria: (1) The subjects had to be between 6 and 16 years of chronological age; (2) Their radiographic films had to have high clarity and good contrast. Using the same inclusion criteria, 100 hand and wrist radiographs from individuals who did not have DS (50 males, 50 females) were selected from the same archives as a control group.
All the hand and wrist radiographs were made with a Philips Oralix X-ray machine operating at 50 kVp and 5 mA, with an exposure time of 0.2 seconds Kodak T - MAT G/RA (Eastman Kodak Corp., São José dos Campos-SP, Brazil) 18-24 cm plain films were used in association with a cassette and Kodak Lanex Regular rare earth screens (Eastman Kodak Co., Rochester, NY). The films were processed in a Macrotec MX-2 automatic processor (Macrotec, São Paulo, Brazil) with Kodak GBX processing chemicals (Eastman Kodak Co., Rochester, NY). The processing time was four minutes.
The sample was split into two groups: films from persons with DS and those without DS. The individuals of each group were divided into A and B subgroups according to their gender. Therefore, a total of four groups were created (Group 1A and Group 2A for females, Group 1B and Group 2B for males).
To prevent any bias during the assessment of skeletal age, the identification tags of the radiographs were covered with dark paper and randomly numbered for later identification. The examiner was also blinded as to the different groups. The skeletal age of all subjects was determined by an experienced oral radiologist according to the method of Greulich & Pyle (1959). This method evaluates the individual's ossification center of the hand and wrist (FIGURE 1), which is then compared to its pair in the atlas of skeletal development of the hand and the wrist.
The authors' suggestion was to begin the assessment of the skeletal maturation by comparing the patient's hand and wrist film with the standard of same gender and nearest chronological age in the atlas. Then the operator compared the film with the adjacent standards, both older and younger than the one of nearest chronological age. The operator then selected the standard that was closest to the patient's film for a more detailed comparison. The individual's skeletal age was established by matching the majority of the ossification centers with those of a certain age in the atlas.
The radiographic images were displayed in a darkened room over a light box and viewed with a dark mask to block excess light. Data were tabulated and submitted for statistical analysis. Simple linear regression analysis was used to compare the relationship between the skeletal age and the chronological age of each group of individuals.
The difference between the chronological age (CA) and the skeletal age (SA) of each individual was calculated to establish whether the skeletal age was delayed or advanced in relation to the chronological age. The mean values of these differences for Group 1A were compared with those of Group 1B by means of Student's *t*-test. The same comparison was made with Groups 2A and 2B. Student's *t*-test was used to compare the mean values for the differences of the chronological age and the skeletal age of Group 1A and Group 2A, etc. These comparisons were made to evaluate whether the skeletal maturation would be the same among individuals of same population (Group 1A _ Group 1B and Group 2A _ Group 2B) and among individuals of same gender but from different populations.

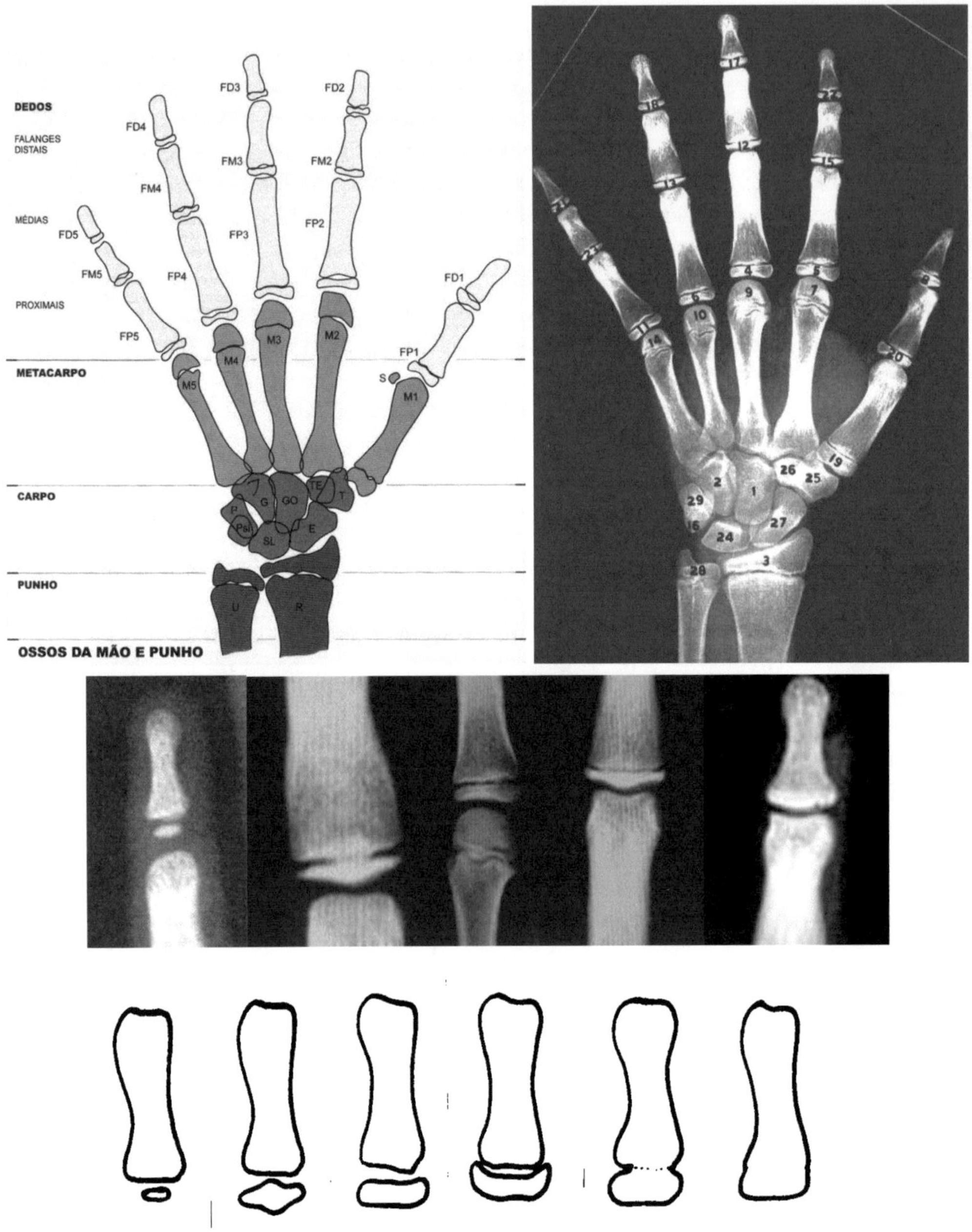

Fig. 1. (A)Anatomy of hand and wrist of bones used to evaluate Greulich & Pyle method (1959). (B) Sequence of ephyfises and diaphesis maturation.

3. Results

The sample of 40 individuals with DS included 21 females (52.5%), mean age of 11.12 ± 3.05 years, and 19 males (47.5%), mean age of 12.43 ± 3.13 years. The control group comprised 100 individuals who did not have DS, 50 females (50%), mean age of 11.26 ± 2.38 years, and

50 males (50%), mean age of 11.02 ± 2.40 years. The mean and the standard deviation of chronological age (CA), skeletal age (SA), and the difference between the CA and the SA in months are shown in Table 1.

Group	Chronological age		Skeletal age		Difference CA-SA	
	Mean	SD	Mean	SD	Mean	SD
1A Females with DS	133.05	36.67	144.19	48.59	-11.14	20.40
2A Females	135.16	28.63	131.16	34.18	4.00	10.14
1B Males with DS	149.16	37.60	164.68	57.21	-15.53	23.90
2B Males	132.28	28.91	126.36	29.40	5.92	12.53

CA= Chronological age , SA= Skeletal age, SD= Standard-deviation, DS= Down syndrome

Table 1. Mean and standard-deviation of the chronological age (CA), skeletal age (SA) and difference of CA and SA for each group (in months).

The skeletal age (SA) of Groups 2A and 2B, individuals without DS was, on average, 4.0 and 5.9 months delayed in relation to the chronological age (CA) (Table 1). However, the SA of Groups 1A and 1B, individuals with DS was, on average, 11.1 and 15.5 months advanced in relation to the CA.
Student's *t*-test results for comparisons of mean values for the differences of the SA and the CA between Groups 1 and 2 are shown in Table 2.

	CA-SA (non-DS individuals x DS individuals)		
	t critical	**Stat t**	***p*-value***
Female	2.06	3.23	< 0.05
Male	2.07	3.72	< 0.05

CA= Chronological age, SA= Skeletal age, SD= Standard-deviation, DS= Down syndrome, *<=0.05

Table 2. The *p*-values for comparisons of the mean values of the differences between the CA and SA for Groups 1A and 2A and groups 1B and 2B.

When the mean values of the CA and SA differences for Groups 1A and 2A were compared, significant statistical differences were found ($p < 0.05$). The same was detected for the comparison of Groups 1B and 2B ($p < 0.05$) (Table 2). Therefore, the subjects with DS had their SA advanced in relation to their CA, when compared to the subjects who did not have DS.

The *t*-test results were used to compare the SA and the CA differences between males and females. When the mean values of the differences of CA and SA for Groups 2A and 2B were compared, no significant statistical differences were detected ($p > 0.54$). The skeletal maturation of non-DS male and female individuals was also similar. In other words, they had, on average, a delayed SA in relation to their CA. No significant statistical differences between the mean values of the differences between SA and CA were found when Groups IA and 1B were compared ($p = 0.40$). Hence, the SA of individuals with DS, males and females, on average, was advanced in relation to the CA (Table 1).

Figure 2 presents a chart with values of the differences between the CA and the SA for each subject in Group 1, and for each subject in Group 2. From the analysis of the results, we verified that there was a tendency of young individuals with DS (around 7 years of age) to have their SA delayed in relation to their CA. However, the SA of these individuals overtook their CA during adolescent maturation. At the age of 15, most individuals had their SA advanced in relation to their CA. Figures 3A, 3B, 3C, 3D show the examples of male and female at 7 years and at 15 years old, with different cases of delayed and advanced SA.

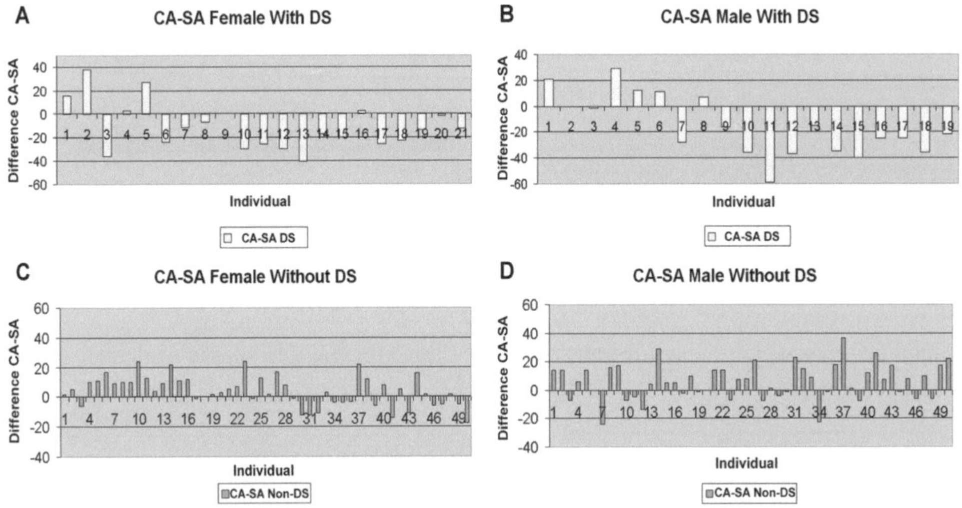

Fig. 2. Charts representing the difference between CA and SA of each subject in each group. A: Group 1A; B: Group 1B; C: Group 2A; D: Group 2B.

The linear regression analysis showed that the duration of skeletal maturation was shorter in individuals with DS when compared to those who did not have DS, as shown by the tendency lines (Figure 2A, C) and by the angular coefficients of the linear regression equations (Table 3). During the early stages of skeletal maturation, the subjects with DS tended to have their SA delayed in relation to their CA. However, during the latter stages of skeletal maturation, these individuals tended to have an advanced SA in relation to their CA (Figure 2B, D). Still, a good correlation between SA and CA was observed in individuals with DS ($R2 > 0.85$) (Table 3).

Figure 5 presents tendency charts (A,C) of the SA in relation to the CA, line charts of the SA, and the CA of each individual without DS (B,D), divided by gender.

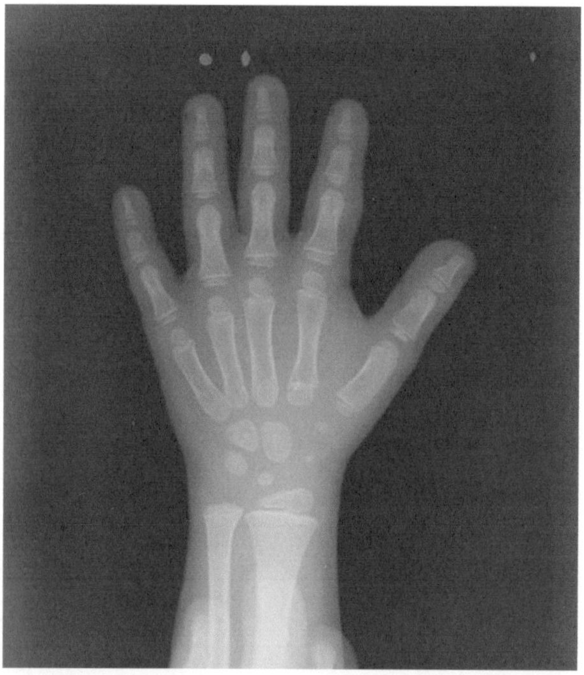

Male - Delayed skeletal age (SA) at 6 years old. Chronological age (CA) 75 = months; Skeletal age (SA) = 54 months

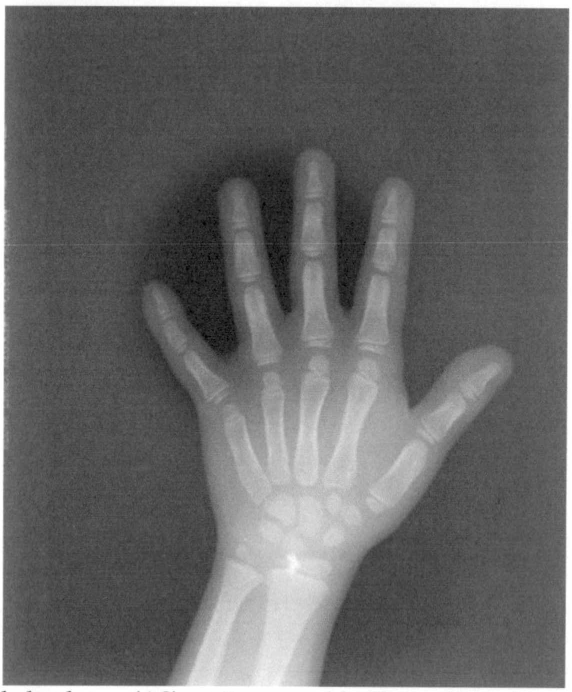

Female - Delayed skeletal age (AS) at 7 years old. Chronological age (CA) 87 = months; skeletal age (SA) = 60 months.

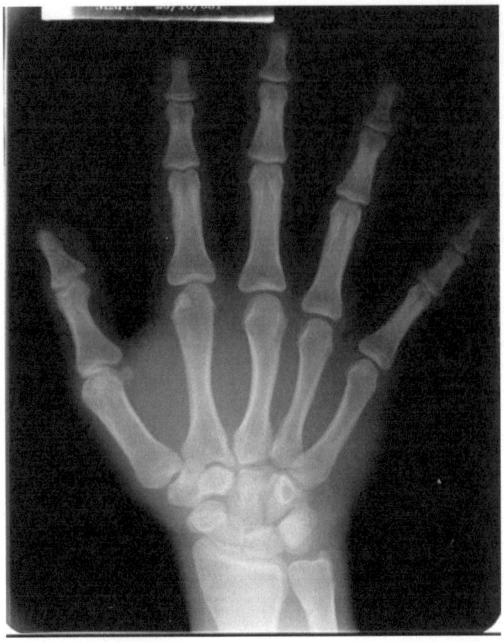

Male - Advanced skeletal age (SA) at 15 years old. Chronological age (CA) 188 months and skeletal age (SA) 228 months

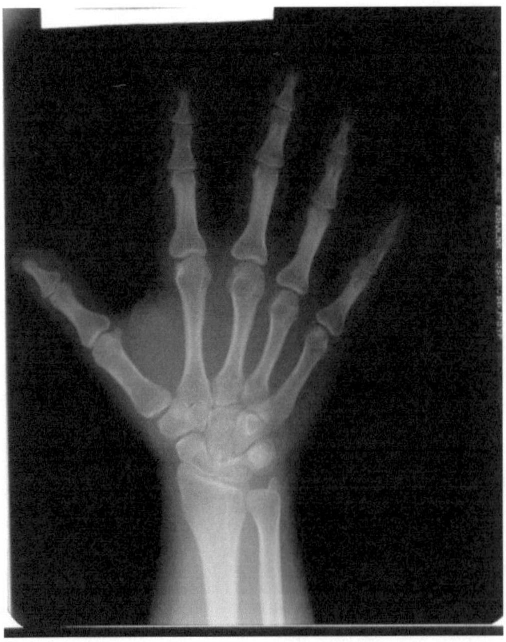

Female - Advanced skeletal age (SA) at 15 years old. Chronological age (CA) 191 months and skeletal age (SA) 204 months

Fig. 3. Examples of skeletal age (SA) evaluated by Greulich & Pyle method, around 7 years and at 15 years, for both, male and female.

Figure 4 presents the tendency charts (A,C) of the SA in relation to the CA, line charts of the SA, and the CA of each subject without DS (B,D), divided by gender.

The SA tended to be similar to the CA in females who did not have DS, as shown in Figure 3 (A,B) and by angular coefficient of the linear regression analysis (Table 3). We also observed a good correlation between the SA and the CA in these individuals (R2 = 0.927). Nevertheless, in males without DS there was a tendency for their SA to be delayed in relation to their CA, as shown in Figure 3 (C,D) and by the angular coefficient of the linear regression analysis (Table 3). A good correlation between the SA and the CA was found in males (R2 = 0.824), although this correlation was lower than the correlation between the SA and the CA for females.

Figure 4 presents tendency charts (A,C) of the SA in relation to the CA, line charts of SA, and the CA of each subject with DS (B,D), divided by gender.

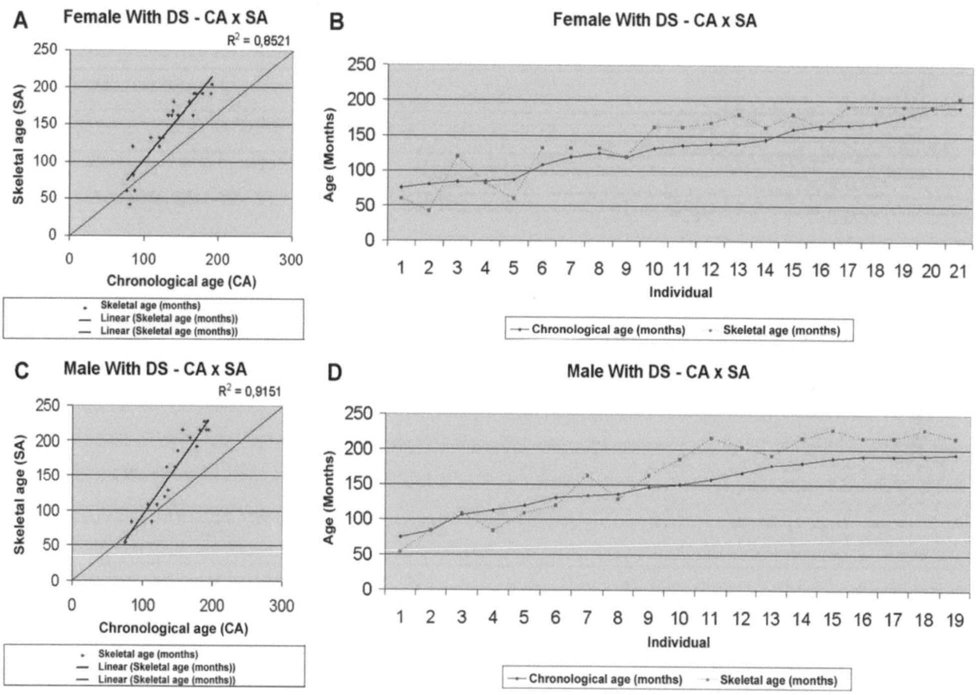

Fig. 4. Group 1A (A, B) and Group 1B (C, D). A and B: Tendency chart representing the skeletal age versus the chronological age. C and D: Line chart of the skeletal age and the chronological age of each subject.

4. Discussion

It is known that DS is a result of a genetic anomaly that causes a number of local and systemic changes whose manifestations are expressed in various degrees. However, to what extent the condition alters the timing of growth and the duration of growth is a subject that needs further study.

In our study, we observed that the skeletal age (SA) of females without DS (Group 2A) and males without DS (Group 2B) was on average 4.0 and 4.92 months delayed in relation to the chronological age (CA) (Table 1). On the other hand, the SA of Groups 1A and 1B was on average 11.14 and 15.53 months advanced in relation to their CA (Table 1).

When the mean values of the differences of CA and SA of Groups 1A and 2A were compared, statistically significant differences were found ($p < 0.05$) (Table 2).

The same was detected for the comparison of Groups 1B and 2B ($p < 0.05$) (Table 2). Therefore, subjects with DS had their SA advanced in relation to their CA (Table 1) when compared to the control subjects.

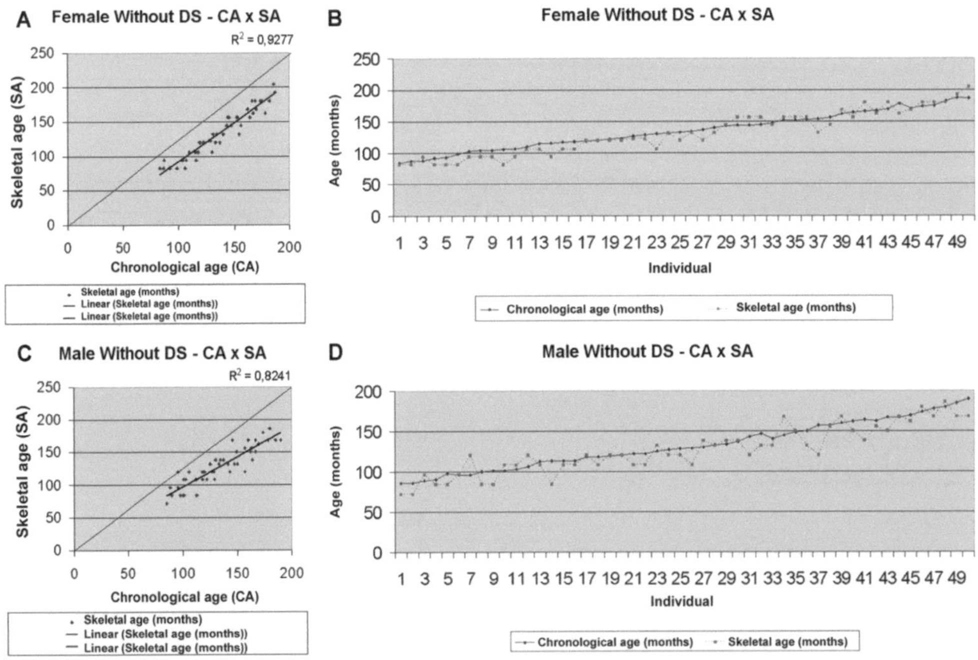

Fig. 5. Group 2A (A, B) and Group 2B (C, D). A and B: Tendency chart representing the skeletal age versus the chronological age. C and D: Line chart of the skeletal age and the chronological age of each subject.

	Male		Female	
	Equation	R^2	Equation	R^2
Group 1	IO=1,45xIC-52,4*	0,92	IO=1,22xIC-18,54*	0,85
Group 2	IO=0,92xIC+4,21*	0,82	IO=1,14xIC-24,25*	0,93

*Y=ax+b, where y=SA; x=CA; a= angular coefficient; b= linear coefficient

Table 3. Results of the linear regression tests for the comparisons between CA and SA in each group.

When the mean values of the differences of CA and SA of Groups 2A and 2B were compared, no significant differences were detected ($p > 0.05$). Therefore, the skeletal maturation of the control subjects (male and female) was similar, which means their SA was delayed in relation to their CA (Table 1).

No statistically significant differences between the mean values of the differences between the SA and the CA were found when Groups 1A and 1B were compared ($p > 0.05$). Therefore, the SA of male and female subjects with DS was advanced in relation to their CA (Table 1).

From the analysis of the results, we verified that there was a tendency for individuals with DS, at about 7 years of age, to have their SA delayed in relation to their CA. However, the SA of these individuals overtook their CA during adolescent maturation. At the age of 15 years, most of these individuals had their SA advanced in relation to their CA (Figure 2). An evaluation of the linear regression analysis showed that the duration of skeletal maturation was shorter for individuals with DS when compared to the controls group(Figure 4A,C), and also from the angular coefficients of the linear regression equations (Table 3). A good correlation between the SA and the CA was observed for subjects with DS ($R2 > 0.80$) (Table 3). Similar results have been reported by Pozsonyi et al. (1964) and statistically Sannomiya et al. (1998).

In female individuals without DS, their SA tended to go along with their CA, as seen (Figure 5A, B) in the angular coefficient of the linear regression analysis (Table 3). We also observed a good correlation between the SA and the CA of the control subjects ($R2 > 0.927$). For male subjects, there was a tendency for their SA to be delayed in relation to their CA, as can be seen in the angular coefficient of the linear regression analysis (Table 3). They also had a good correlation between their SA and their CA ($R2 > 0.824$), although this correlation was lower than the correlation between the SA and the CA of the female subjects.

Thus, contrary to what we expected, in this study the skeletal development of individuals with DS had a shorter period of skeletal maturation when compared to individuals who did not have DS.

Although the SA was delayed in relation to the CA in young individuals with DS, there was a more pronounced period of growth, which caused the skeletal maturation of individuals with DS to be completed earlier. These results have also been reported by Pozsonyi *et al.* (1964) and Sannomiya et al. (1998).

The results of our study are important if patients with DS need orthodontic treatment because the correct time for treatment of skeletal malocclusions depends on the skeletal maturation stage of the individual. Also, the outcome of some treatment modalities, such as palatal expansion for the correction of posterior cross-bites, can be affected by the stage of skeletal development of an individual.

5. Conclusion

Based on the results of this study, we concluded that the skeletal age (SA) of the individuals with DS was delayed in relation to the chronological age (CA) by the age of 7 years (SA < CA) when compared to those who did not have DS. However, at the age of 15 years, their skeletal age was advanced in relation to their chronological age (SA > CA). Therefore, we suggest that individuals with DS had a shorter period of skeletal adolescent development with early maturation when compared to the individuals without DS which end of skeletal maturation is usually around 18 years of age.

6. References

Aguiar, MJB; Leão LL, Souza; MMR, Eiras; LCR, Aguiar FF & Silva MESR. (2007). Síndrome de Down. Belo Horizonte: Faculdade de Medicina da UFMG; S.D. (acess em Mar 15 2011). Available from: http://www.medicina.ufmg.br/down/apresentacao.htm.

Alpöz AR & Eronat C. (1997). Taurodontism in children associated with trisomy 21 syndrome. *J Clin Pediat Dent.* Vol.1, No.22, pp. 37-39.

Ali FE; Al-Bustan, MA; Al-Busairi, WA; Al-Mulla, FA; Esbaita, EY. (2006) Cervical spine abnormalities associated with Down syndrome. *Intern Orthop.* Vol. 30, No. 4, pp. 284-289. [acess em Mar 20 2011]. Available: DOI: 10.1007/s00264-005-0070-y.

Barata, LF & Branco, A. (2010) Os Distúrbios fonoarticulatórios na síndrome de Down e na intervenção precoce. *Rev. CEFAC.* Vol 12, No. 1, pp. 134-139.

Castilho, ARF & Marta, SN. (2010) Evaluation of the incidence of dental caries in patients with Down syndrome after their insertion in a preventive program. *Ciência & Saúde ColetivaVol. 15, Supl. 2, pp.3249-3253.*

Cavalcante, LB; Pires, JR & Scarel-Caminaga. (2009). Doença periodontal em indivíduos com syndrome de Down: enfoque genético. *RGO Porto Alegre* Vol. 57, No.4, pp. 449-453.

Coe, DA; Matson, JL; Russell, DW; Slifer, KJ; Capone, GT & Baglio C. (1999) Behavior problems of children with Down syndrome and life events. *J Autism Dev Disord.* Vol.29, No. 2, pp. 149-156.

Cohen, MM & Winer, RA. (1965) Dental and facial characteristics in Down's syndrome (Mongolism). *J Dent Res. Vol.* 44, Suppl 1, pp. 197-209.

Coelho, CRZ & Loevy, HT. (1982) Odontological aspects of Down's syndrome. *ARS Curandi Odontol. Vol* 8, No. 3, pp. 9-16.

Desai SS. (1997) Down syndrome: a review of the literature. *Oral Surg Oral Med Oral Pathol Oral Radiol Endod. Vol* (84), pp. 279-285.

Greulich, WW; Pyle, SI. (1959) *Radiographic atlas of skeletal development of the hand and wrist.* Stanford: Stanford University Press.

Hayes, A & Batshaw, ML. (1993) Down syndrome. *Pediatr Clin North Am.* Vol. 40, pp.523-535.

Higa, PM & Vargas-Machuca, MV. (2004) Características cràneo-faciales en pacientes con syndrome de Down en dos colegios de educación especial en Lima. *Rev Estomatol Heredian.* Vol. 14, pp. 51-53.

Hill, DA; Gridley, G; Cnattingius, S; Mellemkjaer, L; Linet, M & Adami, H. (2003) Mortality and cancer incidence among individuals with Down syndrome. *Arch Intern Med.* Vol. 163, pp. 705-711.

Ingalls, TH & Butler, RL. (1953) Mongolism, Implications of dental anomalies. *N Eng J Med* Vol. 19, pp. 511-512.

Jara, L; Ondarza, A; Blanco, R & Valenzuela, C. (1993) The sequence of eruption of the permanent dentition in a chilean sample with Down's syndrome. *Archs oral Biol.* Vol.38, pp. 85-89.

Jensen, GM; Cleall, JF & Yip, AS. (1973) Dentoalveolar morphology and developmental changes in Down's syndrome (trisomy 21). *Am J Orthod.* Vol. 64, No. 6, pp.607-618.

Kumasaka, S; Miyagi, A; Sakai, N; Shindo, J & Kashima, I. (1997) Oligodontia: a radiographic comparison of subjects with Down syndrome and normal subjects. *SCD Special Care Dent.* Vol 4, No. 17, pp. 137-141.

Lee, SR; Kwon, HK; Song, KB & Choi, YH. (2004) Dental caries and salivary immunoglobulin A in Down syndrome children. *J Paediatr Child Health.* Vol.40, pp. 530-533.

Mariano, MPK; Krahembull, SMB & Magalhães, MHCG. (1999) Alterações sistêmicas de interesse odontológico na síndrome de Down. *RPG Rev Pós Grad.* Vol. 6, pp.218-221.

Moraes, MEL; Medici-Filho, E; Moraes, LC. (1998) Surto de crescimento puberal: relação entre mineralização dentária, idade cronológica, idade dentária e idade óssea - método radiográfico. *Rev Odontol UNESP.* Vol. 27, pp.111-129.

Moraes, MEL; Bastos, MS; Moraes, LC & Rocha, JC. (2002) Prevalência de cárie pelo índice CPO-D em portadores de síndrome de Down. *PGRO-Pós-Grad Rev Odontol.* Vol. 5, No. 2, pp. 64-73.

Moraes, LC; Medici-Filho, E; Castilho, JCM; Moraes, MEL; Dotto, PP & Dotto, GN. (2004) Ocorrência de taurodontismo em indivíduos portadores de síndrome de Down. *Rev Inst Cienc Saúde.* Vol. 22, No. 4, pp. 317-322.

Moraes, MEL; Bastos, MS; Santos, LRA; Castilho, JCM; Moraes, LC & Medici-Filho, E. (2007a) Dental age in patients with Down syndrome. *Braz Oral Res.* Vol. 21, No. 3, pp. 259-264.

Moraes, MEL; Moraes, LC; Dotto, GN; Dotto, PP; Santos, LRA. (2007b) Dental anomalies in patients with Down syndrome. *Braz Dent J.* Vol. 18, No. 4, pp. 346-350.

Moraes, MEL. (2007c) Instabilidade Atlanto-axial em indivíduos com síndrome de Down por meio de radiografias da coluna cervical. Tese Livre-docência - Faculdade de Odontologia de São José dos Campos.

Murakami, J; Kato, T; Kawai, S; Akiyama, S; Amano, A & Morisaki, I. (2008) Cellular motility of Down syndrome gingival fibroblasts is susceptible to impairment by porphyromonas gingivalis invasion. *J Periodontol* Vol. 79, No. 4, pp. 721-727.

Mustacchi, Z & Rozoni, G. (1990) Síndrome de Down: aspectos clínicos e odontológicos. *São Paulo: CID Ed.* 249p.

Nahas AB. (2004) Síndrome de Down e meu filho. 4ª ed. Florianópolis:[s.n.]; 60p.

Nadel L. (2003) Donw's syndrome: a genetic disorder in biobehavioral perspective. *Genes Brain Behav.* Vol 2, pp. 156-166.

Oliveira, ACB; Ramos-Jorge, ML & Paiva, SM. (2001) Aspectos relevantes à abordagem odontológica da criança com síndrome de Down. *Rev CROMG.* Vol. 1, No. 7, pp.36-42.

Pilcher ES. (1998) Dental care for the patient with Down syndrome. J Down Syndr Res Pract. Vol. 3, No. 5, pp.111-116.

Pozsonyi, J; Gibson, D & Zarfas, DE. (1964) Skeletal maturation in mongolism (Down's syndrome). *J Pediatr.* Vol. 64, pp. 75-78.

Reuland-Bosma, W; van der Reijden, WA & van Winkwlhoff AJ. (2001) Absence of a specific subgingival microflora in adults with Down's syndrome. *J Clin Periodontol.* Vol. 28, No. 11, pp. 1004-1009.

Rey SC. (1991) Principais alterações craniofaciais em portadores de síndrome de Down. *Rev Fac Odontol. FZL* Vol. 3, pp. 59-64.

Ribeiro, LMA; Jacob, CMA; Pastorinho, AC; Kim, CAE; Fomin, ABF & Castro, ABBM. (2003) Avaliação dos fatores associados a infecções recorrentes e/ou em pacientes com síndrome de Down. *J Pediatr.* Vol. 79, No. 2, pp. 141-148.

Santos LRA. (2004) Estudo radiográfico da cronologia da mineralização dos dentes caninos, pré-molares e segundos molares inferiores permanentes em pacientes portadores de síndrome de Down. [Dissertação] São José dos Campos, Faculdade de Odontologia de São José dos Campos, Universidade Estadual Paulista.

Sannomiya, EK; Medici-Filho, E; Castilho, JCM & Grasiozi, MAOC. (1998) Avaliação da idade óssea em indivíduos portadores da sindrome de down, por meio de radiografias da mão e punho. *Rev Odontol UNESP.* Vol. 27, No. 2, pp. 527-536.

Seagriff-Curtin, P; Pugliese, S & Romer, M. (2006) Dental considerations for individuals with Down syndrome. *N Y State Dent J* Vol. 72, No. 2, pp. 33-35.

Schwartzman, JS. (2003) Síndrome de Down. 2ª ed. São Paulo: Mackenzie.

Spitzer, R. (1955) Radiological changes in teeth and skull in mental defectives. *Br J Radiol.* Vol. 28, No. 327, pp. 117-127.

Thompson, C. (1976) The palate in Down's syndrome. *Dent Assit.* Vol. 6, No. 45, pp. 16-20.

Toscano, MDP. (1994) Estágios cronológicos de desenvolvimento dentário em crianças portadoras de síndrome de

Down. Estudo radiográfico [Dissertação de Mestrado]. Araraquara: Faculdade de Odontologia da UNESP.

5

Oral Health in Individuals with Down Syndrome

Ronald H.W. Cheng, Cynthia K.Y. Yiu and W. Keung Leung
Faculty of Dentistry, The University of Hong Kong
China

1. Introduction

John Langdon Down (1866) first described the clinical entity of Down Syndrome (DS) at mid-nineteenth century and one century later, the DS primary cause due to trisomy 21 was reported (Lejeune et al., 1959). Until now, the etiology of Down syndrome remains unknown. DS is predominantly due to non-disjunction of chromosome 21; while translocation of an extra copy of the same chromosome accounted for a small proportion of the condition. A mosaic vary of the situation comes about when the extra chromosome 21 is present in some, but not all, cells of the affect individual.

DS itself is not a disease, however affected individuals have greater risk in acquiring many systemic conditions. Persons with DS are susceptible to upper respiratory tract and chest infections. Approximately 50% have some forms of heart defect, usually ventricular septal defect, some may require antibiotic cover for invasive dental treatment. Alzheimer disease is a problem in later life of DS individuals.

Down syndrome is characterized by central growth deficiency with delayed mental and physical development. All individuals with DS are mentally impaired to some degree, ranging from mild to severe.

There is a unique combination of facial features in DS subjects, regardless of race or ethnicity. Persons with DS are often short with a short neck and underdeveloped or hypoplastic mid-face, with outer canthus of the eye higher than the inner giving rise to slant-eyes appearance. The palpebral fissure is narrow, and there is often a medial epicanthic fold. There may be speckling of the iris (Brushfield's spots), cataracts, eye infections and bi- or uni-lateral strabismus. The mid-face hypoplasia often associates with poorly developed paranasal air sinuses, giving rise to a sloping forehead and a flat face. Class III malocclusion and relatively prognathic mandible are also common observations.

DS is the commonest chromosomal abnormality in live-born infants (Bower et al., 2000). DS has been estimated to occur in approximately 1 in 732 infants in the United States (Sherman et al., 2007). In the United Kingdom, the overall prevalence of DS is 1.08 per 1000 live births from 1985-2004 and one-year survival of live births with DS increased, especially in babies with cardiovascular malformations, reaching almost 100% (Irving et al., 2008). Long-term survival is also improving, and the large majority of people with DS are now expected to live well into adult life, due to better living conditions, better health care and more sophisticated surgical techniques (Glasson et al. 2002). Health care workers, educationists and whoever involved are therefore required to keep up with the current knowledge and development of contemporary DS management strategies.

2. Oral features of Down syndrome individuals

2.1 Soft tissues

Common oral soft tissue manifestations of DS individuals include large and fissured tongue, cracked lips (Figure 1). The tongue in DS is large (macroglossia) relative to the size of the oral cavity. In fact, studies have shown that the tongue size of individuals with DS does not differ significantly from that of the general population (Ardran et al., 1972). It is the oral space, which is small (Guimaraes et al., 2008). There can be marked fissuring of the dorsum of the tongue, and because of poor muscular control, the tongue is often protruded.

A B

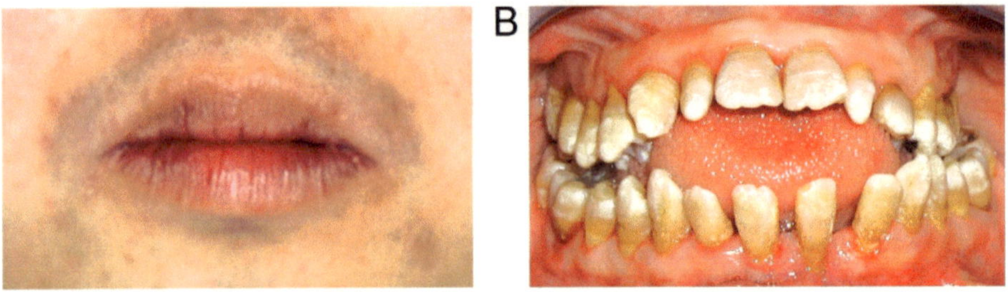

Fig. 1. Common oral soft tissue feature of Down Syndrome individuals. A. cracked lip; B. Large tongue relative to size of oral cavity. Subject also has microdontia or peg-shaped upper lateral incisors.

Generalized orofacial muscles hypotonia e.g. orbicularis, zygomatic, masseter, and temporalis muscles, contributes to poor oral seal, poor suck, poor tongue control, and difficulties with jaw stability. The angle of the mouth is pulled down with elevated upper lip. The lower lip is thick, dry, fissured and everted (Desai, 1997). Persistent mouth opening due to the relatively large tongue in a reduced oral cavity may lead to mouth breathing, drooling, chapped lower lip, and angular cheilitis or infectious lesion at the corner of the mouth. The mucosal lining of the oral cavity is thin because of the reduction in salivary flow rate (Siqueira Jr. & Nicolau, 2002). Chaushu et al. (2002) also argued that drooling in DS individual was due to open mouth posture, protruded tongue and hypotonic orofacial muscle instead of hypersalivation, since they demonstrated a reduced stimulated parotid salivary flow rate.

Tongue appears with bilateral, unilateral or isolated oval depression and is described as raised white scalloped border. This usually is caused by frictional movement against teeth, diastema, tongue thrusting, tongue sucking, clenching or enlarged tongue (Langlais et al., 2009). Geographic and fissured tongue is also seen in DS individuals (Laskaris, 2003). Fissured or scrotal tongue consists of various patterns, lengths and depths: single midline fissure, double fissures, or multiple fissures of the dorsal surface of the anterior two thirds of the tongue (Langlais et al., 2009). This condition is asymptomatic, however it may cause food impaction and subsequently halitosis. Increases in bifid uvula, submucous cleft and cleft palates have been reported in this population (Crespi, 1993).

2.2 Midfacial complex and palate

The development of whole craniofacial complex is retarded and the facial profile is relatively concave. The maxilla in DS individual is deficient in development and the mandible is of normal size or slightly hypoplastic (Boyd et al., 2004). The deficient development in vertical height of the maxilla resulted in overclosure of the mandible and thus projected the lower arch forward relative to upper (Desai, 1997).

DS patients displayed significantly higher frequency of shelf-like or "stair palate" (Skrinjarić et al., 2004). Westerman et al. (1975) compared 40 DS individuals with 44 control subjects and concluded that the palatal dimension were narrower in width, shorter in depth, and lower in height. In fact, the terms high arch and narrow palatal vault (Figure 2) were subjectively described and only partly correct.

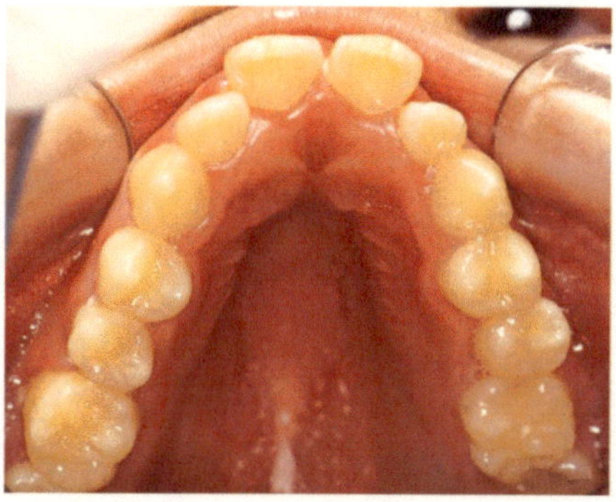

Fig. 2. Deficient maxillary development in Down Syndrome individual leading to narrow palatal vault.

2.3 Malocclusion

Malocclusion or improper meeting of the upper and lower teeth is common in DS individuals and there is a large deviation in occlusal relationship (Lowe 1990). The following factors play an important role in malocclusion: mouth breathing, improper chewing, evidence of bruxism, tooth agenesis, midline deviation in upper arch, anterior open bite, spacing of teeth, dysfunction of temporomandibular joint, delayed eruption and/or exfoliation of both deciduous and permanent dentition, characteristic tongue thrust, hypotonic ligamentary apparatus of temporomandibular joint, developmental disturbances of the mandible (platybasia) and maxilla (midfacial complex), and the jaw relationships (Borea et al., 1990).

2.3.1 Malalignment

Ondarza et al. (1995) analyzed 136 individuals with DS and compared them with mentally impaired individuals and normal Chilean individuals. They showed a higher frequency of malalignments in both the primary and permanent dentition compared with the other groups. The most frequently involved teeth were central incisors, lateral incisors and canines. Anterior and posterior crowding was also often seen in DS individuals (Reuland-Bosma & van Dijk, 1986). Crowding is frequent, especially in maxilla, due to underdevelopment (Figure 3A & B).

Increased in prevalence of canine impaction (15%), and upper canine and first premolar transposition (15%) were also found in DS individuals (Figure 3C & D), which was a phenomenon that could only be explained by genetic anomaly (Shapira et al., 2000).

2.3.2 Jaw relationships

Angle Class III malocclusion was present in two thirds of DS individuals (Boyd et al., 2004).

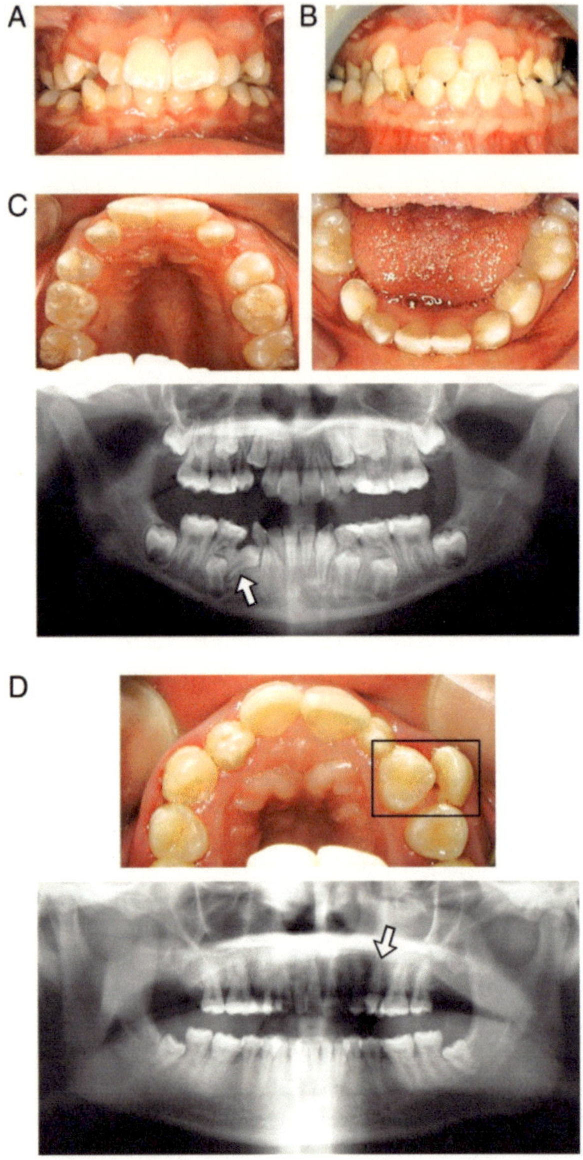

Fig. 3. Malalignment and tooth impaction in Down Syndrome subjects. A. Malaligned mixed dentition; B. Malaligned permanent dentition; C. Impacted lower right first premolar (arrow). Subject also has missing lower left lateral incisor; D. Transpositioned upper left canine and first premolar (box and arrow).

The higher incidence of Class III malocclusion is due to underdevelopment of the midface and not to prognathism. Approximately 69% of them had mandibular overjet. Other findings were anterior open bite, posterior crossbite, anterior crossbite, mesial molar occlusion, sagittal malocclusion (Desai, 1997) (Figure 4). Vigild (1985) recorded in 37 DS cases with 41% mandibular overjet, 54% mesial molar occlusion, 38% open bite and 65% crossbite.

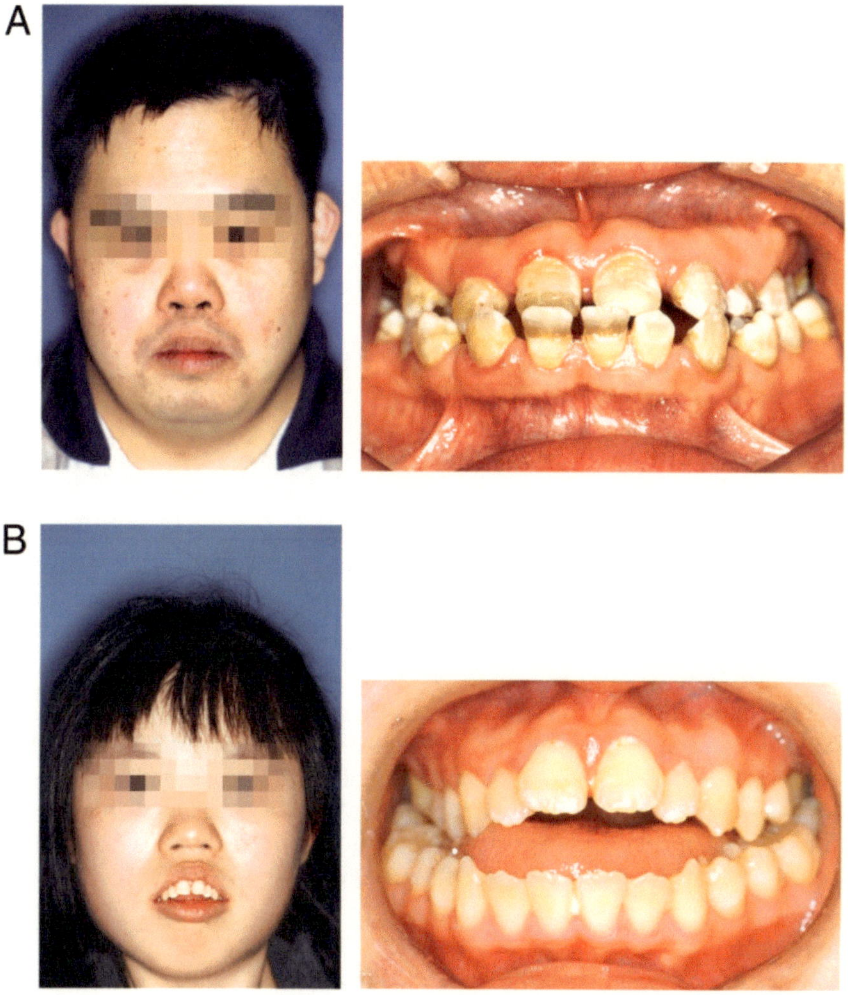

Fig. 4. Common jaw relationships of Down Syndrome subjects. A. Angle Class III malocclusion with posterior cross bite. Also note subject has enamel hypoplasia; B. Angle Class III malocclusion with anterior open bite.

2.4 Hard tissues

Dental features associated with DS individuals include: microdontia of permanent dentition, altered crown morphology and shape, short root, enamel hypoplasia and hypocalcification, thinner enamel and dentine in the permanent dentition, taurodontism, hypodontia and supernumerary teeth, asymmetry and delayed eruption (Desai, 1997) (Figures 1B, 3C, 4A, 5A & 5B).

2.4.1 Microdontia

DS individuals presented with true generalized microdontia in permanent dentition (Lowe, 1990), but in primary dentition, this is less well documented (Bell et al., 2001, Kieser et al., 2003). Clinical crowns are frequently conical, short, and small (Townsend 1983, 1987).

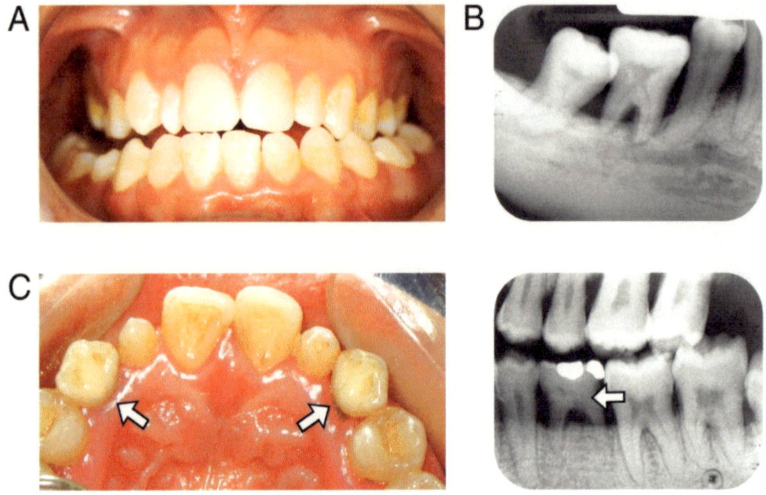

Fig. 5. Dental hard tissue anomalies of Down Syndrome subjects. A. Microdontia or peg-shaped right lateral incisor; B. Short rooted lower right molars. Also note subject has radiographic sign of bone loss around teeth indicating periodontitis; C. Retained primary or deciduous upper canines (arrows) or lower left second primary molar (radiograph, arrow). Please note the corresponding permanent successors in both cases are missing.

Bell et al. (2001) examined the lower incisors dimension of individuals with DS and found that reduced permanent crown size was associated with a reduction in both enamel and dentine thickness and enamel was actually significantly more reduced. Desai (1997) reported that all teeth except the upper first molars and lower incisors were reduced in size, with complete root formation. Peg-shaped lateral incisors (Cheng et al., 2007), shovel incisors and slender canines were frequently seen (Scully, 1976).

2.4.2 Hypodontia

Dental agenesis is a common characteristic in DS individuals, ranges from 30-53%, and the teeth most frequently absent in them are also most often absent in normal population (Kieser et al., 2003).

Both Japanese (Kumasaka et al., 1997) and Brazilian studies (Acerbi et al., 2001), found 60-63% of DS individuals had one or more missing teeth. In a detailed study, Russell and Kjaer (1995) studied 100 DS individuals and compared with Danish normal population. Missing teeth had a 10 times greater frequency in DS individuals than in general population and a higher frequency in males than in females. Agenesis occurred more frequently in the mandible than in the maxilla and most often on the left side. The most frequent absent teeth were lower incisors, followed by upper second premolars, upper lateral incisors, lower second premolars, upper second molars, lower central incisors and canines. As from an earlier U.S. study (Orner, 1971), the author reported that 53% out of 212 DS individuals had missing permanent teeth. The descending frequency of missing teeth were the upper lateral incisors (31%) followed by the lower second premolars (26%), upper second premolars (18%), lower lateral incisors (12%), and lower central incisors (7%).

Due to missing permanent successor, the corresponding primary tooth did not resorb or resorbed so slowly that it could be retained well into adulthood (Figure 5C).

2.4.3 Abnormal crown and root morphology

Enamel hypoplasia and hypocalcification, affecting both primary and permanent dentitions, are relatively common in DS children (Figure 4A). Severity of tooth wear was significantly greater in DS children when compared to unaffected children, with DS children displaying a multifactorial aetiology of tooth wear, including attrition and erosion (Bell et al., 2002). Except for mandibular first premolar, crown and root lengths of permanent teeth are shorter than normal (Kelsen et al., 1999). Taurodontism is frequent finding in persons with DS (Rajić & Mestrović, 1998). Taurodontism together with abnormally short root would reduce extent of periodontal attachment and result in tooth mobility commonly seen in these persons (Figure 5B).

2.4.4 Eruption of primary dentition

Primary dentition in DS individuals usually developed late and subsequently delayed the eruption, particularly upper and lower anterior teeth and first molars. Ondarza et al. (1997) compared 255 Chilean DS individuals against normal population and showed that central incisors, lateral incisors and canines' eruption were delayed significantly. However, they reported the chronologic age of primary tooth eruption within DS individuals was not significantly different.

As usual, central incisors erupted first, and second molars usually last, but in between there was a great deal of variation in the sequence of eruption. The first eruption was usually at the age of 12 to 14 months but could be delayed up to 24 months and taking up to 4 to 5 years of age to complete (Desai, 1997).

2.4.5 Eruption of the permanent dentition

Eruption of permanent dentition is also delayed in DS individuals. 240 Chilean DS individuals were studied (Jara et al., 1993). They had altered eruption sequence but the authors argued that this was not necessarily a consequence of alterations in the time of eruption. Six year old molars and lower incisors could erupt until the age of 8 to 9 years (Desai 1997).

A New Zealand nationwide survey on DS individuals' oral condition was carried out by Cutress (1971a & 1971b). The author found that the chronologic sequence of eruption in DS individuals was similar to the normal population. The least affected teeth were upper and lower first molars and central and lateral incisors. Asymmetries between left and right side mainly affected the canines and premolars. Children with DS maintained a certain similarity in eruption sequence and symmetry compared with normal children.

3. Oral diseases of Down syndrome individuals

3.1 Dental caries

Low prevalence of dental caries or tooth decay in both primary and permanent dentitions of DS individuals has been widely reported (Cutress, 1971a; Orner, 1975; Barnett et al., 1986; Vigild, 1986; Ulseth et al., 1991; Gabre et al., 2001; Bradley & McAlister, 2004; Cheng et al., 2007; Dellavia et al., 2009; Davidovich et al., 2010).Cutress (1971a) examined 416 DS subjects and found lower prevalence of dental caries than normal population, but after adjusting the age of teeth eruption, there were only small and no significant difference between 2 groups. Later in another study (Orner, 1975), when dental caries experience was compared between DS individuals and their siblings, it was found that DS individuals experienced less than one third caries than their unaffected siblings. Similarly, a study by Barnett et al. (1986) in

New Jersey, USA, reported that DS individuals had lower caries prevalence when compared with age matched mentally disabled subjects.
Vigild (1986) reported that DS individuals had less carious lesions but also fewer permanent teeth than those mentally retarded individuals. However, when data was analyzed on the basis of tooth numbers and not on tooth surfaces, the author concluded that individuals with DS were also susceptible to caries.
Ulseth et al. (1991) had also found that while the caries prevalence of adults with DS was lower than Norwegian general population, it was similar to that of people with other disabilities. Comparing with subjects of similar mental status, Bradley and McAlister (2004) reported that among the 71 Irish children with DS, higher prevalence of caries free children was observed than children in special needs or mainstream schools. DS individuals who were caries free had significantly lower *Streptococcus mutans* counts (Shapira et al., 1991) and elevated salivary *Streptococcus mutans* specific IgA concentrations (Lee et al., 2004).
The low caries prevalence had been postulated to be related to delayed eruption, reduced time of exposure to a cariogenic environment, congenitally missing teeth, higher salivary pH and bicarbonate levels, microdontia, spaced dentition, and shallow fissures of the teeth (Desai, 1997; Boyd et al., 2004). Recently, it has been shown that a different salivary environment of electrolytes and pH is manifested in DS children, leading to the lower reported caries rate (Davidovich et al., 2010)

3.2 Periodontal disease

DS individuals usually present with poor oral hygiene and manifested as marginal gingival inflammation, acute and subacute necrotizing gingivitis, advanced chronic periodontitis, loss of attachment in form of gingival recession and increased pocket depth, alveolar bone loss, suppuration or even abscesses, furcation involvement in the molars, increased tooth mobility, and even loss of teeth (Shaw & Saxby, 1986) (Figures 5B & 6).
DS individuals had a prevalence of 60 to 90% percent and increased severity of periodontal disease compared with normal age-matched controls and subjects with other mental disabilities of similar age (Cutress, 1971b; Orner, 1976; Barnett et al., 1986; Reuland-Bosma & van Dijk, 1986;, Modeer et al., 1990; Shapira et al., 1991; Ulseth et al., 1991; Desai, 1997; Gabre et al., 2001; Lopez-Perez et al., 2002; Sakellari et al., 2005; Cheng et al., 2007; Khocht et al., 2010). Obviously the severity of periodontal disease among DS individuals is milder in recent years' reports as better dental care have been employed to take care of them early in their life.
Lopez-Perez et al. (2002) examined 32 DS individuals and age-matched controls and found that there were greater extent of gingivitis and periodontitis in DS group. When comparing with subjects affected by other learning disabilities of similar age distribution, DS individuals exhibited earlier, rapid and generalized periodontal destruction (Saxen et al., 1977; Barnett et al., 1986). In Finland, Saxen et al. (1977) compared panoramic radiographs of DS individuals versus age-matched control and reported that 84% of DS adults showed advanced bone loss of 2.5mm or more as compared with only 27% in the controls. Barnett et al. (1986) examined 30 DS individuals and 30 similar mental status individuals and reported that bone loss was found in 60% of sites of DS individuals versus 9.3% of sites in controls.
Sakellari et al. (2005) investigated the severity of periodontal disease in DS individuals and compared the group with healthy individuals or cerebral palsy patients. They reported that periodontal inflammation and treatment needs were significantly higher in DS individuals. Shaw and Saxby (1986) showed that DS individuals had periodontal bone loss pattern

similar to that of juvenile periodontitis. Lower incisors were reported exhibiting early signs of alveolar bone loss in approximately 35% of DS adolescents (Modeer et al., 1990; Barr-Agholme et al., 1992).

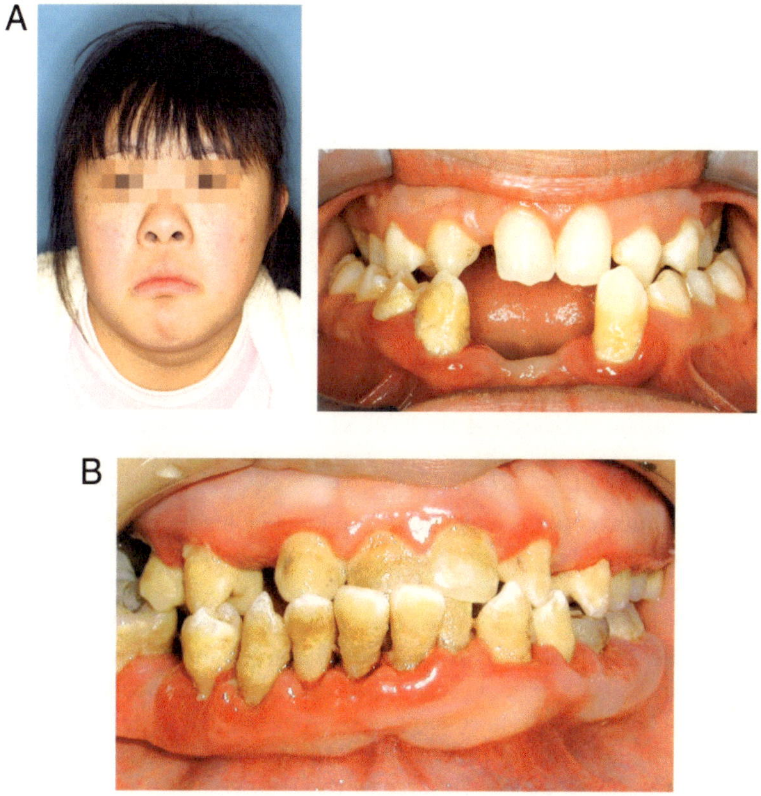

Fig. 6. Periodontal disease in Down Syndrome subject. A. Gingival inflammation in lower dental arch, mixed dentition. Subject also has congenital missing upper lateral incisors and all lower incisors; B. Periodontitis in permanent dentition of an adult DS individual.

There is only one longitudinal study to record the development of periodontal disease in DS adults. After 7 years observation, Agholme et al. (1999) found the prevalence of bone loss increased from 35% to 74% among 33 DS individuals. The severity and progression of the disease, however, was not as rapid as reported in the literature.

Bradley and McAlister (2004) suggested that majority of DS children had poor oral hygiene, but they could not demonstrate the children had earlier onset periodontal disease. At the same time, there was only moderate relationship between dental plaque and periodontal disease severity in DS individuals (Lopez-Perez et al., 2002). Thus, rapid and severe periodontal destruction in those DS individual affected could not be explained by poor oral hygiene alone (Reuland-Bosma & van Dijk, 1986).

4. Management principles for oral diseases in Down syndrome individuals

There are quite a number of distinguished developmental or behavioral features and systemic manifestations associated with DS individuals which could affect oral diseases management. The followings are brief summary regarding how aspects of such features can affect oral health.

4.1 Development, behavior, mental status, cognitive and early aging

Persons with DS certainly have learning disability. Despite the homogeneity of low IQ and delayed mental development, DS individuals have different characters. DS children develop to a plateau in their adolescence which attain overall learning abilities equivalent to unaffected children aged 6 to 8 years. Knowing that oral hygiene of 6-year-old are not as good as 8-12 year-old children (Sandström et al., 2011), the anticipated oral hygiene of DS subjects would not be ideal if no special extra attention is given. Moderate to mild mental retarded individuals are on the other hand, mobile, function and perform well and highly motivated in sheltered workshop (Crespi, 1993). Common characteristics observed in young DS individuals have been described as quiet, passive, natural spontaneity, genuine warmth, penetrating calamity in relating to other people, fond of music, gentleness, patience and tolerance, complete honesty (Desai, 1997). All these together make supervised group oral hygiene approach possible (Shyama et al., 2003). Approximately 30% of the individuals with DS are affected by dementia (Kieser et al., 2003) when they get older. Although the degree of intellectual disability affects the efficacy of supragingival or above the gum line plaque control, sustaining individuals with DS motivation by supervised toothbrushing and systematic oral health care education could achieve good oral hygiene levels (Shyama et al., 2003).

4.2 Systemic anomalies

Medical problems associated with DS have been well noted. In Hong Kong, high prevalence of medical problems was detected in children and teenagers with DS. Among 407 DS individuals, cardiovascular problems were observed in 53%, endocrine problems in 27%, gastrointestinal problems in 11%, haematological problems in 4%, neurological problems in 7%, sleep problems in 9%, skeletal problems in 14%, visual problems in 48% and auditory problems in 34% (Yam et al. 2008). Children with DS have a 10- to 20-fold higher risk of developing leukemia (Lange, 2000). Dental treatment plans for DS subjects therefore need to be formulated upon careful and thorough medical history and appropriate precautionary measures incorporated.

4.3 Cardiac anomalies

Many DS individuals have multiple congenital cardiac defects. The most common are atrioventricular septal defects, following ventricular septal defects, atrial septal defect, patent ductus arteriosus and tetralogy of Fallot (Freeman et al. 1998). There is also an increased incidence of mitral valve disorders which include mitral valve prolapse, mitral insufficiency, deformed mitral valve, and mitral valve absence (van Dyke et al., 1990). The need of antibiotic prophylaxis should be assessed and followed. Severe form of such cardiac complications may associate with increased risk in infection of the myocardium or increased general anesthesia complications. All these can potentially hinder oral health providers in smoothly deliver primary oral health care.

4.4 Atlantoaxial instability

Approximately 13% of DS individuals (Cohen, 1998) have excess movement of the joint between C1 and C2. The presence of 5mm or more space between the posterior aspect of anterior arch of the atlas and the odontoid process is considered atlantoaxial instability and is at a higher risk of spine translocation. Neck of DS individuals during dental treatment should be maintained in a relaxed position in order to avoid that from occurring.

4.5 Nervous system anomalies

DS boys develop gross motor skills better than fine motor skills (Hoffman et al., 1990). Although development of motor function is usually delayed and has restricted coordination, coordination improves with age (Desai, 1997). Daily dental care or plaque control may be a difficult task for DS subjects which predisposing them to periodontal disease.

4.6 Obstructive sleep apnea

Obstructive sleep apnea (OSA) is common and occurs in 50% of children with DS (Mitchell et al., 2003; Shott et al., 2006). Patients with DS have many predisposing factors for OSA, including glossoptosis, hypopharyngeal collapse, recurrent and enlarged adenoid tonsils, enlarged lingual tonsils and relative macroglossia (Donnelly et al., 2004). Dentist plays an important role in recognizing and treatment of sleep-disordered breathing. If left untreated, OSA can further developmental delay, lead to pulmonary hypotension and congestive heart failure. The most effective oral appliances for patients with DS are mandibular advancement devices that fit both the maxillary and mandibular teeth, similar to an orthodontic retainer or athletic mouthguard (Waldman et al., 2009).

4.7 Orofacial dysfunction

Orofacial dysfunction in children with DS is related to mouth breathing, muscle hypotonia and discrepancy between alveolar arches (Faulks et al., 2008a). Early appliance therapy using Castillo-Morales plate had been promising in stimulating the lips and tongue and improving oromotor function (Carlstedt et al., 2003, Backmän et al., 2007). A long-term follow up study of children with DS, being treated with Castillo-Morales plate at a mean age of 13 months for 19 months, showed improved orofacial appearance and function that remain stable after 13 years (Korbmacher et al., 2006). Oromotor therapy may also be combined with functional orthodontic treatment such as palatal expansion with removable appliance, elimination of occlusal interference by grinding and use of composite overlay to free mandibular movement in older DS children (Faulks et al., 2008b).

4.8 Dental diseases

Down syndrome is characterized by abnormalities in learning, memory, and language that lead to mild-to-profound impairment in intellectual functioning. Vision hearing disorders and hypothyroidism can further negatively impact cognitive functioning in children with DS (Lott & Dierssen, 2010). There is often a delay or impairment in language development in DS children. Receptive language is typically stronger than expressive language, and vocabulary is stronger than syntax (Martin et al., 2009). They exhibit phonological-altered spoken communication with more unimodal gestural answer. Dentist should find out from caregiver the patient's level of intellectual and functional abilities and communicate directly with DS individuals using short, clear instructions. The primary caregiver is encouraged to stay with DS individuals during dental treatment to enhance cooperation and communication. Visuo-spatial processing and perception are generally viewed as relative strengths in individuals with DS, therefore preventive advice should be given together with pictures, diagrams and models.

4.8.1 Caries

Various studies have shown a reduced prevalence of caries in DS children when compared with unaffected children (Stabholz et al., 1991; Bradley & McAlister, 2004; Cogulu et al., 2006; Davidovich et al., 2010). It has been reported that young DS children had prolonged use of bottle as a result of feeding problems or behavioral difficulties, with increased risk of developing nursing bottle caries (Randell et al., 1992) (Figure 7). Paired analysis of Candaian DS and non-DS siblings showed that children with DS were less likely to receive caries-preventive treatment, restorative care and more likely to have had a dental extraction (Allison & Lawrence, 2004; Fung et al., 2008). This highlights the importance of early preventive care in children with DS.

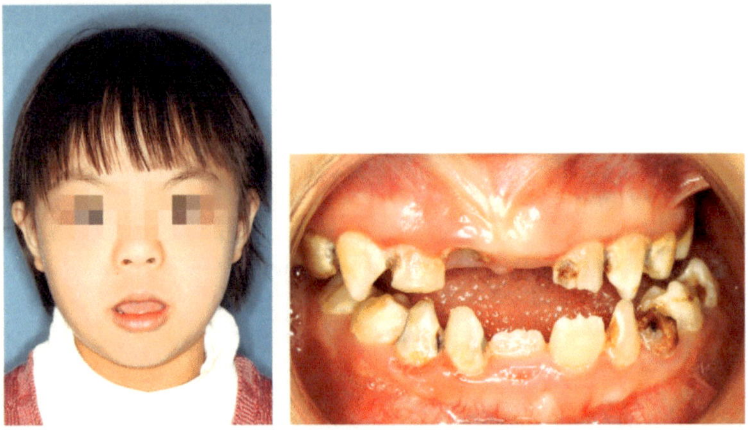

Fig. 7. Dental decay (caries) in Down Syndrome subject. Nursing bottle caries in early mixed dentition. Almost all primary teeth are involved.

The first dental visit of DS children should occur at the 12-18 months of age to monitor tooth development and eruptions. An intensive preventive programme is recommended and should include: regular oral hygiene motivation, dietary counseling, topical fluoride and fissure sealants application. Motor development is usually delayed in younger DS children and may lead to reduced manual dexterity of the children. Parents and caregivers should be educated on the need to help with tooth brushing until the individual has acquired sufficient motor skills (Desai, 1997).

Most DS children are affectionate and cooperative for dental treatment; while some may require treatment under sedation or general anaesthesia. Children with DS exhibit atlantoaxial instability, extreme care is needed during intubation and orientation of head by the paediatric dentist during provision of dental treatment under general anaesthesia.

4.8.2 Periodontitis

Periodontal treatment needs were obviously higher in DS adults than in normal healthy adults (Shapira et al., 1991; Sakellari et al., 2005). Cichon et al. (1998) reported that there was no improvement in clinical and microbiological parameters after a single session of scaling and root planing and oral hygiene instructions. The conventional standard periodontal therapy could not eliminate periodontal pathogens or even had no remarkably effect on subgingival microbiota. The authors attributed these unsatisfactory clinical outcomes to poor plaque control and impaired host defense mechanisms.

However, Sakellari et al. (2001) suggested that a frequent recall program with 3-month period could overcome inadequate supragingival plaque control and subsequently altered subgingival environment after treating five DS individuals with non-surgical periodontal therapy for 6 months. Yoshihara et al. (2005) also advocated providing periodic preventive care to DS individuals in order to suppress the progression of periodontal disease. The authors compared individuals who had frequent dental visit (mean intervals between visits: 3.7 ± 1.3 months) versus those who had visits more than one year apart and revealed that the regular review group had better clinical parameters. Cheng et al. (2008) reported satisfactory healing response on 21 DS individuals treated by non-surgical mechanical periodontal therapy (followed by monthly recalls) and the adjunctive use of chlorhexidine gel for toothbrushing and chlorhexidine mouthwash twice daily.

It appears from the above conflicting and varied findings, conventional periodontal therapy which involves oral hygiene instructions, scaling and root debridement cannot guarantee good gingival healing response. The standard gingival response to debridement is gingival shrinkage. Gingival recession connotes reduction in pocket depth, elimination of excessive sulcular depth. Besides, restoration of normal contour and color of the gingiva, reduction of gingival exudates can be gradually achieved. However, there is still no gold standard available indicating how periodontal disease in DS adults can be best managed and no evidence showing vigorous periodontal treatment may prevent periodontal disease progression or prolong tooth retention.

Appropriate modification of periodontal therapy involves non-surgical periodontal therapy adjuncted with regular use of chemical plaque control agents, and frequent recall schedule in DS adults may be a way forward.

5. Conclusions

DS individuals are basically a group of patients requiring special oral health care services. They have more missing , malaligned teeth and often affected with malocclusion. They have less carious teeth, but experienced more severe and extensive periodontal diseases. Despite the fact that the latter two diseases are preventable, there are inadequate resources in many communities for DS subjects or their caretakers to upkeep their oral health. DS care providers should acquire appropriate level of oral health awareness and communities can consider improving accessibility of DS subjects to oral health care in order to assist maintenance of oral and overall health for this group of special need patients.

6. References

Acerbi, A.G., Claudio de Freitas & Gallottini de Magalhaes MHC. (2001). Prevalence of numeric anomalies in the permanent dentition of patients with Down syndrome. Spec Care Dentist, Vol. 21, No. 2, pp. 75-78, ISSN 1754-4505

Agholme, M.B., Dahllof, G. & Modeer, T. (1999). Changes of periodontal status in patients with Down syndrome during a 7-year period. Eur J Oral Sci Vol. 107, No. 2, pp. 82-88, ISSN 0909-8836

Allison, P.J. & Lawrence H.P. (2004). A paired comparison of dental care in Canadians with Down syndrome and their siblings without Down syndrome. Community Dent Oral Epidemiol, Vol. 32, No. 2, pp. 99-106, ISSN 0301-5561

Ardran, G.M., Harker, P. & Kemp, F.H. (1972). Tongue size in Down's syndrome. J Ment Defic Res Vol. 16, No. 3, pp. 160-166, ISSN 0022-264X

Bäckman, B., Grevér-Sjölander, A.C., Bengtsson, K., Persson, J. & Johansson, I. (2007). Children with Down syndrome: oral development and morphology after use of palatal plates between 6 and 48 months of age. Int J Paediatr Dent, Vol. 17, No. 1, pp. 19-28, ISSN 0960-7439

Barnett, M.L., Press, K.P., Friedman, D. & Sonnenberg, E.M. (1986). The prevalence of periodontitis and dental caries in a Down's syndrome population. J Periodontol, Vol. 57, No. 5, pp. 288-293, ISSN 0022-3492

Barr-Agholme, M., Dahllof, G., Linder, L. & Modeer T. (1992). Actinobacillus actinomycetemcomitans, Capnocytophaga and Porphyromonas gingivalis in subgingival plaque of adolescents with Down syndrome. Oral Microbiol Immunol , Vol. 7, No. 4, pp. 244-248, ISSN 0902-0055

Bell, E.J., Townsend, G.C., Wilson, D., Kieser, J.A. & Hughes, T. (2001). Effect of Down syndrome on the dimensions of dental crowns and tissues. Am J Hum Biol, Vol. 13, No. 5, pp. 690-698, ISSN 1042-0533

Bell, E.J., Kaidonis, J. & Townsend, G.C. (2002). Tooth wear in children with Down syndrome. Aust Dent J, Vol. 47, No. 1, pp. 30-35, ISSN 0045-0421

Borea, G., Magi, M., Mingarelli, R. & Zamboni, C. (1990). The oral cavity in Down syndrome. J Pedodontics, Vol. 14, No. 3, pp. 139-140, ISSN 0145-5508

Bower, C., Leonard, H. & Petterson, B. Intellectual disability in Western Australia. (2000). J Paediatr Child Health, Vol. 36, No. 3, pp. 213–215, ISSN 1034-4810

Boyd, D., Quick, A. & Murray, C. (2004). The Down syndrome patient in dental practice, part II: clinical considerations. N Z Dent J, Vol. 100, No. 1, pp. 4-9, ISSN 0028-8047

Bradley, C. & McAlister, T. (2004). The oral health of children with Down Syndrome in Ireland. Spec Care Dentist, Vol. 24, No. 2, pp. 55-60, ISSN 1754-4505

Carlstedt, K., Henningsson, G. & Dahllöf, G. (2003). A four-year longitudinal study of palatal plate therapy in children with Down syndrome: effects on oral motor function, articulation and communication preferences. Acta Odontol Scand, Vol. 61, No. 1, pp. 39-46, ISSN 0001-6357

Chaushu, S., Becker, A., Chaushu, G. & Shapira, J. (2002). Stimulated parotid salivary flow rate in patients with Down syndrome. Spec Care Dentist, Vol. 22, No. 1, pp. 41-44, ISSN 1754-4505

Cheng, R.H., Leung, W.K., Corbet, E.F. & King, N.M. (2007). Oral health status of adults with Down syndrome in Hong Kong. Spec Care Dentist, Vol. 27, No. 4, pp. 134-138, ISSN 1754-4505

Cheng, R.H., Leung, W.K. & Corbet, E.F. (2008). Non-surgical periodontal therapy with adjunctive chlorhexidine use in adults with down syndrome: a prospective case series. J Periodontol, Vol. 79, No. 2, pp. 379-385, ISSN 0022-3492

Cichon, P., Crawford, L. & Grimm, W.D. (1998). Early-onset periodontitis associated with Down's syndrome clinical interventional study. Ann Periodontol, Vol. 3, No. 1, pp. 370-380.e, ISSN 1553-0841

Cogulu, D., Sabah, E., Kutukculer, N. & Ozkinay, F. (2006). Evaluation of the relationship between caries indices and salivary secretory IgA, salivary pH, buffering capacity and flow rate in children with Down's syndrome. Arch Oral Biol, Vol. 51, No. 1, pp. 23-28, ISSN 0003-9969

Cohen, W.I. (1998). Atlantoaxial instability: what's next? Arch Pediatr Adolesc Med, Vol. 152, No. 2, pp. 119-122, ISSN 1072-4710

Crespi, P.V. Metabolic and genetic jaw diseases. (1993). In: Regezi, Sciubba, editors. Oral pathology clinical pathologic correlations. 2nd edition. Philadelphia: WB Saunders Co, pp. 458-493, ISBN 0721636217.

Cutress, T.W. (1971a). Dental caries in Trisomy 21. Arch Oral Biol, Vol. 16, No. 11, pp. 1329-1344, ISSN 0003-9969

Cutress, T.W. (1971b). Periodontal disease and oral hygiene in trisomy 21. Arch Oral Biol, Vol. 16, No. 11, pp. 1345-1355, ISSN 0003-9969

Davidovich, E., Aframian, D.J., Shapira, J. & Peretz, B. (2010). A comparison of the sialochemistry, oral pH, and oral health status of Down syndrome children to healthy children. Int J Paediatr Dent, Vol. 20, No. 4, pp. 235-241, ISSN 0960-7439

Dellavia, C., Allievi, C., Pallavera, A., Rosati, R. & Sforza, C. (2009). Oral health conditions in Italian Special Olympics athletes. Spec Care Dentist, No. Vol. 29, No. 2, pp. 69-74, ISSN 1754-4505

Desai, S.S (1997). Down syndrome: a of the literature. Oral Surg Oral Med Oral Pathol Oral Radiol Endod, Vol. 84, No. 3. pp. 279-285, ISSN 1079-2104

Donnelly, L.F., Shott, S.R., LaRose, C.R., Chini, B.A. & Amin, R.S. (2004). Causes of persistent obstructive sleep apnea despite previous tonsillectomy and adenoidectomy in children with down syndrome as depicted on static and dynamic cine MRI. AJR Am J Roentgenol, Vol. 183, No. 1, pp. 175-181, ISSN 0361-803X

Down, J.L.H. (1866). Observations on an ethnic classification of idiots. London Hospital Clinical Lectures and Reports, No. 3, pp. 259-262. Reprinted in Arch Neurol. 1971, No. 25, pp. 89-90, ISSN 0003-9942.

Faulks, D., Collado, V., Mazille, M.N., Veyrune, J.L. & Hennequin, M. (2008a). Masticatory dysfunction in persons with Down's syndrome. Part 1: aetiology and incidence. J Oral Rehabil, Vol. 35, No. 11, pp. 854-862, ISSN 0305-182X

Faulks, D., Mazille, M.N., Collado, V., Veyrune, J.L. & Hennequin, M. (2008b), Masticatory dysfunction in persons with Down's syndrome. Part 2: management. J Oral Rehabil, Vol. 35, No. 11, pp. 863-869, ISSN 0305-182X.

Freeman SB, Taft LF, Dooley KJ, Allran K, Sherman SL, Hassold TJ, Khoury MJ, Saker DM. (1998). Population-based study of congenital heart defects in Down syndrome. Am J Med Genet, Vol. 80, No. 3, pp. 213-217, ISSN 1096-8628

Fung, K., Lawrence, H. & Allison, P. (2008). A paired analysis of correlates of dental restorative care in siblings with and without Down syndrome. Spec Care Dentist, Vol. 28, No. 3, pp. 85-91, ISSN 1754-4505

Gabre, P., Martinsson, T. & Gahnberg, L.(2001). Longitudinal study of dental caries, tooth mortality and interproximal bone loss in adults with intellectual disability. Eur J Oral Sci, Vol. 109, No. 1, pp. 20-26, ISSN 0909-8836

Glasson, E.J., Sullivan, S.G., Hussain, R., Petterson, B.A., Montgomery, P.D. & Bittles, A.H. (2002). The changing survival profile of people with Down's syndrome: implications for genetic counselling. Clin Genet, Vol. 62, No. 5, pp. 390-393, ISSN 0009-9163

Guimaraes, C.V., Donnelly, L.F., Shott, S.R., Amin, R.S. & Kalra, M. (2008). Relative rather than absolute macroglossia in patients with Down syndrome: implications for treatment of obstructive sleep apnea. Pediatr Radiol, Vol. 38, No. 10, pp. 1062-1067, ISSN 1432-1998

Hoffman, M.N., Peterson, L.L. & Van Dyke. D.C. Motor and hand function. (1990). In: van Dyke, D.C., Lang, D.J., Heide, F., van Duyne, S. & Soucek, M.J., editors, Clinical perspectives in the management of Down syndrome. New York: Springer-Verlag, pp. 93-101, ISBN 038796987X.

Irving, C., Basu, A., Richmond, S., Burn, J. & Wren, C. (2008). Twenty-year trends in prevalence and survival of Down syndrome. Eur J Hum Genet, Vol. 16, No. 11, pp. 1336-1340, ISSN 1018-4813

Jara, L., Ondarza, A., Blanco, R. & Valenzuela, C. (1993). The sequence of eruption of the permanent dentition in a Chilean sample with Down's syndrome. Arch Oral Biol, Vol. 38, No. 1, pp. 85-89, ISSN 0003-9969

Kelsen, A.E., Love, R.M., Kieser, J.A. & Herbison, P. (1999). Root canal anatomy of anterior and premolar teeth in Down's syndrome. Int Endod J, Vol. 32, No. 3, pp. 211-216, ISSN 0143-2885

Khocht, A., Janal, M. & Turner, B. (2010). Periodontal health in Down syndrome: contributions of mental disability, personal, and professional dental care. Spec Care Dentist, Vol. 30, No. 3, pp. 118-123, ISSN 1754-4505

Kieser, J., Townsend, G. & Quick, A. (2003). The Down syndrome patient in dental practice, part I: pathogenesis and general and dental features. N Z Dent J, Vol. 99, No. 1, pp. 5-9, ISSN 0028-8047

Korbmacher, H.M., Limbrock, J.G. & Kahl-Nieke, B. (2006). Long-term evaluation of orofacial function in children with Down syndrome after treatment with a stimulating plate according to Castillo Morales. J Clin Pediatr Dent, Vol. 30, No. 4, pp. 325-328, ISSN 1053-4628

Kumasaka, S., Miyagi, A., Sakai, N., Shindo, J. & Kashima, I. (1997). Oligodontia: A radiographic comparison of subjects with Down Syndrome and normal subjects. Spec Care Dentist, Vol. 17, No. 4, pp. 137-141, ISSN 1754-4505

Lange, B. (2000). The management of neoplastic disorders of haematopoiesis in children with Down's syndrome. Br J Haematol, Vol. 110, No. 3, pp. 512-524, ISSN 0007-1048

Langlais, R.P., Miller, C.S. & Nield-Gehrig, J.S. (2009). Color Atlas of Common Oral Diseases. 4th edition. Philadelphia: Lipponcott Williams & Wilkins, ISBN 9780781780971.

Laskaris, G. (2003). Diseases of the tongue. In: Color atlas of oral diseases. 3rd edition. Stuttgart; New York: Thieme, pp. 120-129, ISBN 3137170036.

Lee, S.R., Kwon, H.K., Song, K.B. & Choi, Y.H. (2004). Dental caries and salivary immunoglobulin A in Down syndrome children. J Paediatr Child Health, Vol. 40, No. 9-10, pp. 530-533, ISSN 1034-4810

Lejeune, J., Gautier, M. & Turpin, M.R. (1959). Etude des chromosomes somatiques de neuf enfants mongoliens. C R Acad Sci (Paris), Vol. 248, No. 11, pp. 1721-1722, ISSN 0764-4442

Lopez-Perez, R., Borges-Yanez, S.A., Jimenez-Garcia, G. & Maupome, G. (2002). Oral hygiene, gingivitis, and periodontitis in persons with Down syndrome. Spec Care Dentist, Vol. 22, No. 6, pp. 214-220, ISSN 1754-4505

Lott, I.T. & Dierssen, M. (2010). Cognitive deficits and associated neurological complications in individuals with Down's syndrome. Lancet Neurol, Vol. 9, No. 6, pp. 623-633, ISSN 1474-4422

Lowe, G. (1990). Dental problems. In: van Dyke, D.C., Lang, D.J., Heide, F., van Duyne. S. & Soucek, M.J., editors. Clinical perspectives in the management of Down syndrome. New York: Springer-Verlag, pp. 72-79, ISBN 038796987X.

Mitchell, R.B., Call, E. & Kelly, J. (2003). Diagnosis and therapy for airway obstruction in children with Down syndrome. Arch Otolaryngol Head Neck Surg, Vol. 129, No. 6, pp. 642-645 ISSN 0886-4470

Martin, G.E., Klusek, J., Estigarribia, B. & Roberts, J.E. (2009). Language characteristics of individuals with Down Syndrome. Top Lang Disord, Vol. 29, No. 2, pp. 112-132, ISSN 0271-8294

Modeer, T., Barr, M. & Dahllof, G. (1990). Periodontal disease in children with Down's syndrome. Scand J Dent Res, Vol. 98, No. 3, pp, 228-234, ISSN 0029-845X

Ondarza, A., Jara, L., Bertonati, M.I. & Blanco, R. (1995). Tooth malalignments in Chilean children with Down syndrome. Cleft Palate Craniofac J, Vol. 32, No. 3, pp. 188-193, ISSN 1545-1569

Ondarza, A., Jara, L., Munoz, P. & Blanco, R. (1997). Sequence of eruption of deciduous dentition in a Chilean sample with Down's syndrome. Arch Oral Biol, Vol. 42, No. 5, pp. 401-406, ISSN 0003-9969

Orner, G. (1971). Congenitally absent permanent teeth among mongols and their sibs. J Ment Defic Res, Vol. 15, No. Pt 4, pp. 292-302, ISSN 0022-264X

Orner, G. (1975). Dental caries experience among children with Down syndrome and their sibs. Arch Oral Bio, Vol. 20, No. 10, pp. 627-634, ISSN 0003-9969

Orner, G. (1976). Periodontal disease among children with Down's Syndrome and their siblings. J Dent Res, Vol. 55, No. 5, pp. 778-782, ISSN 0022-0345

Rajić, Z. & Mestrović, S.R. (1998). Taurodontism in Down's syndrome. Coll Antropol, Vol. 22 Suppl: pp. 63-67, ISSN 0350-6134

Randell, D.M., Harth, S. & Seow, W.K. (1992). Preventive dental health practices of non-institutionalized Down syndrome children: a controlled study. J Clin Pediatr Dent, Vol. 16, No. 3, pp. 225-229, ISSN 1053-4628

Reuland-Bosma, W. & van Dijk, L.J. (1986). Periodontal disease in Down's syndrome; A review. J Clin Periodontol, Vol. 13, No. 1, pp. 64-73, ISSN 0303-6979

Russell, B.G. & Kjaer, I. (1995). Tooth agenesis in Down syndrome. Am J Med Genet, Vol. 55, No. 4, pp. 466-471, ISSN 1096-8628

Sandström, A., Cressey, J. & Stecksén-Blicks, C. (2011). Tooth-brushing behaviour in 6-12 year olds. Int J Paediatr Dent, Vol. 21, No. 1, pp. 43-49, ISSN 0960-7439

Sakellari, D., Belibasakis, G., Chadjipadelis, T., Arapostathis, K.N. & Konstantinidis A. (2001). Supragingival and subgingival microbiota of adult patients with Down's syndrome. Changes after periodontal treatment. Oral Microbiol Immunol, Vol. 16, No. 6, pp. 376-382, ISSN 0902-0055

Sakellari, D., Arapostathis, K.N. & Konstantinidis, A. (2005). Periodontal conditions and subgingival microflora in Down syndrome patients. A case-control study. J Clin Periodontol, Vol. 32, No. 6, pp. 684-690, ISSN 0303-6979

Saxen, L., Aula, S. & Westermarack, T. (1977). Periodontal disease associated with Down's Syndrome: An orthopantomographic evaluation. J Periodontol, Vol. 48, No. 6, pp. 337-340, ISSN 0022-3492

Shott, S.R., Amin, R., Chini, B., Heubi, C., Hotze, S. & Akers, R. (2006). Obstructive sleep apnea: Should all children with Down syndrome be tested? Arch Otolaryngol Head Neck Surg, Vol. 132, No. 4, pp. 432-436, ISSN 0886-4470

Scully, C. (1976). Down syndrome and dentistry. Dental Update, Vol. 3, No. 4, pp. 193-196, ISSN 0305-5000

Shapira, J., Stabholz, A., Schnrr, D., Sela, M.N. & Mann, J. (1991). Caries levels, Streptococcus mutant counts, salivary pH and periodontal treatment needs of adult Down syndrome patients. Spec Care Dentist, Vol. 11, No. 6, pp. 248-251, ISSN 1754-4505

Shapira, J., Chaushu, S. & Becker, A. (2000). Prevalence of tooth transposition, third molar agenesis and maxillary canine impaction in individuals with Down syndrome. Angle Orthod, Vol. 70, No. 4, pp. 290-296, ISSN 0003-3219

Shaw, L. & Saxby, M.S. (1986). Periodontal destruction in Down syndrome and in juvenile periodontitis: how close a similarity? J Periodontol, Vol. 57, No. 11, pp. 709-713, ISSN 0022-3492

Sherman, S.L., Allen, E.G., Bean, L.H. & Freeman, S.B. (2007). Epidemiology of Down syndrome. Ment Retard Dev Disabil Res Rev, Vol. 13, No. 3, pp. 221-227, ISSN 1080-4013

Shyama, M., Al- Mutawa, S.A., Honkala, S. & Honkala, E. (2003). Supervised toothbrushing and oral health education program in Kuwait for children and young adults with Down syndrome. Spec Care Dentist, Vol. 23, No. 3, pp. 94-99, ISSN 1754-4505

Siqueira Jr, W.L. & Nicolau, J. (2002). Stimulated whole saliva components in children with Down syndrome. Spec Care Dentist, Vol. 22, No. 6, pp. 226-230, ISSN 1754-4505

Skrinjarić, T., Glavina, D. & Jukić, J. (2004). Palatal and dental arch morphology in Down syndrome. Coll Antropol, Vol. 28, No.2, pp. 841-847, ISSN 0350-6134

Stabholz, A., Mann, J., Sela, M., Schurr, D., Steinberg, D. & Shapira, J. (1991). Caries experience, periodontal treatment needs, salivary pH, and Streptococcus mutans counts in a preadolescent Down syndrome population. Spec Care Dentist, Vol. 11, No. 5, pp. 203-208, ISSN 1754-4505

Townsend, G.C. (1983). Tooth size in children and young adults with trisomy 21 (Down syndrome). Arch Oral Biol, Vol. 28, No. 2, pp. 159-166, ISSN 0003-9969

Townsend, G.C. (1987). A correlative analysis of dental crown dimensions in individuals with Down syndrome. Hum Biol, Vol. 59, No. 3, pp. 537-548, ISSN 0018-7143

Ulseth, J.O., Hestnes, A., Stovner, L.J. & Storhaug, K. (1991). Dental caries and periodontitis in persons with Down Syndrome. Spec Care Dentist, Vol. 11, No. 2, pp. 71-73, ISSN 1754-4505

van Dyke, D.C., Lang, D.J., Miller, J.D., Heide, F., van Duyne, S. & Chang, H. (1990). Common medical problems. In: van Dyke, D.C., Lang, D.J., Heide, F., van Duyne, S. & Soucek, M.J., editors. Clinical perspectives in the management of Down syndrome. New York: Springer-Verlag, pp. 3-14, ISBN 038796987X.

Vigild, M. (1985). Prevalence of malocclusion in mentally retarded young adults. Community Dent Oral Epidemiol, Vol. 13, No. 3, pp. 183-184, ISSN 0301-5561

Vigild, M. (1986). Dental caries experience among children with Down's syndrome. J Ment Defic Res, Vol. 30, No. Pt3, pp. 271-276, ISSN 0022-264X

Waldman, H.B., Hasan, F.M. & Perlman, S. (2009). Down syndrome and sleep-disordered breathing: the dentist's role. J Am Dent Assoc, Vol. 140, No. 3, pp. 307-312, ISSN 0002-8177

Westerman, G.H., Johnson, R. & Cohen, M.M. (1975). Variations of palatal dimensions in patients with Down's syndrome. J Dent Res, Vol. 54, No. 4, pp. 767-771, ISSN 0029-845X

Yam WK, Tse PW, Yu CM, Chow CB, But WM, Li KY, Lee LP, Fung EL, Mak PP, Lau JT. (2008). Medical issues among children and teenagers with Down syndrome in Hong Kong. Downs Syndr Res Pract, Vol.12, No. 2, pp. 138-140, ISSN 1753-7606

Yoshihara, T., Morinushi, T., Kinjyo, S. & Yamasaki, Y. (2005). Effect of periodic preventive care on the progression of periodontal disease in young adults with Down's syndrome. J Clin Periodontol, Vol. 32, No. 6, pp. 556–560, ISSN

Part 3

Neoplastic Disease

6

Infections and Acute Leukemia in Children with Down Syndrome

Juan Manuel Mejía-Aranguré et al.*
Unidad de Investigación Médica en Epidemiología Clínica, Hospital de Pediatría, Instituto Mexicano del Seguro Social (IMSS).
División de Laboratorios de Vigilancia e Investigación Epidemiológica, IMSS.
Mexico

1. Introduction

Down syndrome (DS), or trisomy 21, is a genetic alteration caused by the presence of an extra chromosome 21. In different parts of the world, the incidence of DS varies from 0.3 to 3.4 per 1000 births, with a ratio of 1:1000 births being reported principally in America and Europe (Canfield et al., 2006; Hassold et al., 1996; Wahab et al., 2006; Webb et al., 2007). DS is associated with cardiovascular diseases; deficiencies of the digestive, immune, and endocrine systems; hematological problems; and also early onset of Alzheimer disease (Freeman et al., 2008; Holland et al., 2000; Linabery et al., 2008; Van Cleeve & Cohen, 2006; Wiseman et al., 2009).

Compared to children without this syndrome, children with DS have ten- to twenty-fold higher risk of developing acute leukemia (AL) (Fong & Brodeur, 1987; Malinge et al., 2009; Ross et al., 2005a; Taub, 2001); it is estimated that approximately 1–2% will develop leukemia (Hasle et al., 2000; Malinge et al., 2009; Taub, 2001). Of those children with DS who develop leukemia, 60% is classified as having acute lymphoblastic leukemia (ALL) and 40%, with acute myeloblastic leukemia (AML). Of those with AML, the most common type is M7, or acute megakaryoblastic leukemia (AMKL), found in 62% of this group of children (Hitzler & Zipursky, 2005). Approximately 10% of children with DS are born with a transitory myeloproliferative syndrome (TMS) that, in some cases, spontaneously disappears during the first few months of life; nevertheless, approximately, 20% of these children irreversibly develop AML. Children with DS have up to 500-fold higher risk of developing AMKL during the first four years (Hasle et al., 2000, 2001; Malinge et al., 2009; Zipursky, 2003).

Because the high incidence of AL in children with DS is strong evidence of the participation of chromosome 21 in the development of AL, investigation has been directed toward the

---

*María Luisa Pérez-Saldivar, Janet Flores-Lujano, Carolina Bekker Méndez, Sandra Pinto-Cardoso, David Aldebarán Duarte-Rodríguez, Arturo Fajardo-Gutiérrez
Unidad de Investigación Médica en Epidemiología Clínica, Hospital de Pediatría, Instituto Mexicano del Seguro Social (IMSS).
División de Laboratorios de Vigilancia e Investigación Epidemiológica, IMSS.Mexico
Histocompatibility & Immunogenetics (H&I) laboratory, National Health Service Blood and Transplant (NHSBT)UK

search for a gene, or genes, on chromosome 21 which may cause an interruption of cellular differentiation and mark the onset of AL. Research has been focused specifically on the study of the relation that exists between TMS and its developing into AMKL in patients with DS (Gamis & Hilden, 2002; Roy et al., 2009; Taub & Ravindranath, 2002; Zwaan et al., 2010). Study of this model has permitted the identification of the genes that provoke mutations that cooperate in the malignant transformation of hematopoietic precursor cells. One of these genes is *GATA1* (Hitzler et al., 2003; Vyas & Roberts, 2006; Zwaan et al., 2010), which codes for a transcription factor of chromosome X which codes for the signaling of zinc which is essential for the differentiation of erythrocytes and magakaryocytes in the hematopoietic cell line. Mutation in this gene causes the production of the short protein, GATA1s, having an altered capacity of transactivation, thus contributing to the uncontrolled proliferation of immature megakaryocytes (Cantor, 2005; Hitzler et al., 2003; Wechsler et al., 2002). It has been found that mutation occurs in utero and, therefore, acts as an early pathological event, prior to the onset of TMS; however, in the absence of trisomy 21, such mutation is not sufficient for the induction of leukemia. Another transcription factor RUNX1, encoded by a gene on chromosome 21, plays a very important role in the development of AML (Hitzler & Zipursky, 2005; Izraeli et al., 2007). RUNX1 is essential for the differentiation of megakaryocyte progenitors and is responsible for the reduction of platelets (Migas et al., 2011; Speck & Gilliland, 2002). The function of *RUNX1* is commonly interrupted by chromosomal translocations that have been associated with different types of AL. These include the translocation t(8;21) that generates the fusion gene *RUNX1/CBFA2T1* or *AML1/ETO*, which is associated with 40% of the AML type M2; the translocation t(12;21), called fusion gene *ETV6/RUNX1* or *TEL/AML1*, which is associated with 20% of ALL of the pro-B-cell precursors; and the gene that codes for CBFβ and that is the target of chromosomal aberrations such as inv(16) and t(16;16) in AML type M4 (Karrman et al., 2006; Zuna et al., 2011). Although it had been thought that GATA1 and RUNX1 were exclusive, it was later shown that RUNX1 cooperates with GATA1 during megakaryocytic differentiation, playing a very important role in predisposing a patient with DS to develop AMKL (Elagib et al., 2003). Nevertheless, in a recent study by the Children's Oncological Group (COG), it was found that children with DS had significantly fewer *ETV6/RUNX1* abnormalities than did children without DS (Maloney et al., 2010). Other genes that undergo mutations are *Janus Kinase 2* (*JAK2*) and *Janus Kinase 3* (*JAK3*) (Malinge et al., 2009); these genes are located on chromosome 9p24 and activate the encoding of tyrosine kinase, which has been reported in the majority of patients with myeloproliferative disorders. This type of mutation brings about a dysregulation of the activity of the kinase and a phosphorylation of tyrosine (Meydan et al., 1996; Mullighan et al., 2009). However, it has been shown that patients with DS who have this mutation have a better response to chemotherapeutic treatment. Other potential candidates include the transcription factors of the family of proto-oncogenes, such as ETS, ERG, and GABPα, which have been shown to be expressed and to functionally participate in megakaryocytic differentiation (Wiseman et al., 2009). The dysregulation of the proto-oncogene *EGR* has been observed in different types of cancer; *EGR* is over-expressed in AML, just as the proto-oncogene *ETS2* is over-expressed in AMKL; this dysregulation directly affects the cell cycle by regulating the expression of genes that require DNA synthesis and the degradation of the inhibitors of the cell cycle. It appears to a critical regulator of the development of lymphocytes in the precursors of B cells (Holterman et al., 2010; Sashida et al., 2010).

From the foregoing and from other reports in the literature, the mechanisms that predispose children with DS to develop AL are augmented by chromosome fragility, alteration of DNA repair mechanisms, immunological alterations, and the increase of viral replication (Robison, 1992; Xavier & Taub, 2010). If it is true that trisomy 21 can increase the proliferation of normal lymphoid progenitors, then for the children with DS (who already have a genetic susceptibility) to develop leukemia, this proliferation must be accompanied by additional events such as exposure of these children to environmental risks (Levanon et al., 2001; Rabson, 2010; Ross, 1999). Several environmental factors have been studied in children with DS: exposure in utero to X-rays; post-natal exposure to ionizing radiation, certain chemicals (such as pesticides and benzene), or to electromagnetic fields (EMF); habits of the parents, such as alcohol consumption and tobacco use before and during the pregnancy, or vitamin consumption; and viral infections of the mother during the pregnancy or of the child after birth.

2. Environmental factors associated with development of AL in children with DS

There have been relatively few studies concerning the association between exposure to environmental factors and the development of AL in children with DS; a brief description of the findings of these studies is germane to the current discussion.

Linabery et al. (2006) and the COG carried out a case-control study to determine if there were an association between exposure to radiation (X-rays) and the development of AL in children with DS. Of the 158 children with DS and AL who were identified from the registration files of COG, 97 had ALL and 61 had AML); the controls, 173 healthy children with DS, were selected from the same primary-care hospitals or clinics where the cases were treated in a normal fashion before their being diagnosed with AL. Three periods of possible exposure to radiation were studied; these were prior to conception, in utero, and postnatal. Data for the variable of the study was obtained by means of a telephone interview with the parents. In this interview, the parents were asked about any episodes of exposure to radiation (X-rays) during these periods. The results showed that there was no association between exposure to radiation and the development of ALL and AML in children with DS. The limitations of this study are due to the manner in which the exposure was measured and to the fact that the type of radiation, the radiation dose, and the part of the body exposed were not taken into account. In addition, it is probable that there had been a bias in the identification of the controls: not all the primary-care physicians furnished a list of potential controls; therefore, the authors had to seek a care center different than the one that had treated the case.

Data from these same groups of children were used in another case-control study conducted by the COG to determine if exposure of the mother to pesticides in the home was associated with the risk of AML or ALL in their children with DS. Positive associations with the development of ALL were found for exposure to pesticides in the home (odds ratio (OR): 2.25; 95% confidence interval (CI): 1.13, 4.49); to a pesticide (OR: 2.18; 95% CI: 1.08, 4.39); and to a chemical (OR: 2.72; 95% CI: 1.17, 6.35). No statistically significant association for AML was found in children with DS. The notable limitation in this study is that a third of the mothers and physicians were unable to provide data for the potential controls, so that another physician was consulted (Alderton et al., 2006).

Another case-control study concerned the relation between parental habits (smoking tobacco and alcoholism by the father) prior to the pregnancy or the passive exposure of the child to tobacco smoke and the development of leukemia by the child with DS. In this study, the sample size was 27 children with DS who had leukemia (ALL = 22; AML = 5) and 58 controls who were recruited from institutions of special education for children with DS. The parents of the case children and control children were interviewed concerning the frequency of their exposure to tobacco in the year prior to the pregnancy and during the pregnancy and concerning the passive exposure of the child to tobacco smoke prior to diagnosis (Mejía-Aranguré et al., 2003). Risk of the child with DS to develop AL was associated with the father's having smoked during the year prior to the pregnancy (OR: 3.57; 95% CI: 0.82, 20.27); with the father's having consumed alcohol in the year prior to the pregnancy (OR: 3.10; 95% CI 1.12, 8.62; and with the child with DS having been passively exposed to tobacco smoke (OR: 3.39; 95% CI: 1.09, 10.48). Although the sample size was small, important associations were encountered. However, it is probable that there was a bias in the selection of the control group.

Another of the factors that have generated numerous studies is the relation of the exposure of children to magnetic fields (MF) and the development of AL. This study was carried out with children with DS: 42 children had DS and ALL, with 124 healthy children with DS as controls. The controls were recruited from institutions providing special education to children with DS. The principal variable of exposure was measured in the home of the child by means of a gausometer, in addition to visual inspection of the wiring around the house. For each of the children, the parents were interviewed by health-care personnel at the attending health-care center. The data so obtained indicated that there was a positive association when there had been an exposure to MF >6.00 mG (OR: 3.7; 95% CI: 1.05, 13.1). It is interesting to note that, despite the few number of cases, the risk was found to be high, thus showing that, for children with a high susceptibility to environmental exposures that carry a risk, such factors become evident even though few individuals are studied. Nonetheless, it is probable that this study contains the same selection bias as the previous study (Mejía-Aranguré et al., 2007).

Puumala et al. (2007) conducted a case-control study to determine whether the reproductive history of the mother or infertility treatment was associated with a risk for the children with DS to develop ALL or AML. As mentioned earlier in this section, of the 158 cases captured by COG, 97 were diagnosed with ALL and 61, with AML; the 173 controls were healthy children with DS. To measure the variable of exposure, a telephone interview was carried out, evaluating the reproductive history and infertility treatment. The results were null; only an association between AML in children with DS was reported when an infertility treatment had been performed one year prior to the pregnancy (OR: 2.22; 95% CI: 1.14, 4.33). The possible limitations to this study are that the controls were recruited from the same clinic from which the cases had been recruited; however, a list of potential controls was not always available. Also, there could have been a memory bias when measuring the principal variable.

Ross et al. (2005b) studied the consumption of vitamins close to the time of conception and its association with the development of AL in children with DS. This case-control study utilized the same 158 children with DS and AL (97 cases with ALL; 61 with AML) that had been identified by COG and 173 healthy children with DS as controls. The mother of each child was interviewed by telephone to obtain information concerning the consumption of these supplements prior to the pregnancy and both before and after realizing that she was pregnant. A decrease in the risk of leukemia was observed when the vitamins had been taken as supplements during the periconception period (OR: 0.63; 95% CI: 0.39, 1.00). When stratified by type of leukemia, the risk of ALL was reduced (OR: 0.51; 95% CI: 0.30, 0.89); this was not found for AML (OR: 0.92; 95% CI: 0.48, 1.76). Consumption of vitamins during the periconception period after the realization of the pregnancy was associated with an increase in the risk of leukemia (OR: 1.61; 95% CI: 1.00, 2.58), for both ALL and AML. It should be pointed out that there was a possible confusion bias due to the increased risk of consuming vitamins by the mother after becoming pregnant; therefore, an underlying biological process could confound the study.

The role of infections in the etiology of leukemia and DS also has been under intensive study. By means of a case-control study using the same group of patients taken from the COG registry (the number of patients, recruitment of the controls, and measurement of the variable were given in more detail in foregoing paragraphs), the Children's Oncology Group (COG) evaluated the association between both the mother's state of health and episodes of infections during the pregnancy and the development of AL. The results obtained showed that the health problem most frequently encountered during pregnancy was vaginal bleeding, which had an associated reduction in the risk for AL for all the cases (OR: 0.57; 95% C: 0.33,0.99). The mother's having undergone amniocentesis was associated with an increase in the risk for AML (OR: 2.06; 95% CI: 0.90,4.69). One of the biases in this study is that of memory, due to the length of time between the pregnancy and the study interview (Ognjanovic et al., 2009).

In a case-control study that used this same group of children (details of the COG study, including cases, controls, and interview are given in foregoing paragraphs), Canfield et al. (2004) studied whether early infections in children with DS, as well as infections that the mothers underwent during pregnancy, played a role development of AL. In this study, it was found that there was a negative association between the risk of AL and any infection during the first two years of life: OR: 0.55: 95% CI: 0.33,0.92 for combined AL; OR: 0.53; 95% CI: 0.29,0.97 for ALL; and OR: 0.59; 95% CI: 0.28,1.25 for AML.

Similarly, Flores-Lujano et al. (2009) investigated whether either infections or breastfeeding was associated with risk of AL in children with DS. In this case-control study, the sample size was 57 children with DS and AL (45 ALL and 12 AML), with 218 healthy children with DS as controls. The controls were recruited from centers of special education for children with DS. Health-care personnel carried out the interviews in the health-care centers and in the special education institutions. In these interviews, questions specifically focused on infections and hospitalization in the first year of life and on breastfeeding. Although a statistically significant association was not found for these factors and general AL, hospitalization for an infection during the first year of life increased the risk (OR: 3.57; 95% CI: 1.59,8.05). Together with the foregoing results, this indicates that alteration of the immunological micro-environment could increase the risk for the development of AL in children with DS. A characteristic of these children is their having a higher frequency of infections than children without DS. This aspect should be investigated in greater depth.

3. Infection and leukemia in children

3.1 Infections and space-time clustering of children with childhood leukemia

The theme of viral infections and childhood leukemia has been approached through cluster analysis. The findings are interpreted in both a time and space context. Due to studies of this type, possible evidence has been postulated that support the idea of an infectious etiology in childhood leukemia (Francis et al, 2011; McNally et al, 2009). Studies of this type describe geographical and historical units, not individuals or populations per se. Though the results of such studies make reference to individuals and populations, the interpretations given have to be placed on a time line or in a geographical territory.

Under the foregoing terms, a cluster consists of a group of persons, who group together, whether temporally, geographically, or both temporally and geographically. When found to cluster simultaneously both temporally and geographically, this phenomenon is known as space-time clustering.

McNally and Eden (2004) commented that if infections are implicated in the etiology of childhood leukemia, then the geographic distribution of those children would demonstrate a space clustering within a determined time frame (McNally & Eden, 2004); that is to say, that they would form a space-time clustering.

With the premise that a space-time clustering can show evidence of an infectious etiology for children with leukemia, we performed a revision of the publications that concern this theme by availing ourselves of the information retrieval system provided by Pub Med, PubMed is a free database maintained by the United States National Library of Medicine at the National Institutes of Health. We compared the number of cluster-analysis studies in general with that of studies that specifically dealt with space-time clustering. Then, we further refined the search to retrieve the space-time studies that concerned children with leukemia. Finally, we made a brief description of the type and number of the publications that had been done concerning space-time clustering and children with leukemia (Table 1; Fig. 1).

Key word	**Number of publications**
Cluster analysis	59761
Cluster analysis + Leukemia	1292
Cluster analysis + Childhood + Leukemia	168
Space-time clustering	1801
Space-time clustering + Leukemia	124
Space-time clustering + Childhood + Leukemia	61

Table 1. Number of publications retrieved by iterative searches of PubMed database by using distinct key words. (Access date: 4 March 2011)

The key words (cluster analysis, space-time clustering; leukemia; childhood) utilized in PubMed were chosen because they are medical subject headings (MeSH), a controlled vocabulary for indexing articles in PubMed. These predetermined terms are used in the PubMed database to avoid omission of some study related to the theme of the search. We did not select any other limitation to annotate the search. The quantity of publications (59,761) retrieved when the term "cluster analysis" was used as the sole search word shows that this type of study is used widely. However, it should be noted that this number includes not only studies *of* clustering, but also studies *by* clustering.

When "space-time clustering" was used as the search term, the results were distinct: 1801 publications were retrieved. Of the 124 space-time clusterings concerning leukemia, approximately one half (61) dealt with childhood leukemia. These publications started in 1968 with a study, presented at a symposium, which was published in Nippon Ketsueki Gakkai Zasshi (Hirayama, 1968). In 1969, Glass & Mantel (1969) published a study concerning children in Los Angeles, California, in which mortality data were used in an exceptional way.

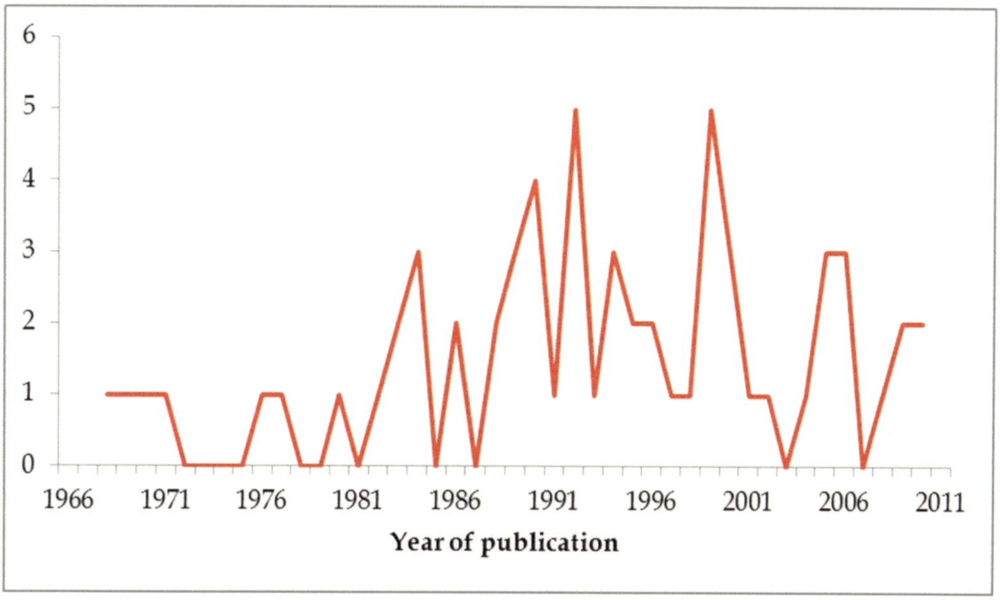

Fig. 1. Quantity of publications, retrieved by iterative searches of PubMed (see text), concerning both space-time clustering and childhood leukemia

The annual publication rate of such studies increased slowly until reaching a maximum in 1991; thereafter they started to decline. However, since the end of the last century, there appeared new peaks, notably in 1999, 2005, and 2009, thus showing a possibly renewed interest in performing this type of study.

The reason that such studies are performed may be due to the fact that populations worldwide live within a demarked time and geographical area. Infections are processes that are also limited to a time, to a space, and to a population. These studies cannot demonstrate solid support for any relation, but their consistency can provide a very strong argument. The two principal hypotheses of the concept of the infectious etiology of childhood leukemia, those postulated by Greaves (1988) and by Kinlen (1988), have been consistently supported by these cluster analysis studies and their results inspire other researchers to continue studies on this possible relation.

3.2 Viral theories of cancer and leukemia

In the first half of the last century, the viral theory of cancer and leukemia was almost in disrepute. So much so, that there was great difficulty in obtaining funds or laboratory facilities for research projects dealing with the hypothetical virus origin of cancer (Gross, 1974). In 1951, it was demonstrated that a transmissible virus causes mouse leukemia (Gross, 1951a). In those experiments, when inoculated into newborn mice of a non-leukemic inbred strain, filtrates prepared from leukemic mouse tissues were found to induce leukemia or lymphosarcomas. Complicated genetic theories had been used to explain the phenomenon of the development of "spontaneous" leukemia in successive generations of mice of certain inbred lines, such as AK or C58. However, the correct explanation was provided by the demonstration that mouse leukemia virus is transmitted, in a latent form, from one generation to another directly through the embryos (Gross, 1951b), probably through the germinal cells (Ahmed, 2005). The activation of the virus may not occur during the lifespan of the carrier host and the host may remain in good health, even though it carries the virus and transmits it to its progeny. A variety of tumors and leukemias in several animal species were found to be caused by filterable viruses, transmissible by inoculation of newborn host. The mouse-leukemia virus induces leukemia not only in mice but also in rats; it can be transmitted from rat-to-rat filtrates (Gross, 1963). Cat leukemia was found to be caused by a virus transmissible by filtrates not only from cats but also from dogs (Jarrett et al., 1964; Rickard et al., 1973, as cited in Dutcher & Chieco-Bianchi, 1973). It is still not understood why certain tumors and leukemias, such as mammary tumors in mice or leukemia in mice, cats, or chickens, contain virus particles and can be readily transmitted to other hosts by filtered extracts; similar tumors and lymphomas, which develop naturally in other species such as dogs, rats, and humans, do not seem to contain virus particles. This may be due to improper experimental methods; for example, no virus particles had been found in bovine lymphosarcoma until these leukemic cells were placed into short-term tissue cultures (Gillet et al., 2007).

In 1969, in an apparent attempt to elucidate the role of viruses in the etiology of cancer, Todaro and Huebner (1972) proposed the "oncogene" theory, suggesting that most cells of vertebrates carry, as an essential part of their natural evolutionary inheritance, "oncogenic information" (the oncogene), and that cancer results from the destruction of the normal "repressor system" that keeps both the oncogenic and virogenic information in check in the normal adult cell. In other words, "endogenous virogenes" (genes for the production of type-C viruses) and oncogenes (the portion of the virogene responsible for transforming a normal cell into a tumor cell) were maintained in an unexpressed form by "repressors" in normal cells. Agents, such as radiation, chemical carcinogens, or the normal process of aging, could activate the genes and may transform cells by "switching on" the endogenous oncogenic information (Huebner & Todaro 1969; Todaro & Huebner, 1972). Gross (Gross, 1963; Jarrett, 1964; Rickard et al., 1973, as cited in Dutcher & Chieco-Bianchi, 1973) pointed out that there is a fundamental difference between the vertical theory and the oncogene theory (Gross, 1963). The concept of vertical transmission of oncogenic viruses assumes that, at some point, the oncogenic viruses entered the animal host from outside and, since that time, have been passed from one generation to the other as a latent infection (Jarrett, 1964), whereas the "oncogene" theory postulates that the genome responsible for producing the infectious virus is part of the inherited genetic material of all cells of normal vertebrates. Gross furthered commented that, in the former case, the oncogene theory would be very similar to the original concept of vertical transmission of latent oncogenic viruses, with only some significant changes in terminology and with the assumption that latent oncogenic viruses are present in almost all somatic cells of vertebrates. If the oncogene theory assumes that infectious viruses can be produced from normal endogenous components of healthy, normal not infected cells, then such a concept would be untenable, without returning to the old concept of spontaneous generation of infectious agents (Rickard et al., 1973, as cited in Dutcher & Chieco-Bianchi, 1973).

3.2.1 Kinlen's hypothesis

Infection has been causally linked to some leukemias in animals and in adult humans and has often been considered as a basis for childhood leukemia. If childhood leukemia does have such an origin, the lack of an appreciable space-time clustering suggest that the infection is spread mainly by trivially infected subjects, rather than by children with leukemia. In 1990, Kinlen suggests that childhood leukemia represents a rare response to a much commoner, perhaps an unidentified mild or subclinical, infection, the transmission of which is facilitated when large number of people come together, particularly when they are from a variety of origins (Kinlen et al., 1990). This hypothesis was discussed in a study that showed a significant increase in childhood leukemia in a rural district in Scotland. This area, located at a distance from a conurbation and having no nuclear power installation in the vicinity, experienced a large influx of people during the 1950's (Kinlen, 1988) . Kinlen mentions that, when evaluating the findings, it is crucial to take into consideration the factors that are likely to increase the scale of contacts between susceptible people and the carriers of an unrecognized infection. Such factors, in the presence of that infection, may promote the development of leukemia and probably an epidemic of the infection itself, producing discernible long-term effects. Contact between those infected and susceptible individuals is the basis for the spread of any infection. That the total number of potential contacts is of great importance has been shown in occupational studies of infections such as influenza (Oxford et al., 2005) and tuberculosis (Hewitt &Stewart, 1951), as well as in the description of outbreaks of many other infections. New contacts between members of different communities must have occurred on an unusual scale both directly and indirectly as new towns rapidly grew in this area (Kinlen, 1988). Kinlen added that the greater the diversity in geographic origins among sizeable groups of residents, the more likely it is that appreciable differences in herd immunity will be found among different subgroups. The rate of progress of an epidemic is primarily regulated by the number of susceptible people and by the rate of contact between those infected and susceptible people (Fox et al.,1971). The best-known cluster of childhood leukemia is that in Niles, Illinois, USA, which consisted of eight cases during 1957–60, seven of whom were pupils of a single parish school. The population of Niles grew from 3587 in 1950 to 20 393 in 1960, with most of the increase occurring in 1955–60 and in the parish that later experienced the leukemia cluster (Heath & Hasterlik, 1990). The increased opportunity for new contacts, both in the crowed parish school (class size of 50) and in the adjoining church, could have favored both transmission of an infectious agent and repeated exposure to infected individuals.

3.2.2 Greaves' hypothesis

Greaves (1986) proposed that, at its peak incidence at about ages 3 and 4 years, ALL is due not to specific viruses, but to mutations that may delay exposure to various non-specific infective agents as well as to other immunological challenges (Greaves, 1986). Kinlen (1990) implied that, as this hypothesis is difficult to test epidemiologically, it would be problematic to distinguish definitively such effects from those of specific agents, as are observed in the majority of infection-based illnesses (Kinlen, 1990).

Kinlen (1990) concluded that their findings provide support not only for infection being a basis for childhood leukemia (not only the lymphatic type), but also specifically for an infection being promoted by greater levels of social contact, particularly among people from communities that previously has been widely separated. In locales where an excess of childhood leukemia has been recorded, the dynamics of herd immunity in such communities, taken as a whole, must be given greater attention.

Furthermore, Greaves and Chan suggest that much of the variation reported in the literature is a consequence of selective under-reporting and premature death in places where socio-economic conditions are poor (Den Otter et al., 1986). They also pointed out that the rate of lymphocyte proliferation in early childhood will be influenced by the pattern of exposure to micro-organisms, which will vary with social, environmental, and geographical factors. The idea of spontaneous mutations is not new. In one study, Den Otter et al. (1987) attempted to calculate both the incidence of the so-called "endogenous malignancy" and the number of mutations required for carcinogenesis by using measured mutant frequencies (Gross, 1951). Morris (1989) referred to the Den Otter study when he proposed an improved mathematical formula for application specifically to the incidence of lymphoid malignant (Morris, 1989). Morris concluded that his mathematical model showed that, if an increased mutation rate affects a subset of cell divisions, then the number of cell generations affected is more important than the absolute number of cell divisions affected. He is aware that the model he proposed fails to explain the age distribution of ALL without an additional assumption of a fallible mechanism that normally would eliminate malignant-clones. In this case, the activation of one growth-control gene by the loss of two regulatory genes would be enough for neoplasia.

3.2.3 Alexander's hypothesis

The Leukaemia Research Fund Data Collection Survey (DCS) is a specialist registry of leukemias and lymphomas, which collects high-quality incidence data for about half of England and Wales. The DCS published an atlas for 1984–88 (Alexander et al., 1991), in which the incidence of childhood ALL recorded by the registry was related both to aspects of community lifestyle from the 1981 census of England and Wales and to the Ordnance Survey digitized 1/625000 map data. The main findings were tested by applying them to the Yorkshire Region Children's Tumor Registry (YRCTR) for 1974–83. Although Yorkshire is in the DCS area, the two data sets are independent because the time periods do not overlap. Alexander considered these data and found that the association between ALL and radon persisted after adjustment for lifestyle factors (Cartwright et al, 1990). It was observed that higher rates of leukemias in children and young people had been reported in areas of higher socio-economic class and socio-economic status. These considerations led to the hypothesis that the incidence of childhood ALL was higher in communities that were isolated, were of higher socio-economic status, and had substantial numbers of commuting individuals. The relevant factors and classifications by each individually were selected in advance of the inspection of incidence data. The findings did not support any association between childhood ALL and commuting-to work distances. However, there was significant evidence that incidence increases, particularly for the childhood peak-age range, with distance from built-up areas. Further analysis of the DCS data showed that the highest rates of childhood ALL were found in those "middle-class" towns and villages which were farthest from urban conurbations. Initial confirmation was given by YRCTR data, with a similar two-fold difference in risk in both data sets. Alexander suggested that the interpretation of the findings and those of Kinlen (Kinlen,1988,1990) and of Cook-Mozaffari et al. (Cook-Mozaffari et al.,1989) was that the lifestyle in isolated communities, i.e., those of higher economic status, is conducive to an unusual exposure to some specific infectious agent or to general infections. This exposure can, in turn, increase the risk of childhood leukemia.

In contrast, Greaves model proposes that no specific agent is involved, but that the reduced exposure to antigenic challenge in infancy leads to greater proliferation of pre-malignant clones that can experience a second malignant change as a result of later infection (Greaves & Chan, 1986). Alexander mentioned that, if it is the timing of exposure to infections that is relevant, then the results found would strongly support the first part of Greaves hypothesis, when it can be shown that the children in the isolated communities experience reduced antigenic challenge in infancy. Therefore, the earliest social grouping may provide an environment particularly conducive to the spread of infections (Davis, 1986) which, Greaves suggests, would facilitate the second malignant event. The authors conclude that their findings tend to favor Greaves model, but further investigations of these communities will be straightforward and have the potential to refine the infection-as-causal-agent models for the etiology of childhood ALL. Possible interpretations include germ-cell damage prior to conception (Fairlie, 2009; Gardner et al., 1990), synergism between viruses and radiation (Pinkel & Nefzger, 1959), and some unknown extra factor.

3.3 Infection during the first year of life and childhood leukemia. Epidemiological evidence

Epidemiological studies have been performed to determine whether an infection during the first year of life is a factor that influences the causality of childhood AL, and specifically ALL. Kinlen and Greaves (1988) proposed that infections may be involved in reducing the risk of developing AL. For that reason, epidemiological studies have evaluated the relation between early infections and childhood AL. The infections that have been evaluated include otitis media, common colds, respiratory tract infections, streptococcus-caused infections, influenza, asthma, gastrointestinal diseases, infections causing diarrhea or vomiting, and infections that may have been recurrent in an early stage or that may have required hospitalization, such as exanthema-like diseases typical of infancy. These studies have demonstrated that exposure to such infections permit the stimulation and maturation of the immunological system of the child, thus reducing the risk that, when challenged by a later infection, the child's immune system would respond in an aberrant manner, resulting in AL. Given that the lymphoid leukemic cells represent a clonal expansion of white cells, these act in the human body as the first line of defense against infectious agents, that normally are regulated by lymphocytes, monocytes, and neutrophils, which in turn neutralize and eliminate the pathogenic agent. Therefore, if there is a aberrant or abnormal response to an infection, it could occasion in the child an excessive proliferation of mutated cells as the immunological response to the late infection, or else it could fails to halt the proliferation of malignant cells (Chan et al., 2002; Dockerty et al., 1999; Greaves & Alexander, 1994; Greaves, 1988; Greaves, 2006; Jourdan-Da et al., 2004; Kinlen, 1988; McNally & Eden, 2004; Ma et al., 2005a; Ma et al., 2009; Neglia et al., 2000; Perillat et al., 2002a; Rudant et al., 2010; Urayama et al., 2011; van Steensel et al., 1986).
The majority of studies carried out to evaluate this association have been epidemiological designs of the case-control type. Such studies have shown that, when children had been exposed to common infections during the first year of life, there was a reduction in the risk of developing AL. However, not all the studies have shown this association; thus, early infection as a causal agent of childhood AL remains a controversial issue. Nevertheless, the importance of early infection during the first year of life, whether resulting in a reduction or an increase in the risk of developing AL, has not been discarded (Table 2)(Cardwell et al., 2008; Chan et al., 2002; Dockerty et al., 1999; Jourdan-Da et al., 2004; McNally & Eden, 2004; McArthur et al., 2008; Ma et al., 2005a; Ma et al., 2009; Neglia et al., 2000; Perillat et al., 2002b; Petridou et al., 2001; Roman et al., 2007; Rosenbaum et al., 2000; Rudant et al., 2010; Shüz et al., 1999; Urayama et al., 2011; van Steensel et al., 1986;).
Some researchers have opted not only to evaluate the relation between early infections and AL by determining the involvement not only of common infections, but also of the

Author, Year (Country)	Van Steensel et al., 1986 (The Netherlands)	Schüz et al., 1999 (Germany)	Dockerty et al., 1999 (New Zealand)	Neglia et al., 2000 (USA)
Design of study	Case-control study (1973–1980)	Case-control study in two parts (1980–1994)	Case-control study (1991–1995)	Case–control study (1 January 1989 and 15 June 1993)
Size of sample	492 cases, 480 controls; age: 0-14 years	1184 cases, 2588 controls; age: 0-14 years	121 cases, 303 controls; age: 0-14 years	1842 cases, 1986 control; age: <15 years of age
Data collection	Mailed questionnaire; addressed to diagnosis	Telephone interviews of parents	Mothers interviewed at home; standardized questionnaires and serological tests	Structured interview
Variables	Breast feeding; birth order; family size; social class; number of rooms in household; infections; hospitalization or consultation for infections; primary infections (measles, chickenpox, mumps, or rubella); periods of fever	First-born child; duration of breastfeeding; deficit in social contacts; routine immunizations; infections; tonsillectomy or appendectomy; allergy of the child; allergy of the mother	Social class, marital status, ethnic group, educational level of parent; home ownership; length of gestation; age of mother at child's birth; weight of child at birth; exposure of mother to X-rays during the first trimester; exposure of child to X-rays or radiotherapy before onset of illness. Tobacco smoking by mother in first trimester or before pregnancy	Interview of mother; gender; age; race; educational level of mother; educational level of father; family income; immunophenotype class.
Odds ratio and relevant results	Common colds RR: 0.8, (95% IC: 0.6-1.0); periods of fever RR: 0.9;(95% IC: 0.7-1.2); primary infections RR: 0.8; (95% IC: 0.4-2.0); these variables were adjusted by birth order, family size, social class, and residential space. Infectious diseases requiring hospitalization RR: 0.6; (95% IC: 0.4-1.0).	Routine immunizations between 0-3 years of age OR: 3.2; (95% IC: 2.3-4.6); tonsillectomy or appendectomy (at least one) OR: 1.4; (95% IC: 1.1-1.9); child with allergy OR: 0.6; (95% IC: 0.5-0.8). Having had tonsillectomy or appendectomy increased child's risk of developing leukemia, whereas allergies showed a protective effect.	A positive relation was found between the infection caused by influenza during the first year of life and the risk for developing leukemia OR: 6.8; (95% CI 1.8-25.7). No other variable was related to acute leukemia.	Neither attendance at, nor time remaining in day care was associated with the risk of developing leukemia. For children with 1–4 episodes of ear infections or sustained infections, the association with development of acute leukemia was not statistically significant.

Table 2. Summary of reviewed articles concerning the epidemiology of early infection and acute childhood leukemia

Author, Year (Country)	Infante et al., 2000 (Quebec, Canada)	Rosenbaum et al., 2000 (New York, USA)	Perillat et. al., 2002b (France)	Chan et al., 2002 (Hong Kong)
Design of study	Case-control study (1989-1995	Case-control study	Case-control study	A population based, case-control study (November 1994 and December 1997)
Size of sample	491 cases 491 control age: 0-9 years	255 cases, 760 controls; age: 0-14 years; 31 county region (cases); (1980-1991)	280 incident cases; 288 hospital controls	116 cases, 788 controls; Age: 2-14 years; the Hong Kong Paediatric Haematology and Oncology Study Group
Data collection	Structured questionnaire administered to mothers by telephone	Standarized questionnaires mailed to the parents	Standarized face-to-face interviews of the mothers	Standarized, face-to face interviews
Variables	Educational level of mother; family income at the time of child's diagnosis; mother's age; father's age; tobacco smoking by mother; infections during pregnancy; child's birth order; attendance at day care or nursery; principal feeding method (breast or bottle); length of breastfeeding; history of recurrent infections of mother; use of antibiotics during pregnancy	Sex; race; educational level of mother; birth order; feeding status at birth (breast, bottle); age at diagnosis; day care or preschool program; family outcome; maternal employment during the pregnancy.	Diagnosed categories (acute leukaemia classification and immunophenotype); sex; age; ethnic origin; hospital where case capture; educational level of mother; occupation of mother at time interview, socio-professional categories; place of residence; birth order; number of siblings; day care; age at start of day care; repeated infections before age 2 years; surgical operation for early ear-nose-throat infections before age 2 years; breastfeeding.	Medical history (infectious illnesses) in the first year of life; breastfeeding; day care/social contacts of index and siblings; own household environment; community environment.
Odds ratio and relevant results	Early attendance at daycare or at nursery and breastfeeding were protective factors against the development of acute leukemia OR: 0.49,	Children who attended day care for >36 months, compared with those that did not, had a lower risk for developing	An inverse association was found between the development of acute leukemia and attendance at day care OR: 0.6; (95% CI: 0.4-1.0), repeated (≥4 per year) early common	Child had rubella and/or fever during first year of life lowered the risk OR: 0.33; (95% CI: 0.16-0.68); change of residence during

	(95% CI: 0.31-0.77) and OR: 0.68; (95% CI: 0.49-0.95), respectively.	leukemia OR: 1.32, (95% CI: 0.70-2.52); attendance at day care for 1-18 months OR: 1.74; (95% CI: 0.89-3.42) or for 19-36; OR: 1.32; (95% CI: 0.64-2.71).	infections before the age of 2 years OR: 0.6 (95% CI: 0.4-1.0), and surgery for infection of nose, ear, or throat before age of 2 years OR: 0.5 (95% CI: 0.2-1.0). Statistically significant interaction was found between attendance at day care and repeated common infections.	first year of life presented a lower risk of child's developing leukemia OR; 0.47; (95% CI:0.23-0.98), whereas with such change during second year, the risk increased, OR: 3.92; (95% CI: 1.47-10.46).

Table 2. (cont'd)

Author, Year (Country)	Jourdan-Da et al. 2004 (France)	Rosenbaum P et al., 2005 (New York, USA)	Ma et al., 2005b (USA)	Roman et al., 2007 (United Kingdom)
Design of study	Case-control study (1995-1998)	Population-based case-control study (1980-1991)		Population-based, case-control study (1991-1996)
Size of sample	473 cases, 567 population-based controls	255 cases, 760 control; age: 0-14 years	294 incident cases, 376 controls; age: 0-14 years	455 cases, 1031 controls; age: 0-14 years
Data collection	Questionnaire	Questionnaire	Personal interview of parents	Interview of parents
Variables	Gender; age at diagnosis; region of residence at diagnosis; socio-professional categories; educational level of mother; educational level of father; birth weight; term of pregnancy; birth order; mother's age at birth; Down syndrome; breastfeeding; infections in the first year of life.	Sex; race; birth year; mother's educational level; family income; maternal smoking; infant feeding at birth; birth order; attended day care before 25 months of age; year of diagnosis leukemia; age at diagnosis leukemia; allergies; history of allergies; common infections (colds, otitis media, influenza, croup, bronchiolitis, pneumonia, vomiting, diarrhoea)	Age; gender; household income; mother's educational level; mother's age at birth; birth weight; birth order; duration of breast feeding; day-care attendance; infections during infancy	Sex; age; diagnoses of infectious disease
Odds ratio and relevant results	Strong association found if child had gastrointestinal illnesses; attendance	Results showed that infection late in the first year of child's life is	Attendance at day care and infections during infancy is associated with a decrease in the	Cases had more episodes of infection than did controls, which was

	at day care lowered risk OR: 0.6; (95% CI: 0.4-0.8); no association found for breastfeeding; birth order (4th or later) showed significant association with increased risk of acute lymphoblastic leukemia OR: 2.0; (95% CI: 1.1-3.7); child's prior episode of asthma was associated with a lower risk of developing acute lymphoblastic leukemia OR: 0.5; (95% CI: 0.3-0.9).	associated with an increment in the risk of developing leukemia.	risk of developing acute lymphoblastic leukemia within the white Hispanic population OR: 0.42; (95% IC: 0.18-0.99 and OR: 0.32; (95% IC: 0.14-0.74), respectively; corresponding data for the Hispanic population, even for those living in the same area, did not agree.	more notable in the neonatal period (≤1 month): 18% of controls and 24% of cases with leukemia were diagnosed with an average of <1 infection OR: 1.4; (95% CI: 1.1-1.9; $p<0.05$). Cases with ≥1 episodes of infection in the neonatal period tended to be diagnosed with acute lymphoblastic leukemia at a relatively young age.

Table 2. (cont'd)

Author, Year (Country)	MacArthur, et al., 2008 (British Columbia and Quebec, Canada)	Cardwell et al., 2008 (United Kingdom)	Urayama et al., 2010 (USA)	Rudant J et al., 2010 (France)
Design of study	Population-based, case-control study (January 1,1990 and December 31,1994	Nested case-control (cohort) study	Case-control study (1995-1999)	National registry-based, case-control study ESCALE (2003-2004)
Size of sample	399 cases, 399 controls; age: 0-14 years	62 cases, 2215 matched controls	669 cases, 977 controls; age: 1-14 years	765 incident cases, 1,681 controls.
Data collection	Standardized personal interviews in the home of child	Data-based		Questionnaire, interviews by telephone
Variables	Gender; age; mother's age; father's age; numbers of live births; annual household income; mother's education; father's education; ethnicity; vaccinations; illness and infections; breastfeeding; allergies; immunosuppressant medication for child; vitamins; antibiotics for child.	Sex; age; consultations; numbers of consultations; antibiotics prescriptions; common infections.	Gender; mother's age at child's birth; mother's educational level; annual household income; birth weight; breast-fed; mother's smoking; day-care attendance; history of common infections as child; ethnicity.	Mother's educational level; parental professional category; place of residence at diagnosis; mother's age at child's birth; number of children of age <15 years in the household; birth order; breastfeeding; duration of breastfeeding; early

				common infections; surgical operation for ear-nose-throat infections; history of allergies; contact with animals; farm visit before age of 2 years
Odds ratio and relevant results	No association found between early infections and acute leukemia; vitamin use was associated with a risk of developing acute leukemia OR; 1.66; (95%CI: 1.18-2.33); with use of immunosuppressors by child, there was a decrease in risk of leukemia OR: 0.37; (95% CI: 0.16-0.84); breastfeeding >6 months had a protective effect against development of leukemia ($p < 0.05$).	One or more infections in the first year of life reduced the risk of leukemia OR: 10.5; (95%CI: 0.69-1.59; $p = 0.83$) and of acute lymphoblastic leukemia OR: 1.05; (95%CI: 0.64-1.74; $p = 0.84$).	When variables were evaluated separately, both attendance at day care at 6 months of age and birth order reduced the risk of leukemia OR: 0.90; (95% CI: 0.82-1.00 and OR: 0.68; (95% CI: 0.50-0.92), respectively) in a white non-Hispanic population, but not in a Hispanic population; however, if these children had ear infections, then the risk of developing acute leukemia was reduced OR: 0.45, (95%CI: 0.25-0.79).	Negative associations were found for children with repeated common infections OR: 0.7; (95% CI: 0.6-0.9); with a history of asthma or eczema OR: 0.7; (95% CI: 0.4-1.0) and OR: 0.7; (95% CI: 0.6-0.9), respectively; with attendance at day care before 1 year of age OR: 0.8; (95% CI: 0.6-1.1); and with prolonged breastfeeding OR: 0.7; (95% CI: 0.5-1.0).

Table 2. (cont'd)

Author, Year (Country)	Urayama et al., 2011 (USA)
Design of study	Observational studies (1993-2008)
Size of sample	14 case-control study
Data collection	Searches of Pub Med database and bibliographies of publications.
Variables	NA
Odds ratio and relevant results	Attendance at day care is associated with a reduced risk of acute lymphoblastic leukemia OR: 0.76; (95%CI: 0.67-0.87).

Table 2. (cont'd)

environment in which the child may have been exposed to diverse infectious agents. Such is the case of attendance in a day care, taking this as a proxy variable to evaluate said infections. Given that in such environment, the child may be in very close contact to those with childhood diseases or other common diseases. This close contact would permit the child to become ill with greater or lesser ease; at the same time, the child's immune system would be stimulated, sooner or later, by such infections (Chan et al., 2002; Dockerty 1999; Jourdan-Da et al., 2004; Ma et al., 2005b; Ma et al., 2009; Perillat et al., 2002b; Rosenbaum et al., 2000; Urayama et al., 2010, Urayama et al., 2011).

Urayama et al. performed two epidemiological studies in the USA, one was a case-control study (Urayama et al., 2010) and the other, a meta-analysis (Urayama et al., 2011). In the meta-analysis, the objective was to evaluate the association between the stay in day care during infancy and the risk of developing AL. Specifically, they evaluated whether early exposure to infection protected the child from AL, concluding that exposure of a child to common infections at an early age reduced the risk of developing AL (OR: 0.76; 95% CI: 0.67–0.87) (Urayama et al., 2010; 2011).

Studies carried out by Dockerty et al. (1999), Infante et al. (2000), Jourdan-Da et al. (2004), Ma et al. (2005b), and Perillat et al. (2002b) also supported these results. They showed that, if a child attends day care at an early age, the risk of developing leukemia is reduced. On the other hand, reports have been published that show no association between these infections or attendance in day care and the development of AL, or that show that rather than being a protective factor these variables are in fact risk factors for developing leukemia. Examples of such studies are those of Cardwell (2008), Dockerty (1999), and Neglia et al. (2000).

3.4 Breastfeeding and acute leukemia. Epidemiological evidence

Some epidemiological studies have evaluated breastfeeding as a possible protective factor. Given that it stimulates the immune response of the child, breast milk should be considered as the primary vaccine that the child receives during the first months of life, protecting the child from infections during this stage. Breast milk contains IgA antibodies against microorganisms and food antigens to which the mother has been exposed; in addition, the milk provides the child with immunoglobulins IgG and IgM, which stimulate phagocytosis and which prevent contact between microorganisms and epithelial cells of the host. The milk also contains B- and T-cell lymphocytes that are converted into lymphopoietic cells derived from the thymus and the spleen or equivalent tissue; these lymphocytes synthesize antibodies IgA, IgG, and IgM. By protecting the child from infections during the first year of life, breast milk can have an impact on the morbidity and mortality caused by diseases. Children fed exclusively with breast milk have fewer infections than do those who were never breastfed (Field, 2005; Macías et al., 2006; Parker, 2001; Reverón, 1995).

These epidemiological findings are supported by several case-control studies which showed that breastfeeding plays an important role in reducing the risk for developing AL during infancy, as breastfeeding can influence the immune response to an infection, modulating the system's response to a challenge (Altinkaynak et al., 2006; Bener et al., 2001; Beral et al., 2001; Davis, 1998; Field, 2005; Guise et al., 2005; Infante et al., 2000; Ip et al., 2007; Kwan et al., 2004; Perillat et al., 2002a; Shu et al., 1995, 1999; Stuebe, 2009).

Meta-analyses of case-control studies have been performed in order to evaluate the role of breastfeeding. Guise et al. (2005) performed a systematic review of articles, published in different electronic databases, with the aim of evaluating the evidence concerning the effect of breastfeeding on the risk of developing childhood AL. These authors reviewed 111 citations, of which they identified 32 articles that had access to the complete article. They concluded that, in at least half the articles that they reviewed, the results support the idea that breastfeeding reduces the risk of developing AL. Kwan et al. (2004) carried out a meta-analysis in order to quantify the findings concerning duration of breastfeeding and the risk of developing ALL and/or AML. They identified 14 case-control studies in which breastfeeding that lasted <6 months or >6 months was evaluated. Breastfeeding for >6 months was found to reduce the risk of developing ALL (OR; 0.76; 95% CI: 0.68–0.84) and AML (OR: 0.85; 95% CI: 0.73–0.98); with breastfeeding for <6 months, this reduction was not lost. Ip et al. (2007) also performed a systematic review to evaluate this association between breastfeeding and AL. They evaluated case-control three studies, the results of which showed that breastfeeding for >6 months is associated with a reduction in the risk of developing ALL (OR: 0.80; 95% CI: 0.71–0.91). (Guise et. al., 2005; Kwan et al., 2004).

3.5 Breastfeeding and acute leukemia in children with DS

Very few studies have evaluated the effect of early infections and breastfeeding in children with DS. One such study was carried out by Canfield et al. (2004) in which they evaluated the relation between early infections and the development of AL, while also evaluating breastfeeding in children with DS. Children with AL diagnosed between January 1997 and October 2002 were recruited through the COG. As mentioned in section 2, the sample size was 158 children with both DS and leukemia and 173 healthy children with DS as controls. For the children with DS who had had infections during the first two years of life, the risk of developing AL was reduced (OR: 0.55; 95% IC: 0.33–0.92), as compared to the children who had been infection-free during that period (Canfield et al., 2004).

In contrast, the results of a study carried out in Mexico City in children with DS did not support the findings of Canfield. In this study evaluating whether breastfeeding and infections during the first year of life demonstrated an association with the development of AL in children with DS, it was found that breastfeeding showed a protective effect, while early infection showed a factor risk of developing AL (OR: 0.84; 95% CI: 0.43-1.61 and OR: 1.70; 95% CI: 0.82-3.52, respectively); however, these effects were not statistically significant. This study also evaluated hospitalization for these infections. The results showed that if a child >6 years of age presented an infection and in addition was hospitalized for said infection, the risk for developing AL was increased (OR: 3.57; 95% CI: 1.59–8.05); therefore, these results do not support the hypothesis, proposed by Greaves, that infections are a protective factor against the development of this disease (Flores et al., 2009).

4. Conclusions

The fact that our results agreed with reports in the literature that maternal breastfeeding during the first six months of life appeared to be a protective effect in the development of AL in children under six years of age should be underscored. The natural practice of breastfeeding does not put either the children or their mothers at risk and does not increase the expenses for the family or for society; therefore, independent of the strength of the mother-child bond that it fosters, breastfeeding should be encouraged as a measure that may lower the risk of children suffering AL during the first years of life (Guise et al, 2005). However, serious infections appeared to be an important risk factor in the development of AL in children over six years of age, especially for children from a low socio-economic background.

The role of infectious agents involved in these groups should be investigated if these are involved in the genesis of AL, above all, in those that occur in children older than six years. To date, the study of children with DS, a population with an elevated susceptibility for AL, has proved to be a very efficient design in the search for environmental factors associated with the development of AL. By using this design in several studies, we have identified associations important to the genesis of ALs, even when the sample size was not very large. The rationale to continue to use this design is that, if ALs result from the interaction of susceptibility to the disease and exposure to different environmental factors, then the search for the effect of these environmental factors in a non-susceptible population will always lead to erroneous results, because the population not susceptible to ALs will not develop the disease no matter how long they are exposed to such environmental factors. This design is an effective and efficient tool for use in studies elucidating the epidemiology of AL. However these results only apply to one population with like susceptibility for developing AL than children with DS.

5. Acknowledgments

This work was supported by a grant (FIS/IMSS/PROT/056) from the Fondo de Investigación en Salud, México, and of projects financed by grants (2007-1-71223/FIS/IMSS/PROT/592 & CB-2007-1-83949/FIS/IMSS/PROT/616) from the Consejo Nacional de Ciencia y Tecnología, México, through its division for the dissemination of the results of scientific investigation. We thank Veronica Yakoleff for translation of the original Spanish manuscript, editorial revision, and for helpful comments.

6. References

Ahmed, N. (2005). The vertical transmission of human immunodeficiency virus type 1: molecular and biological properties of the virus. *Critical Reviews in Clinical Laboratory Science*, Vol.42, No.1, (2005), pp.1-34, ISSN 1549-781X.

Alderton, LE.; Spector, LG.; Blair, CK.; Roesler, M; Olshan, AF.; Robison, LL. & Ross, JA. (2006). Child and maternal household chemical exposure and the risk of acute leukemia in children with Down's syndrome: a report from the Children's Oncology Group. *American Journal of Epidemiology*, Vol.164, No.3, (August 2006), pp. 212-221, ISSN 0002-9262.

Alexander, F.; Ricketts, T.; McKinney, P. & Cartwright, R. (1991). Community lifestyle characteristics and lymphoid malignancies in young people in the UK. *European Journal of Cancer*, Vol.27, No.11, (November 1991), pp.1486-1490, ISSN 0959-8049.

Altinkaynak, S.; Selimoglu, M.; Turgut, A.; Kilicaslan, B. & Ertekin, V. (2006). Breast-feeding duration and childhood acute leukemia and lymphomas in a sample of Turkish children. *Journal of Pediatric Gastroenterology and Nutrition*, Vol.42, No.5, (May 2006), pp.568-572, ISSN 1536-4801.

Bener, A.; Denic, S. & Galadari, S. (2001). Longer Breast-feeding and protection against childhood leukaemia and lymphomas. *European Journal of Cancer*, Vol.37, No.2, (January 2001), pp.234-238, ISSN 0959-8049.

Beral, V.; Fear, N.; Alexander, F. & Appleby, P. (2001). Breastfeeding and childhood cancer. UK Childhood Cancer Study Investigators. *British Journal of Cancer*. Vol.85, No.11, (November 2001), pp.1685-1694, ISSN 1532-1827.

Canfield, KN.; Spector, LG.; Robison, LL.; Lazovich, D.; Roesler, M.; Olshan, AF.; Smith, FO.; Heerema, NA.; Barnard, DR.; Blair, CK. & Ross JA. (2004). Childhood and maternal infections and risk of acute leukaemia in children with Down syndrome: a report from the Children's Oncology Group. *British Journal of Cancer,* Vol.91, No. 11, (November 2004), pp. 1866-1872, ISSN 1532-1827.

Canfield, MA.; Honein, MA.; Yuskiv, N.; Xing, J.; Mai, CT.; Collins, JS.; Devine, O.; Petrini, J.; Ramadhani, TA.; Hobbs, CA. & Kirby, RS. (2006). National estimates and race/ethnic-specific variation of selected birth defects in the United States, 1999-2001. *Birth Defects Research. Part A, Clinical and Molecular Teratology,* Vol. 76, No. 11, (November 2006), pp.747-756, ISSN 1542-0760.

Cantor, AB. (2005). GATA transcription factors in hematologic disease. *International Journal of Hematology,* Vol.81, No.5, (June 2005), pp. 378-384, ISSN 0925-5710.

Cardwell, C.; McKinney, P.; Patterson, C. & Murray, L. (2008). Infections in early life and childhood leukaemia risk: a UK case-control study of general practitioner records. *British Journal of Cancer,* Vol.99, No.9, (November 2008), pp.1529-33, ISSN 1532-1827.

Cartwright R, Alexander F, McKinney P, Ricketts T, Hayhoe F, Clayton D. (1990). *Leukaemia and Lymphoma: an atlas of distribution within areas of England and Wales 1984-1988.* (1st Edition), Leukaemia Research Fund, ISBN 0-950223050, London.

Chan, L.; Lam, T.; Li, C.; Lau, Y.; Li, C.; Yuen, H.; Lee, C.; Ha, S.; Yuen, P.; Leung, N.; Patheal, S.; Greaves, M. & Alexander, F. (2002). Is the timing of exposure to infection a major determinant of acute lymphoblastic leukaemia in Hong Kong?. *Paediatric and Perinatal Epidemiology,* Vol.16, No.2, (April 2002), pp.154-165, ISSN 1365-3016.

Cook-Mozaffari, P.; Darby, S.; Doll R. Forman, D.; Hermon, C.; Pike, MC. & Vincent, T. (1989). Geographical variation in mortality from leukaemia and other cancers in England and Wales in relation to proximity to nuclear installations. 1969-1978. *British Journal of Cancer,* Vol.59, No.3, (March 1989), pp. 476-485, ISSN 1532-1827.

Davis, S. Case aggregation in young adult Hodgkins disease. (1986). Etiologic evidence from a population experience. *Cancer,* Vol.57, No.8,(April 1986), pp.1602-1612, ISSN 1097-0142.

Davis, K. (1998). Review of the evidence for an association between infant feeding and childhood cancer. *International Journal of Cancer supplement,* Vol.11, Issue supplement 11, (March 1998), pp. 29-33, ISSN 0898-6924.

Den Otter, W.; Kotten, J. & Derkinderen, D. (1986). A new model of oncogenesis. *Anticancer Research,* Vol.6, No. 3 pt B, (May-June 1986), pp. 509-514, ISSN 1476-069X.

Den Otter, W.; Kotten, JW. & Derkinderen, DJ. (1987). Carcinogenesis revisited. *Cancer Investigation,* Vol.5, No.1, (1986), pp.69-74, ISSN 1532-4192.

Dockerty, J.; Skegg, D.; Elwood, J.; Herbison, G.; Becroft, D. & Lewis, M. (1999). Infections, vaccinations, and the risk of childhood leukaemia. *British Journal of Cancer,* Vol.80, No.9, (July 1999), pp.1483-1489, ISSN 1532-1827.

Elagib, KE.; Racke, FK.; Mogass, M.; Khetawat, R.; Delehanty, LL. & Goldfarb, AN. (2003). RUNX1 and GATA-1 coexpression and cooperation in megakaryocytic differentiation. *Blood,* Vol.101, No.11, (June 2003), pp. 4333-4341, ISSN 1528-0020.

Fairlie, I. (2009). Commentary: childhood cancer near nuclear power stations. *Environmental Health,* Vol.8, No.23, (September 2009), pp.43, ISSN 0250-7005.

Field, CJ. (2005). The immunological components of human milk and their effect on immune development in infants. *The Journal of Nutrition,* Vol.13, No.1, (January 2005), pp.1-4, ISSN 1541-6100.

Flores, J.; Perez, M.; Fuentes, E.; Gorodezky, C.; Bernaldez, R.; Del Campo, M.; Martinez, A; Medina, A.; Paredes, R.; De Diego, J.; Bolea, V.; Rodriguez, M.; Rivera, R.; Palomo, M.; Romero, L.; Perez, P.; Alvarado, M.; Salamanca, F.; Fajardo, A. & Mejía, J. (2009). Breastfeeding and early infection in the aetiology of childhood leukaemia in Down syndrome. *British Journal of Cancer*, Vol.101, No.5, (September 2009), pp.860-864, ISSN 1532-1827.

Fong, CT. & Brodeur, GM. (1987). Down's syndrome and leukemia: epidemiology, genetics, cytogenetics and mechanisms of leukemogenesis. *Cancer Genetics and Cytogenetics,* Vol.28, No.1, (September 1987), pp. 55-76, ISSN 0165-4608.

Fox, JP.; Elveback, L.; Scott, W.; Gatewood, L. & Ackerman, E. (1971). Herd immunity; basic concept and relevance to public health immunization practices. *American Journal of Epidemiology,* Vol.94, No.3, (September 1971), pp.179-189, ISSN 1476-6256.

Francis, S.; Selvin, S.; Yang, W.; Buffler, P. & Wiemels, J. (2011). Unusual Space-Time Patterning of the Fallon, Nevada Leukemia Cluster: Evidence of an Infectious Etiology. *Chemico-biological interactions,* DOI:10.1016/j.cbi.2011.02.019, (February 2011), ISSN 0009-2797.

Freeman, SB.; Bean, LH.; Allen, EG.; Tinker, SW.; Locke, AE.; Druschel, C.; Hobbs, CA.; Romitti, PA.; Royle, MH.; Torfs, CP.; Dooley, KJ. & Sherman, SL. (2008). Ethnicity, sex, and the incidence of congenital heart defects: a report from the National Down Syndrome Project. *Genetics in Medicine,* Vol.10, No.3, (March 2008), pp. 173-180, ISSN 1530-0366.

Gamis, AS. & Hilden, JM. (2002). Transient myeloproliferative disorder, a disorder with too few data and many unanswered questions: does it contain an important piece of the puzzle to understanding hematopoiesis and acute myelogenous leukemia? *Journal of Pediatric Hematology/Oncology: official Journal of the American Society of Pediatric Hematology/Oncology,* Vol.24, No.1, (January 2002), pp. 2-5, ISSN 1536-3678.

Gardner, M.; Snee, M.; Hall A. et al.(1990). Results of case control study of leukaemia and lymphoma among young people near Sellafield nuclear plant in West Cumbria. *British Medical Journal,* Vol.300, No.6722, (February 1990), pp.423-429, ISSN 0959-8138.

Gillet, N.; Florins, A.; Boxus, M.; Burteau, C.; Nigro, A.; Vandermeers, F.; Balon, H.; Bouzar, AB.; Defoiche, J.; Burny, A.; Reichert, M.; Kettmann, R. & Willems, L. (2007). Mechanisms of leukemogenesis induced by bovine leukemia virus: prospects for novel anti-retroviral therapies in human. *Retrovirology,* Vol.4, No.16, (March 2007), pp.18, ISSN 1742-4690.

Glass, A. & Mantel, N. (1969). Lack of time-space clustering of childhood leukemia in Los Angeles County, 1960-1964. *Cancer Research,* Vol.29, No.11 (November 1969), pp. 1995-

Greaves, M. & Chan, L. (1986). Is spontaneous mutation the major "cause" of childhood acute lymphoblastic leukemia. *British Journal of Haematology,* Vol.64, No.1, (September 1986), pp. 1-13, ISSN 0007-1048.

Greaves, M. (1988). Speculations on the cause of childhood acute lymphoblastic leukaemia. *Leukemia,* Vol.2, No.2, (February 1988), pp. 120–125, ISSN 0887-6924.

Greaves, M. & Alexander, F. (1994). Epidemiological characteristics of childhood acute lymphocytic leukemia. *Leukemia,* Vol.8, No.10, (October 1994), pp.1793-1794, ISSN 0887-6924.

Greaves, M. (2006). Infection, immune responses and the aetiology of childhood leukemia. *Nature Reviews Cancer,* Vol.6, No.3, (March 2006), pp.93-203, ISSN 1474-1768

Gross, L. (1951a). Pathogenic properties, and "vertical" transmission of the mouse leukemia agent. *Proceedings of the Society for Experimental Biology and Medicine,* Vol.78, No.1, (October 1951), pp. 342-348, ISSN 1525-1373.

Gross, L. (1951b) "Spontaneous" leukemia developing in C3H mice following inoculation in infancy, with AK-leukemic extracts, or AK-embryos. *Proceedings of the Society for Experimental Biology and Medicine,* Vol.76, No.1, (January 1951), pp. 27-32, ISSN 1525-1373.

Gross, L. (1963) Serial cell-free passage in rats of the mouse leukemia virus. Effect of thymectomy. *Proceedings of the Society for Experimental Biology and Medicine,* Vol.112, (April 1963), pp. 939-945, ISSN 1525-1373.

Gross, L. (1974). Facts and Theories on Viruses Causing Cancer and Leukemia (Veritical transmission/oncogenic viruses /oncogene theory/protovirus hypotheisis). *Proceedings of the National Academy of Sciences of the United States of America,* Vol. 71, No.5, pp. 2013-2017, ISSN 0027-8424.

Guise, J.; Austin, D. & Morris, C. (2005). Review of case-control studies related to breastfeeding and reduced risk of childhood leukemia. *Pediatrics,* Vol.116, No.5, (November 2005), pp. 724-731, ISSN 1098-4275.

Hasle, H.; Clemmensen, IH. & Mikkelsen, M. (2000). Risks of leukaemia and solid tumours in individuals with Down's syndrome. *Lancet,* Vol.355, No.9199, (January 2000), pp. 165-169, ISSN 1474-547X.

Hasle, H. (2001). Pattern of malignant disorders in individuals with Down's syndrome. *The Lancet Oncol*ogy, Vol.2, No.7, (July 2001), pp. 429-436, ISSN 1470-2045.

Hassold, T.; Abruzzo, M.; Adkins, K.; Griffin, D.; Merrill, M.; Millie, E.; Saker, D.; Shen, J. & Zaragoza, M. (1996). Human aneuploidy: incidence, origin, and etiology. *Environmental and Molecular Mutagenesis,* Vol.28, No.3, (1996), pp. 167-175, ISSN 1098-2280.

Heath, C. & Hasterlik, R. (1990). Leukemia among children in a suburban community 1963. *CA: A Cancer Journal for Clinicians,* Vol.40, No.1, (Jan-Feb 1990), pp. 27-50, ISSN 1542-4863.

Hewitt, D. & Stewart, A. (1951). Measuring the risk of infection at work. *British Journal of Social Medicine,* Vol.5, No.4, (October 1951), pp. 209-222, ISSN 0366-0842.

Hirayama, T. (1968). [Symposium: Epidemiology of leukemia in Japan. An epidemiological study of leukemia in Japan with special reference to the problem of time-space clustering] [Japanese]. *Nippon Ketsueki Gakkai Zasshi,* Vol.31, No.5 (October 1968), pp.737-47. ISSN 0001-5806.

Hitzler, JK.; Cheung, J.; Li, Y.; Scherer, SW. & Zipursky, A. (2003). GATA1 mutations in transient leukemia and acute megakaryoblastic leukemia of Down syndrome. *Blood,* Vol.101, No.11, (June 2003), pp. 4301-4304, ISSN 1528-0020.

Hitzler, JK. & Zipursky, A. (2005). Origins of leukaemia in children with Down syndrome. *Nature Reviews Cancer,* Vol.5, No.1, (January 2005), pp. 11-20, ISSN 1474-1768.

Holland, AJ.; Hon, J.; Huppert, FA. & Stevens, F. (2000). Incidence and course of dementia in people with Down's syndrome: findings from a population-based study. *Journal of Intellectual Disability Research,* Vol.44, No.Pt2, (April 2000), pp. 138-146, ISSN 1365-2788.

Holterman, CE.; Franovic, A.; Payette, J. & Lee, S. (2010). ETS-1 oncogenic activity mediated by transforming growth factor alpha. *Cancer Research,* Vol.70, No.2, (January 2010), pp. 730-740, ISSN 1538-7445.

Huebner, R. & Todaro, G. (1969). Oncogenes of RNA tumor viruses as determinants of cancer. *Proceedings of the National Academy of Sciences of the United States of America,* Vol.64, No.3, (November 1969), pp. 1087-1094, ISSN 0027-8424.

Infante, C.; Fortier, I. & Olson, E. (2000). Markers of infection, breast-feeding and childhood acute leukemia. *British Journal of Cancer,* Vol.83, No.11, (December 2000), pp.1559-1564, ISSN 1532-1827.

Ip, S.; Chung, M.; Raman, G.; Chew, P.; Magula, N.; DeVine, D.; Trikalinos, T. & Lau, J. (2007). Breastfeeding and maternal and infant health outcomes in developed countries. *Evidence Report/Technology Assessment,* No.153, (April 2007), pp.1-186, ISSN 1530-4396.

Izraeli, S.; Rainis, L.; Hertzberg, L.; Smooha, G. & Birger, Y. (2007). Trisomy of chromosome 21 in leukemogenesis. *Blood Cells, Molecules & Diseases,* Vol.39, No.2, (September-October 2007), pp. 156-169, ISSN 1079-9796.

Jarrett, W.; Martin, W.; Crighton, G.; Dalton, R. & Stewart, M. (1964) Transmission experiments with leukemia (lymphosarcoma). *Nature,* Vol.202, (May 1964), pp. 566-567, ISSN 1476-4687.

Jourdan-Da, N.; Perel, Y.; Méchinaud, F.; Plouvier, E.; Gandemer, V.; Lutz, P.; Vannier, J.; Lamagnére, J.; Margueritte, G.; Boutard, P.; Robert, A.; Armari, C.; Munzer, M.; Millot, F.; De Lumley, L.; Berthou, C.; Rialland, X.; Pautard, B.; Hémon, D. & Clavel, J. (2004). Infectious diseases in the first year of life, perinatal characteristics and childhood acute leukaemia. *British Journal of Cancer,* Vol.90, No.1, (January 2004), pp.139-145, ISSN 1532-1827.

Karrman, K.; Forestier, E.; Andersen, MK.; Autio, K.; Borgström, G.; Heim, S.; Heinonen, K.; Hovland, R.; Kerndrup, G. & Johansson, B; Nordic Society of Paediatric Haematology and Oncology (NOPHO) and the NOPHO Leukaemia Cytogenetic Study Group (NLCSG). (2006). High incidence of the ETV6/RUNX1 fusion gene in paediatric precursor B-cell acute lymphoblastic leukaemias with trisomy 21 as the sole cytogenetic change: a Nordic series of cases diagnosed 1989-2005. *British Journal of Haematology,* Vol.135, No. 3, (November 2006), pp. 352-354, ISSN 1365-2141.

Kinlen, L. (1988). Evidence for an infective cause of childhood leukaemia: comparison of a Scottish new town with nuclear reprocessing sites in Britain. *Lancet,* Vol.2, No.8624, (December 1988), pp. 1323-1327. ISSN 1474-547X.

Kinlen, LJ.; Clarke, K. & Hudson, C.(1990). Evidence from population mixing in British New Towns 1946-85 of an infective basis for childhood leukaemia. *Lancet,* Vol. 336, No.8715, (September 1990), pp.557-582, ISSN 1474-547X.

Kwan, L.; Buffler, P.; Abrams, B. & Kiley, V. (2004). Breastfeeding and the risk of childhood leukemia: a meta-analysis. *Public Health Reports,* Vol.119, Nov.6, (November-December 2004), pp.521-535, ISSN 0033-3549.

Levanon, D.; Glusman, G.; Bangsow, T.; Ben-Asher, E.; Male, DA.; Avidan, N.; Bangsow, C.; Hattori, M.; Taylor, TD.; Taudien, S.; Blechschmidt, K; Shimizu, N.; Rosenthal, A.; Sakaki, Y.; Lancet, D. & Groner Y. Architecture and anatomy of the genomic locus encoding the human leukemia-associated transcription factor RUNX1/AML1. *Gene* 2001; Vol.262, No.1-2, (January 2001), pp. 23-33, ISSN 0378-1119.

Linabery, AM.; Olshan, AF.; Gamis, AS.; Smith, FO.; Heerema, NA.; Blair, CK. & Ross JA; Children's Oncology Group. (2006). Exposure to medical test irradiation and acute leukemia among children with Down syndrome: a report from the Children's Oncology Group. *Pediatrics,*Vol.118, No.5, (November 2006), pp. e1499-e1508, ISSN 1098-4275.

Linabery, AM.; Blair, CK.; Gamis, AS.; Olshan, AF.; Heerema, NA. & Ross JA. (2008). Congenital abnormalities and acute leukemia among children with Down syndrome: a Children's Oncology Group study. *Cancer Epidemiology, biomarkers & prevention: a publication of the American Association for Cancer Research, cosponsored by the American Society of Preventive Oncology,* Vol.17, No.10, (October 2008), pp. 2572-2577, ISSN 1538-7755.

Ma, X.; Metayer, C.; Does, M. & Buffler, P. (2005a). Maternal pregnancy loss, birth characteristics, and childhood leukemia (United States). *Cancer Causes & Control,* Vol.16, No.9, (November 2005), pp.1075-1083, ISSN 1573-7225.

Ma, X.; Buffler, P.; Wiemels, J.; Selvin, S.; Metayer, C.; Loh, M.; Does, M. & Wiencke, J. (2005b). Ethnic difference in daycare attendance, early infections, and risk of childhood acute lymphoblastic leukemia. *Cancer Epidemiology, Biomarkers & Prevention,* Vol.14, No.8 (August 2005), pp.1928-1934, ISSN 1538-7755.

Ma, X.; Urayama, K.; Chang, J.; Wiemels, J. & Buffler, P. (2009). Infection and pediatric acute lymphoblastic leukemia. *Blood Cells, Molecules & Diseases,* Vol.42, No.2, (March-April 2009), pp.117-120, ISSN 1096-0961.

MacArthur, A.; McBride, M.; Spinelli, J.; Tamaro, S.; Gallagher, R. & Theriault, G. (2008). Risk of childhood leukemia associated with vaccination, infection, and medication use in childhood: the Cross-Canada Childhood Leukemia Study. *American Journal of Epidemiology,* Vol.167, No.5, (March 2008), pp.598-606, ISSN 1476-6256.

Macías, S.; Rodríguez, S.; & Ronayne, P. (2006). Leche materna: composición y factores condicionantes de la lactancia. *Archivos Argentinos de Pediatría,* Vol.104, No.5, (Septiembre-Octubre 2006), pp.423-430, ISSN 1668-3501.

Malinge, S.; Izraeli, S. & Crispino, JD. (2009). Insights into the manifestations, outcomes, and mechanisms of leukemogenesis in Down syndrome. *Blood,* Vol.113, No.12, (March 2009), pp. 2619-2628, ISSN 1528-0020.

Maloney, KW.; Carroll, WL.; Carroll, AJ.; Devidas, M.; Borowitz, MJ.; Martin, PL.; Pullen, J.; Whitlock, JA.; Willman, CL.; Winick, NJ.; Camitta, BM. & Hunger, SP. (2010). Down syndrome childhood acute lymphoblastic leukemia has a unique spectrum of sentinel cytogenetic lesions that influences treatment outcome: a report from the Children's Oncology Group. *Blood,* Vol.116, No.7, (August 2010), pp. 1045-1050, ISSN 1528-0020.

McNally, R. & Eden, T. (2004). An infectious aetiology for childhood acute leukaemia: a review of the evidence. *British Journal of Haematology,* Vol.127, No.3, (November 2004), pp. 243-263., ISSN 1365-2141.

McNally, R.; Bithell, J.; Vincent, T. & Murphy, M. (2009). Space-time clustering of childhood cancer around the residence at birth. *International Journal of Cancer,* Vol.124, No. 2, (January 2009), pp. 449-455, ISSN 1097-0215.

Mejía, JM.; Fajardo, A.; Flores, H.; Martínez, MC.; Salamanca, F.; Palma, V.; Paredes, R.; Bernáldez, R.; Ortiz, A.; Martínez, A. & Gorodezky, C. (2003). Environmental factors contributing to the development of childhood leukemia in children with Down's syndrome. *Leukemia,* Vol.17, No.9, (September 2003), pp. 1905-1907, ISSN 1476-5551.

Mejia, JM.; Fajardo, A.; Perez, ML.; Gorodezky, C.; Martinez, A.; Romero, L.; Campo, MA.; Flores, J.; Salamanca, F. & Velasquez, L. (2007). Magnetic fields and acute leukemia in children with Down syndrome. *Epidemiology,* Vol.18, No.1, (January 2007), pp. 158-161, ISSN 1531-5487.

Meydan, N.; Grunberger, T.; Dadi, H.; Shahar, M.; Arpaia, E.; Lapidot, Z.; Leeder, JS.; Freedman, M.; Cohen, A.; Gazit, A.; Levitzki, A. & Roifman, CM. (1996). Inhibition of acute lymphoblastic leukaemia by a Jak-2 inhibitor. *Nature,* Vol.379, No. 6566, (February 1996), pp. 645-648, ISSN 1476-4687.

Migas, A.; Savva, N.; Mishkova, O. & Aleinikova, OV. (2011). AML1/RUNX1 gene point mutations in childhood myeloid malignancies. *Pediatrics Blood and Cancer,* DOI: 10.1002/pbc.22980, (February 2011), ISSN 1545-5017.

Morris, J. (1989). A mutational theory of leukaemogenesis. *Journal of Clinical Pathology,* Vol.42, No.4, (April 1989), pp.337-340, ISSN 1472-4146.

Mullighan, CG.; Zhang, J.; Harvey, RC.; Collins-Underwood, JR.; Schulman, BA.; Phillips, LA.; Tasian, SK.; Loh, ML.; Su, X.; Liu, W.; Devidas, M.; Atlas, SR.; Chen, IM.; Clifford, RJ.; Gerhard, DS.; Carroll, WL.; Reaman, GH.; Smith, M.; Downing, JR.; Hunger, SP. & Willman, CL. (2009). JAK mutations in high-risk childhood acute lymphoblastic leukemia. *Proceedings of the National Academy Science of the United States of America,* Vol.106, No.23, (June 2009), pp. 9414-9418, ISSN 1091-6490.

Neglia, J.; Linet, M.; Shu, X.; Severson, R.; Potter, J.; Mertens, A.; Wen, W.; Kersey, J. & Robison, L. (2000). Patterns of infection and day care utilization and risk of childhood acute lymphoblastic leukaemia. *British Journal of Cancer,* Vol.82 No.1, (January 2000), pp.234-240, ISSN 1532-1827.

Ognjanovic, S.; Puumala, S.; Spector, LG.; Smith, FO.; Robison, LL.; Olshan, AF. & Ross JA. (2009). Maternal health conditions during pregnancy and acute leukemia in children with Down syndrome: A Children's Oncology Group study. *Pediatric Blood & Cancer,* Vol.52, No.5, (May 2009), pp. 602-608, ISSN 1545-5017.

Oxford, J.; Manuguerra, C.; Kistner, O.; Linde, A.; Kunze, M.; Lange, W.; Schweiger, B.; Spala, G.; Rebelo de Andrade, H.; Pérez Breña, PR.; Beytout, J.; Brydak, L.; Caraffa de Stefano, D.; Hungnes, O.; Kyncl, J.; Montomoli, E.; Gil de Miguel, A.; Vranckx, R. & Osterhaus, A. (2005). A new European perspective of influenza pandemic planning with a particular focus on the role of mammalian cell culture vaccines. *Vaccine,* Vol.23, No.46-47, (November 2005):5440-5449, ISSN 0264-410X.

Parker, L. (2001). Breast-feeding and cancer prevention. *European Journal of Cancer,* Vol.37, No.2, (January 2001), pp.55-8, ISSN 09-59-8049 81.

Perillat, F.; Clavel, J.; Jaussent, I.; Baruchel, A.; Leverger, G.; Nelken, B.; Philippe, N.; Schaison, G.; Sommelet, D.; Vilmer, E. & Hemon, D. (2002a). Breast-feeding, fetal loss and childhood acute leukemia. *European Journal of Pediatrics,* Vol.161, No.4, (April 2002), pp.235-237, ISSN 1432-1076.

Perrillat, F.; Clavel, J.; Auclerc, M.; Baruchel, A.; Leverger, G.; Nelken, B.; Philippe, N.; Schaison, G.; Sommelet, D.; Vilmer, E. & Hémon, D. (2002b). Day-care, early common infections and childhood acute leukaemia: a multicentre French case-control study. *British Journal of Cancer,* Vol.8, No.86 (April 2002), pp.1064-1069, ISSN 1532-1827.

Petridou, E.; Dalamaga, M.; Mentis, A.; Skalkidou, A.; Moustaki, M.; Karpathios, T.; Trichopoulos, D. & Childhood Haematologists-Oncologists Group. (2001). Evidence on the infectious etiology of childhood leukemia: the role of low herd immunity (Greece). *Cancer Causes & Control,* Vol.12, No.7, (September 2001), pp.645-52, ISSN 1573-7225.

Pinkel, D. & Nefzger, D. (1959). Some epidemiological features of childhood leukaemia in the Buffalo, NY area. *Cancer,* Vol.12, No.2, (March-April 2008), pp.351-358, ISSN 1097-0142.

Puumala, SE.; Ross, JA.; Olshan, AF.; Robison, LL.; Smith, FO. & Spector LG. (2007). Reproductive history, infertility treatment, and the risk of acute leukemia in children with down syndrome: a report from the Children's Oncology Group. *Cancer,* Vol.110, No.9, (November 2007), pp. 2067-2074, ISSN 1097-0142.

Rabson, AB. (2010). Trisomy 21 leukemias: finding the hits that matter. *Oncogene,* Vol.29, No. 46, (November 2010), pp. 6099-6101, ISSN 1476-5594.

Riveron, R. (1995). Valor inmunológico de la leche materna. *Revista Cubana de Pediatría,* Vol. 67, No.2, pp.1-16, ISSN 0034-7531.

Robison, LL. (1992). Down syndrome and leukemia. *Leukemia,* Vol.6, Suppl.1, pp. 5-7, ISSN 1476-5551.

Roman, E.; Simpson, J.; Ansell, P.; Kinsey, S.; Mitchell, C.; McKinney, P.; Birch, J.; Greaves, M.; Eden, T. & United Kingdom Childhood Cancer Study Investigators. (2007). Childhood acute lymphoblastic leukaemia and infections in the first year of life: A report from the United Kingdom Childhood Cancer Study. *American Journal of Epidemiology,* Vol.165, No.5, (March 2007), pp.496–504, ISSN 1476-6256.

Rosenbaum, P.; Buck, G. & Brecher, M. (2000). Early child-care and preschool experiences and the risk of childhood acute lymphoblastic leukemia. *American Journal of Epidemiology,* Vol.152 No.12, (December 2000), pp.1136-1144, ISSN 1476-6256.

Rosenbaum, P.; Buck, G. & Brecher, M.; (2005). Allergy and infectious disease histories and the risk of childhood acute lymphoblastic leukaemia. *Paediatric and Perinatal Epidemiology,* Vol.19, No.2, (March 2005), pp.152-164, ISSN 1365-3016.

Ross, JA. (1999). Epidemiologic studies of childhood leukemia: where do we go from here? *Medical and Pediatric Oncology,* Vol.32, No.1, (January 1999), pp. 65-67, ISSN 1096-911X.

Ross, JA.; Spector, LG.; Robison, LL. & Olshan, AF. (2005a). Epidemiology of leukemia in children with Down syndrome. *Pediatric Blood & Cancer,* Vol.44, No.1, (January 2005), pp. 8-12, ISSN 1545-5017.

Ross, JA.; Blair, CK.; Olshan, AF.; Robison, LL.; Smith, FO.; Heerema, NA. & Roesler, M. (2005b). Periconceptional vitamin use and leukemia risk in children with Down syndrome: a Children's Oncology Group study. *Cancer,* Vol.104, No.2, (July 2005), pp. 405-410, ISSN 1097-0142.

Roy, A.; Roberts, I.; Norton, A. & Vyas, P. (2009). Acute megakaryoblastic leukaemia (AMKL) and transient myeloproliferative disorder (TMD) in Down syndrome: a multi-step model of myeloid leukaemogenesis. *British Journal of Haematology,* Vol.147, No.1, (October 2009), pp. 3-12, ISSN 1365-2141.

Rudant, J.; Orsi, L.; Menegaux, F.; Petit, A.; Baruchel, A.; Bertrand, Y.; Lambilliotte, A.; Robert, A.; Michel, G.; Margueritte, G.; Tandonnet, J.; Mechinaud, F.; Bordigoni, P.; Hémon, D. & Clavel, J. (2010). Childhood acute leukemia, early common infections, and allergy: The ESCALE Study. *American Journal of Epidemiology,* Vol.172, No.9, (November 2010), pp.1015-1027, ISSN 1476-6256.

Sashida, G.; Bazzoli, E.; Menendez, S.; Liu, Y. & Nimer, SD. The oncogenic role of the ETS transcription factors MEF and ERG. *Cell Cycle,* Vol.9, No. 17, (September 2010), pp. 3457-3459, ISSN 1551-4005.

Schüz, J.; Kaletsch, U.; Meinert, R.; Kaatsch, P. & Michaelis, J. (1999). Association of childhood leukaemia with factors related to the immune system. *British Journal of Cancer,* Vol.80, No.3-4, (May 1999), pp.585-90, ISSN 1532-1827.

Shu, X.; Clemens, J.; Zheng, W.; Ying, D.; Ji, B. & Jin, F. (1995). Infant breastfeeding and the risk of childhood lymphoma and leukaemia. *International Journal of Epidemiology,* Vol.24, No.1, (February 1995), pp. 27-32, ISSN 1464-3685 83.

Shu, X.; Linet, M.; Steinbuch, M.; Wen, W.; Buckley, J.; Neglia, J.; Potter, J.; Reaman, G. & Robison, L. (1999). Breast-feeding and risk of childhood acute leukemia. *Journal*

National Cancer Institute, Vol.91, No.20, (October 1999), pp.1765-1772, ISSN 1460-2105 77.

Speck, NA. & Gilliland, DG. (2002). Core-binding factors in haematopoiesis and leukaemia. *Nature Reviews Cancer,* Vol.2, No.7, (July 2002), pp. 502-513, ISSN 1474-1768.

Stuebe, A. (2009). The risks of not breastfeeding for mothers and infants. *Reviews in Obstetrics and Gynecology,* Vol.2 No.4, (Fall 2009), pp.222-231, ISSN 1941-2797.

Taub, JW. (2001). Relationship of chromosome 21 and acute leukemia in children with Down syndrome. *Journal of Pediatric Hematology/Oncology,* Vol.23, No.3, (March-April 2001), pp. 175-178, ISSN 1536-3678.

Taub, JW. & Ravindranath, Y. (2002). Down syndrome and the transient myeloproliferative disorder: why is it transient? *Journal of Pediatric Hematology/Oncology: official Journal of the American Society of Pediatric Hematology/Oncology,* Vol.24, No.1, (January 2002), pp. 6-8, ISSN 1536-3678.

Todaro, GJ. & Huebner, RJ. (1972) N.A.S. symposium: new evidence as the basis for increased efforts in cancer research. *Proceedings of the National Academy of Sciences of the United States of America,* Vol.69, No.4, (April 1972), pp. 1009-1015, ISSN 0027-8424.

Urayama, K.; Buffler, P.; Gallagher, E.; Ayoob, J.; Ma, X. (2010). A meta-analysis of the association between day-care attendance and childhood acute lymphoblastic leukaemia. *International Journal of Epidemiology,* Vol.39, No.3 (June 2010), pp.718-732, ISSN 1464-3685 64.

Urayama, K.; Ma, X.; Selvin, S.; Metayer, C.; Chokkalingam, A.; Wiemels, J.; Does, M.; Chang, J.; Wong, A.; Trachtenberg, E. & Buffler, P. (2011). Early life exposure to infections and risk of childhood acute lymphoblastic leukemia. *International Journal of Cancer,* Vol.128, No.7, (April 2011), pp.632-643, ISSN 1811-9735.

Van Cleve, SN. & Cohen, WI. (2006). Part I: clinical practice guidelines for children with Down syndrome from birth to 12 years. *Journal of Pediatric Health Care: official publication of National Association of Pediatric Nurse Associates &Practitioners,* Vol.20, No.1, (January-February 2006), pp. 47-54, ISSN 0891-5245.

van Steensel, H.; Valkenburg; H. & van Zanen G. (1986). Childhood leukemia and infectious diseases in the first year of life: a register-based case-control study. *American Journal of Epidemiology,* Vol.124 No.4, (October 1986), pp.590-594, ISSN 1476-6256.

Vyas, P. & Roberts, I. (2006). Down myeloid disorders: a paradigm for childhood preleukaemia and leukaemia and insights into normal megakaryopoiesis. *Early Human Development,* Vol.82, No.12, (December 2006), pp. 767-773, ISSN 0378-3782.

Wahab, AA.; Bener, A. & Teebi, AS. (2006). *Clinical Genetics,* Vol.69, No.4, (April 2006), pp. 360-362, ISSN 0009-9163.

Webb, D.; Roberts, I. & Vyas, P. (2007). Haematology of Down syndrome. *Archives of Disease in Childhood Fetal and Neonatal Edition,* Vol.92, No.6, (November 2007), pp. F503-F507, ISSN 1468-2052.

Wechsler, J.; Greene, M.; McDevitt, MA.; Anastasi, J.; Karp, JE.; Le Beau, MM. & Crispino, JD. (2002). Acquired mutations in GATA1 in the megakaryoblastic leukemia of Down syndrome. *Nature Genetics,* Vol.32, No. 1, (September 2002), pp. 148-152, ISSN 1546-1718.

Wiseman, FK.; Alford, KA.; Tybulewicz, VL. & Fisher, EM. (2009). Down syndrome—recent progress and future prospects. *Human Molecular Genetics,* Vol.18, No.R1 (April 2009), pp.R75-R83, ISSN 1460-2083.

Xavier, AC. & Taub, JW. (2010). Acute leukemia in children with Down syndrome. *Haematologica,* Vol.95, No.7, (July 2010), pp. 1043-1045, ISSN 1592-8721.

Zipursky, A. (2003). Transient leukaemia--a benign form of leukaemia in newborn infants with trisomy 21. *British Journal of Haematology,* Vol.120, No.6, (March 2003), pp. 930-938, ISSN 1365-2141.

Zuna, J.; Madzo, J.; Krejci, O.; Zemanova, Z.; Kalinova, M.; Muzikova, K.; Zapotocky, M.; Starkova, J.; Hrusak, O.; Horak, J. & Trka, J. (2011). ETV6/RUNX1 (TEL/AML1) is a frequent prenatal first hit in childhood leukemia. *Blood,* Vol.117, No.1, (January 2011), pp. 368-369, ISSN 1528-0020.

Zwaan, CM.; Reinhardt, D.; Hitzler, J. & Vyas, P. (2010). Acute leukemias in children with Down syndrome. *Hematology/Oncology Clinics of North America,* Vol.24, No.1, (February 2010), pp. 19-34, ISSN 0889-8588.

7

Unique Myeloid Leukemias in Young Children with Down Syndrome: Cell Origin, Association with Hematopoietic Microenvironment and Leukemogenesis

Jun Miyauchi
Department of Pathology and Laboratory Medicine, Tokyo Dental College Ichikawa General Hospital, Ichikawa, Chiba-ken Japan

1. Introduction

Patients with Down syndrome (DS) are at 10- to 36-fold higher risk of developing leukemia (Roy et al., 2009). In children with DS aged 4 years or older, acute lymphoblastic leukemia (ALL) is the predominant type of leukemia just as it is in the general pediatric population, whereas acute myeloid leukemia (AML) is more common than ALL in patients with DS less than 4 years of age. Interestingly, acute megakaryoblastic leukemia (AMKL), a rare subtype of AML in non-DS patients, comprises 62-86% of AML cases in children with DS (Hitzler, 2007; Roy et al., 2009), which will be referred to as AMKL-DS hereafter. Furthermore, hematological abnormalities that are indistinguishable from AMKL-DS occur in about 10% of neonates with DS but spontaneously disappear within several months of life. This disorder has been given a variety of names, including transient leukemia (TL), transient myeloproliferative disorder (TMD) and transient abnormal myelopoiesis (TAM). In 20-30% of patients with TL, AMKL-DS develops later through the stage of myelodysplastic syndrome (MDS) within 4 years. These disorders, namely, TL, MDS and AMKL-DS, in young children with DS have many unique features and had been considered a disease entity that was called "Myeloid leukemias of Down syndrome", then later renamed "Myeloid proliferations related to Down syndrome" in the current World Health Organization (WHO) Classification published in 2008. This review summarizes recent data on clinical, cellular and molecular biological aspects of these myeloid neoplasms with special reference to the origin of neoplastic cells, the organs where they arise and multistep model of leukemogenesis.

2. Transient leukemia (TL)

2.1 Clinical features

TL is a disorder of neonates with DS, with median age at diagnosis being 7 days (range, 1-65 days) (Massey et al., 2006). Clinical manifestations in symptomatic cases include hepatosplenomegaly, effusions, bleeding and skin rash, but there are no overt signs of symptoms related to TL in other cases. TL is usually found as a result of a routine medical checkup or incidental blood examination performed because of another unrelated illness. The patients remain well and the disease gradually disappears within the first 3 months of life in most cases without any therapy and the prognosis is generally good. However, severe life-threatening complications occur in approximately 15% of patients (Hitzler, 2007). These include two major forms; 1) liver dysfunction caused by infiltration of leukemic blasts and liver fibrosis, leading to progressive obstructive jaundice and liver failure; and 2) cardiopulmonary disease, manifesting as hydrops-like symptoms, including pulmonary edema, pleural or pericardial effusions and ascites (Zipursky, 2003). Leukemic blasts are usually present in the effusions. Other serious complications include hyperviscosity due to massive leukocytosis and hepatosplenomegaly that impairs spontaneous respiration. These patients with severe complications have benefitted from treatment with low-dose cytarabine (Ara-C) (Al-Kasim et al., 2002; Dormann et al., 2004; Klusmann et al., 2008). Furthermore, in 20 to 30% of patients with TL that has spontaneously regressed, AMKL-DS later develops within 4 years of life. In rare cases, however, complete regression of TL does not occur and regrowth of blasts with acquired additional cytogenetic abnormalities directly leads to AMKL-DS.

Laboratory investigations usually demonstrate marked leukocytosis with varying proportions of circulating blasts (Massey et al., 2006). The bone marrow contains increased numbers of blasts but, interestingly, the ratio of blasts in the marrow is often lower than that in the peripheral blood, a peculiar finding for AML because the marrow is usually packed with blasts when a large number of blasts are present in the blood. This phenomenon is considered due to the fetal liver origin of TL, as described below in more detail, and the marrow is only secondarily involved by the disease process. The bone marrow may also contain dysplastic mature megakaryocytes and exhibit features similar to those of MDS that precedes the onset of AMKL-DS (Zipursky et al., 1999).

TL may occur in utero and cause intrauterine fetal death as a result of non-immune hydrops fetalis and cardiac dysfunction due to leukemic cell infiltration into the pericardial or cardiac muscular tissues (Zipursky et al., 1996; Heald et al., 2007; Ishigaki et al., 2011) or visceral fibrosis (Becroft & Zwi, 1990; Ruchelli et al., 1991; Becroft, 1993). Prenatal diagnosis of TL can be made by ultrasonographical detection of hydrops or hepatosplenomegaly followed by chromosomal analysis and hematological examination of fetal blood obtained by umbilical cord centesis (Gray et al., 1986; Zerres et al., 1990; Foucar et al., 1992; Smrcek et al., 2001; Robertson et al., 2003). Accurate estimation of the frequency of TL in fetuses and neonates is difficult because stillbirths with TL may be missed due to the low autopsy rate of stillbirths, or fetuses with TL may spontaneously recover in utero and because TL in neonates without complications may disappear without being noticed. It is roughly estimated that TL occurs in about 20% of patients with DS, including about half of those dying in utero (Zipursky, 2003), but the true incidence of TL needs to be clarified based on prospective population-based studies. TL also occurs in phenotypically normal individuals with trisomy 21 mosaicism (Brodeur et al., 1980; Kalousek & Chan, 1987). In these patients, leukemic blasts always have trisomy 21, indicating that trisomy 21 is an essential prerequisite for TL.

2.2 Characteristics of leukemic blasts

Light microscopically, the blasts of TL may be morphologically undifferentiated (Fig. 1a) or exhibit features of megakaryoblasts with cytoplasmic blebs, similar to AMKL-DS blasts (Fig. 1b), or micromegakaryocytes. Although myeloperoxidase (MPO) is negative, flow cytometric cell surface marker analysis of blasts demonstrates expression of antigens related to multiple hematopoietic cell lineages, including megakaryocytes (CD41, CD42b, CD61), granulocytes (CD13, CD33, CD38), erythroid cells (glycophorin, CD71), stem cells (CD34, CD117) and, in addition, certain characteristic lymphoid markers (CD7 and CD56) (Yumura-Yagi et al., 1992; Langebrake et al., 2005; Massey et al., 2006). Electron microscopic examination demonstrates that the leukemic cells in TL are more heterogeneous than those in AMKL-DS, exhibiting features of megakaryoblasts with varying degree of megakaryocytic differentiation (Fig. 2a), granulocytic precursors (Fig. 2b), including basophils, and erythroid cells (Bessho et al., 1988; Eguchi et al., 1989; Eguchi et al., 1992). The megakaryocytic nature of blasts can be demonstrated by the presence of platelet specific granules (α granules), platelet demarcation membrane and/or positive reaction for platelet peroxidase (PPO) that is present in the perinuclear space and rough endoplasmic reticulum but not in the Golgi apparatus and α granules (Fig. 2a). Some blasts may possess peculiar cytoplasmic granules with internal membranous structures (Fig. 2a, inset), which are called θ granules because of their resemblance to the Greek letter theta (θ) (Bessho et al., 1988; Eguchi et al., 1989; Eguchi et al., 1992). These structures are known to be present in immature precursors of not only megakaryocytic, but also erythroid (Coulombel et al., 1987) and mast cell/basophil (Parkin et al., 1980) lineages. Extreme basophilia in a phenotypically normal newborn with TL, whose leukemic cells showed a chromosome 21 abnormality, has been reported (Worth et al., 1999). These data indicate that the blasts of TL are derived from multipotential hematopoietic progenitors, not restricted to megakaryocytic lineage, and are consistent with the multilineage differentiation potential of TL blasts seen *in vitro* as described below (section 2.4).

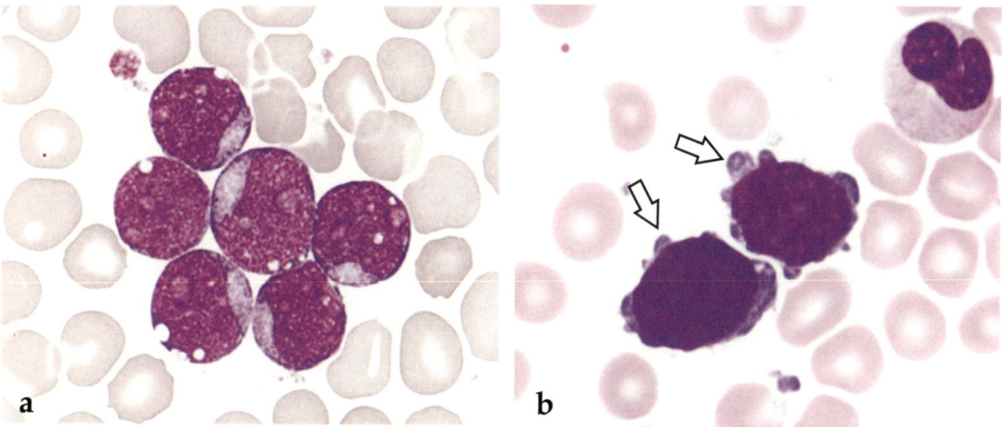

Fig. 1. Morphology of leukemia cells in TL and AMKL-DS. (a) Blasts of TL in the peripheral blood with primitive morphology. (b) Blasts of AMKL-DS in the bone marrow. Note the presence of cytoplasmic bleb (arrow), indicating megakaryoblastic nature.

By utilizing allele-specific polymorphism of genomic markers that reside on the X chromosome and inactivation pattern of one of the X chromosomes in female cells, it has been shown that the blasts of TL are monoclonal populations of cells in the majority of cases (Kurahashi et al., 1991; Miyashita et al., 1991; Massey et al., 2006), indicating that TL is a neoplastic disorder and not a reactive leukemoid reaction, although later works with *GATA1* gene analysis demonstrated that TL in some cases may contain oligoclonal populations of neoplastic cells (see section 4.2). Spontaneous regression of TL does not rule

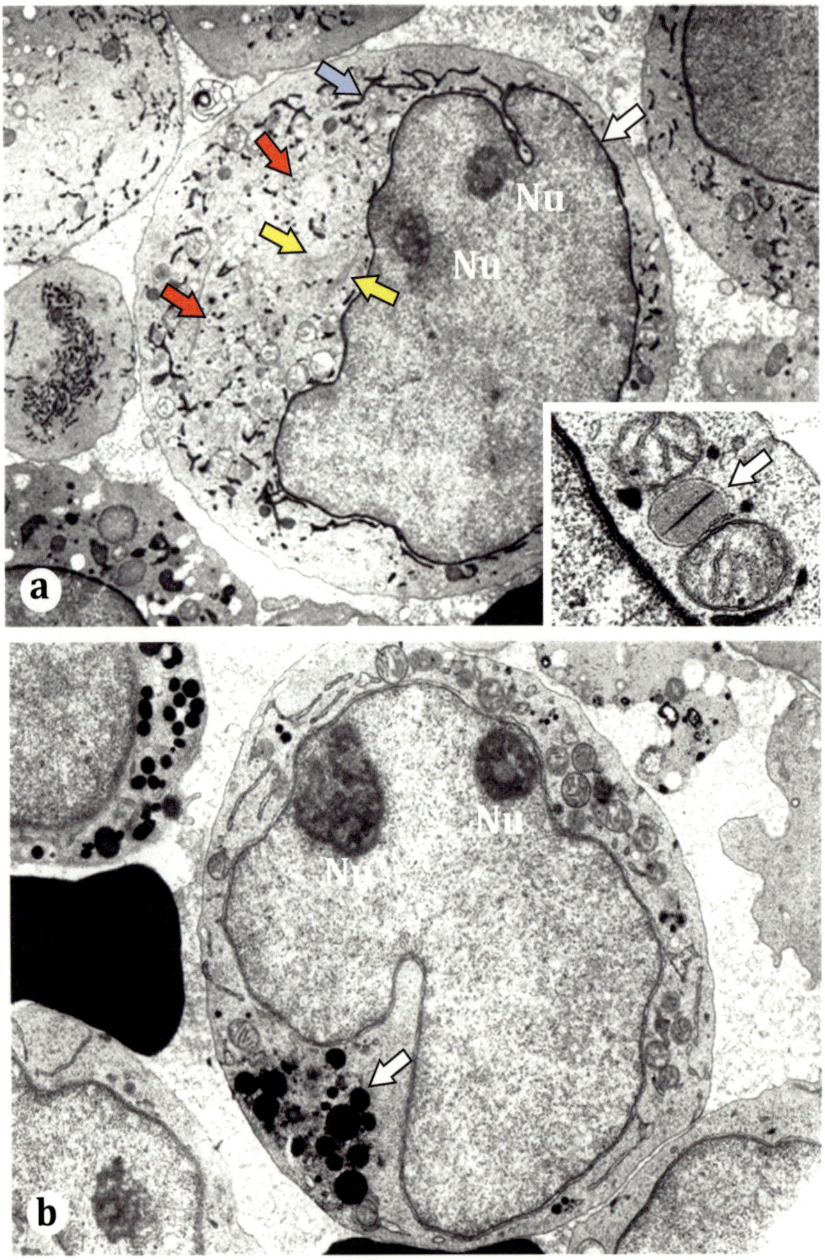

Fig. 2. Electron microscopic appearance of blasts in TL. (a) PPO reaction is positive in the perinuclear space (white arrow) and rough endoplasmic reticulum (blue arrow) but not in α granules (red arrow) and the Golgi apparatus (yellow arrow), indicating megakaryoblastic nature. (Inset) Higher magnification of a θ granule (arrow). (b) A few MPO-positive granules are present (arrow) but other organelles are negative for MPO in this cells, indicating abnormal, minimal myeloid differentiation. Nu, nucleolus.

out the leukemic nature of this disease, since 1) spontaneous regression can be seen in other unquestionable malignant neoplasms, such as neuroblastoma in infants; 2) blasts that are indistinguishable from AMKL-DS blasts appear in the blood and infiltrate in the tissues; and 3) TL can be a fatal disorder in severe cases due to tissue infiltration of blasts in major organs, such as the liver and heart. Based on these data, in addition to other cellular and molecular biological characteristics as described below, TL is now considered a special type of preleukemia or a very unusual form of leukemia with self-limiting growth potential.

2.3 Chromosomal analysis

Chromosomal abnormalities seen in blasts of TL usually include only trisomy 21 in both patients with DS and those with trisomy 21 mosaicism and no other chromosomal abnormalities are present in most cases. This is an important point in the differential diagnosis of TL from AMKL-DS, which usually shows a variety of clonal chromosomal abnormalities (Hayashi et al., 1988). In rare cases, however, abnormalities other than trisomy 21 are found in TL blasts, including additional chromosomes 12 and 14, deletion of a chromosome, der(X;15)(p10;q10), an extra C chromosome and polyploidy with 57 chromosomes (Zipursky, 2003). These abnormalities usually disappear along with spontaneous remission of TL and are usually absent in the blasts of AMKL-DS that has later arisen in the same patients and developed other chromosomal abnormalities. However, in some cases, they may be present in subsequent AMKL-DS blasts (Kitoh et al., 2009), evidence that AMKL-DS develops in some of the clones of TL blasts.

2.4 Differentiation capability of leukemic blasts

When TL blasts are cultured in the presence of hematopoietic growth stimulants, such as phytohemagglutinin-stimulated leukocyte conditioned medium (PHA-LCM) or recombinant hematopoietic growth factors, mature or maturing hematopoietic cells of various lineages appear, including basophils, neutrophils, eosinophils, monocytes and erythroid cells (Suda et al., 1987). However, it was uncertain whether these cells were all derived from TL blasts rather than coexisting normal hematopoietic progenitors in the samples examined. We have recently demonstrated that TL blasts are capable of differentiating into basophil/mast cell lineages when cultured in the presence of interleukin-3, stem cell factor (SCF) or granulocyte-macrophage colony-stimulating factor (GM-CSF) (Fig. 3a), and into megakaryocytes in the presence of thrombopoietin (TPO) (Fig. 3b), by demonstrating that the differentiated cells that appeared after culture carried the same *GATA1* mutations as the TL blasts did before culture (Miyauchi et al., 2010) (see section 4.2). Consistent with these *in vitro* data, massive increase of basophils in the peripheral blood of a patient with TL has been reported (Worth et al., 1999) and another case demonstrating pericardial effusion containing predominantly basophils has been described (Zipursky et al., 1997). We recently reported pathological findings on autopsy of a stillbirth with TL, in which numerous megakaryoblasts and dysplastic megakaryocytes were present in the liver and blood vessels, whereas leukemic blasts infiltrating into the peripheral tissues, including pericardium, expressed MPO (Ishigaki et al., 2011). These findings are consistent with the *in vitro* data described above and indicate that blasts in TL are not simply megakaryoblasts but derived from more primitive hematopoietic progenitors that are capable of differentiating into several myeloid lineages *in vivo*, possibly depending on the hematopoietic microenvironment. The differentiation capability of TL blasts into mature blood cells is unique for AML and might be somehow associated with the spontaneous remission of this disorder. Although TL blasts express some markers of the erythroid lineage and, in fact, erythroblasts at various stages of differentiation appeared in culture of TL blasts in the presence of erythropoietin and SCF in combination, these cells expressed full-length GATA1 but not aberrant GATA1s protein (see section 4.2) and, therefore, it was shown that these differentiated erythroid cells were derived from coexisting normal erythroid progenitors (Miyauchi et al., 2010).

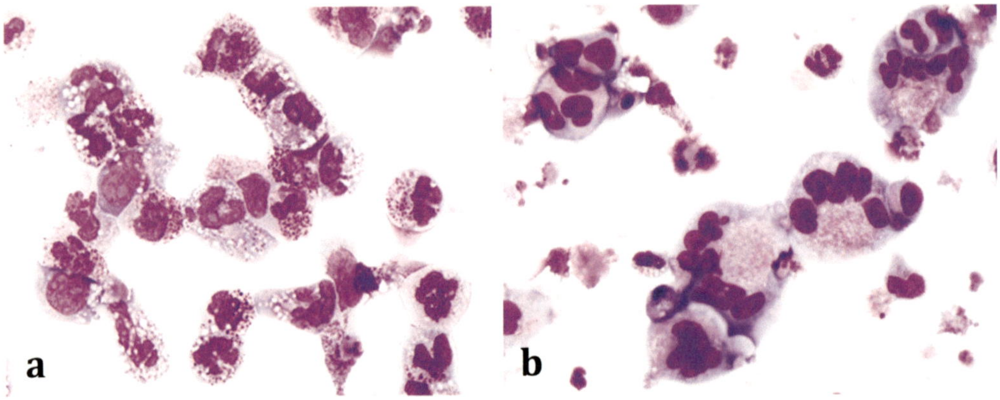

Fig. 3. Morphology of TL blasts after culture in the presence of hematopoietic growth factors. (a) Basophils that appeared in culture with GM-CSF. (b) Mature megakaryocytes that appeared in culture with TPO.

2.5 Origin of leukemic progenitors and association with hematopoietic microenvironment

Although most patients with TL show a favorable prognosis, serious complications develop in some cases as described above. While myelofibrosis is one of the characteristic features of AMKL-DS (Fig. 4a, b), autopsy cases of patients with TL have demonstrated that these patients often exhibit unusual diffuse sinusoidal liver fibrosis (Fig. 4c, d), but not myelofibrosis (Becroft & Zwi, 1990; Ruchelli et al., 1991; Miyauchi et al., 1992; Yagihashi et al., 1995; Schwab et al., 1998; Shiozawa et al., 2004). It has been shown that leukemic blasts in AMKL produce cytokines, including platelet-derived growth factor (PDGF), platelet factor 4 and transforming growth factor β (TGFβ) that stimulate fibroblasts in the bone marrow causing myelofibrosis (Breton-Gorius et al., 1982; Roberts et al., 1986; Sunami et al., 1987; Terui et al., 1990). Since blasts in TL have features similar to those of megakaryoblasts in AMKL-DS and TL is a disorder of neonates and fetuses, it appears that TL is a very unusual form of neoplasia originating from the fetal liver, the major organ of hematopoiesis during the fetal stage, and that leukemic blasts that arise in the fetal liver produce cytokines that stimulate fibroblasts to induce liver fibrosis in the same manner as myelofibrosis in AMKL-DS. Proliferation of dysplastic megakaryocytes and blasts, including megakaryoblasts, in the liver has been shown in autopsy cases of fetuses with TL (Ruchelli et al., 1991; Becroft, 1993; Ishigaki et al., 2011) and production of TGFβ by TL blasts in the liver has been immunohistochemically demonstrated (Arai et al., 1999). The presence of unique hematopoietic progenitors originating from the yolk sac and fetal liver that are sensitive to

GATA1s transgene to cause hyperproliferation of megakaryocytes only during certain fetal developmental stages has been demonstrated by experiments using knock-in mice (Li et al., 2005) (see section 4.2), indicating that these cells are likely the target of leukemic progenitors in TL.

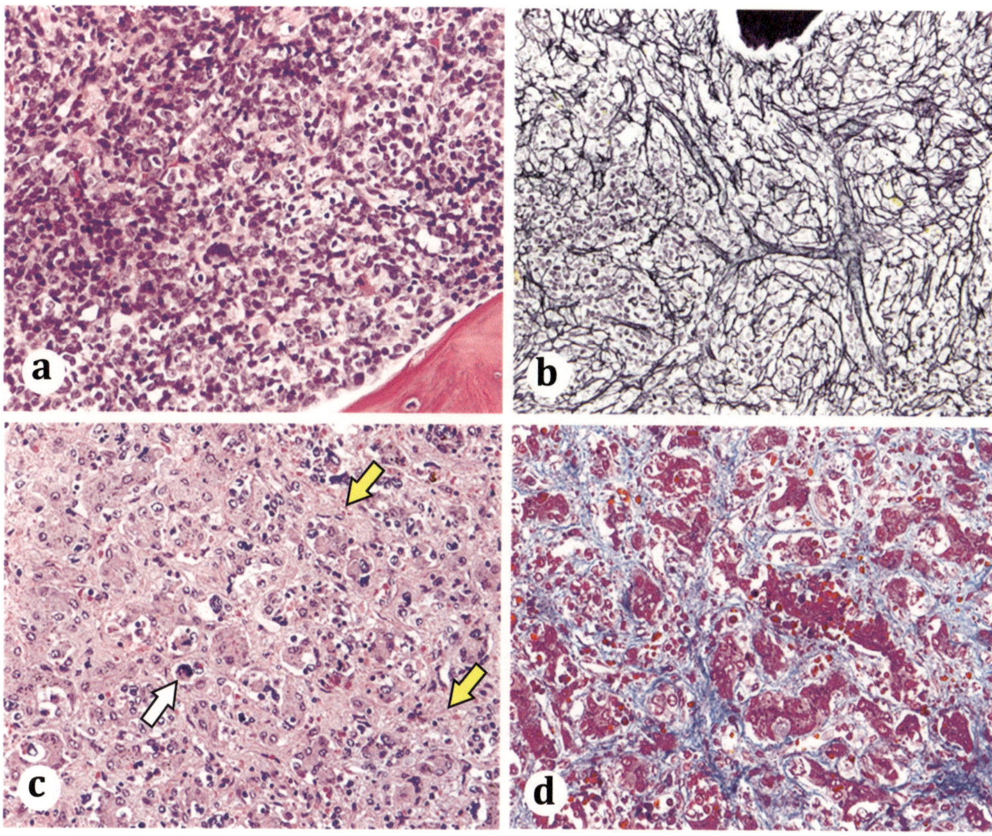

Fig. 4. Histopathology of the bone marrow and liver in patients with AMKL-DS and TL. (a) The bone marrow in a patient with AMK-DS is packed by monotonous blasts, a finding consistent with acute leukemia (H-E stain). (b) Silver impregnation staining of the marrow demonstrates increase of reticulin fibers (myelofibrosis), which is one of the characteristic findings of AMKL. (c) The liver in a patient with TL after regression (H-E stain). Perisinusoidal fibrosis is present (yellow arrow) accompanied by marked distortion of hepatic cords. Atypical megakaryocytes are also seen (white arrow). (d) Azan stain clearly demonstrates perisinusoidal fibrosis of the liver (stained in blue).

2.6 Mechanism of spontaneous remission

The mechanism underlying spontaneous remission of TL is largely unknown, but several plausible explanations have been proposed. First, if the target cells of origin in TL are fetal hematopoietic progenitors of limited lifespan, the growth and differentiation of which are governed by genetic mechanisms controlling fetal hematopoiesis, a developmental switch in genetic control from fetal to adult hematopoiesis after birth may cease the proliferation of leukemic blasts ("intrinsic theory") (Ahmed et al., 2004; Li et al., 2005). Second, if TL is an unusual form of leukemia occurring in the fetal liver, but not in the bone marrow, and the growth of blasts in TL is dependent exclusively on the microenvironment of the fetal liver, a transition of the major site of hematopoiesis from the liver to the bone marrow after birth and cessation of the hepatic hematopoiesis would prevent the growth of TL blasts and cause regression of the disease ("environmental theory") (Miyauchi et al., 1992; Gamis & Hilden, 2002; Ahmed et al., 2004). Other possible mechanisms that may also explain spontaneous remission of TL include the capability of differentiation of TL blasts (Suda et al., 1987). As described above, blasts in TL can differentiate into mature blood cells of at least several lineages *in vitro* and *in vivo*. According to changes in environmental factors that control fetal and adult hematopoiesis after birth, differentiation of TL blasts might be induced, leading to cessation of the growth of TL blasts. Self-induced apoptosis of TL blasts possibly mediated by increased expression of superoxide dismutase, which has been linked to increased apoptosis in DS models and the gene of which is located on chromosome 21, has also been proposed as a cause of spontaneous regression (Taub et al., 2004). Further studies are required to clarify which hypotheses, alone or in combination, are responsible or whether other mechanisms participate in the spontaneous remission of TL.

3. Megakaryoblastic leukemia in Down syndrome (AMKL-DS)

3.1 Clinical features

Patients with DS are susceptible to AMKL, which comprises about 62-86% of AML in DS patients (Hitzler, 2007; Roy et al., 2009). Since AMKL is an infrequent subtype of AML in non-DS patients, the incidence of AMKL-DS compared to that of AMKL in non-DS patients has been estimated to be about 500 times higher. AML in older patients with DS is only rarely AMKL, does not demonstrate *GATA1* mutations (see section 4.2) and is a disease distinct from AMKL-DS.

AMKL-DS has many unique features compared with AMKL in non-DS patients. First, it often occurs in patients with a history of TL within the first 4 years of life after TL has resolved or, rarely, during the process of incomplete remission of TL, although cases of AMKL-DS without preceding TL have also been documented (Ahmed et al., 2004). Second, while AMKL in non-DS is clinically aggressive and the prognosis is poor, AMKL-DS shows a very high remission rate and favorable prognosis, with survival probability ranging between 70 and 90%, in response to chemotherapy (Hitzler, 2007). The cause of favorable prognosis of AMKL-DS is thought, at least in part, to be due to the high sensitivity of leukemic blasts to chemotherapy such as Ara-C. Third, AMKL-DS in 20-60% of patients is preceded by a prolonged period of cytopenia (usually several months to even years of thrombocytopenia) accompanied by proliferation of dysplastic megakaryocytes in the bone marrow, which corresponds to the MDS phase, before the onset of AMKL-DS (Zipursky et al., 1994). This preceding MDS phase is not present in other forms of AMKL in non-DS patients and is unique to AMKL-DS.

3.2 Common and distinct features of leukemic blasts in AMKL-DS and TL

Besides the difference in age of onset, there are many other differences as well as common features between AMKL-DS and TL. Blasts in AMKL-DS and TL exhibit great similarity in cytological characteristics, including morphology, cytochemistry and cell surface antigen expression. Blasts in AMKL-DS exhibit megakaryoblastic morphology in both light and electron microscopic observation likewise the case of TL (Fig. 1b). Flow cytometric analysis of blasts in AMKL-DS also shows almost identical antigen expression to that of TL blasts, except for a somewhat lower expression of CD34 and CD56 in AMKL-DS than in TL. In contrast to the blasts of TL, in which trisomy 21 is the sole chromosomal abnormality in most cases, blasts in AMKL-DS usually show a variety of chromosomal abnormalities besides constitutional trisomy 21, with additional chromosome 8 or 21 being most frequent. Although hepatic fibrosis is often seen in TL patients with severe liver dysfunction, fibrosis of the bone marrow (myelofibrosis) is one of the characteristic features of AMKL-DS (Fig. 4a, b), indicating that AMKL arises in the bone marrow whereas TL may arise in the fetal liver, organs that are the major sites of hematopoiesis after and before birth, respectively. In contrast to the benign and self-limiting clinical course of TL, AMKL-DS is potentially a lethal disorder, which does not exhibit spontaneous remission and requires chemotherapy, although the cure rate and prognosis is better than those of AMKL in non-DS patients. *GATA1* gene mutations are present in nearly all patients with AMKL-DS as in the case of TL (see section 4.2).

4. GATA1 and its role in leukemogenesis

4.1 Structure and function of GATA1

GATA1 is a member of the six GATA family of zinc-finger transcription factors (GATA1 to GATA6), which share a highly conserved zinc finger domain that recognizes the consensus nucleotide sequence motif (A/T)GATA(A/G) (Cantor, 2005). GATA1 plays important roles in hematopoiesis in a lineage-specific manner for erythroblasts, megakaryocytes, mast cells and eosinophils. Mutations of the *GATA1* gene, which resides on the X chromosome at Xp11.23, have been shown to play a critical role in leukemogenesis of DS-related myeloid leukemias. The full length GATA1 protein (molecular weight: approximately 50kD) contains three well characterized domains; two zinc finger domains (N-terminal and C-terminal zinc fingers) and a transcriptional activation domain at the N-terminal portion of the protein (Fig. 5). The C-terminal zinc finger is required for DNA binding, while the N-terminal zinc finger stabilizes this interaction and mediates interactions with a cofactor Friend of GATA1 (FOG1) (Tsang et al., 1997). The full-length GATA1 protein is produced by translation from methionine at codon 1 (Met1) on exon 2 (n.b., exon 1 is not coding) (Fig. 5). In some type of cells, another shorter isoform of GATA1 (molecular weight: approximately 40kD), referred to as GATA1s, is physiologically produced in a much smaller amount by alternative splicing from Met84 on exon 3 of the full GATA1 mRNA (Calligaris et al., 1995) (Fig. 5). GATA1s lacks N-terminal activation domain and has reduced transactivation potential, but it retains two zinc fingers and, therefore, can bind DNA and interact with FOG1. GATA1s is produced in a variety of cell lines and normal fetal liver and is thought to be important for embryonic development.

4.2 *GATA1* gene mutations in TL and AMKL-DS

Mutations affecting the *GATA1* gene in patients were first reported by Wechsler et al. (2002) exclusively in leukemic cells of AMKL-DS, and subsequently many groups of investigators reported *GATA1* mutations in nearly all patients with TL, MDS and AMKL in DS patients (Greene et al., 2003; Groet et al., 2003; Hitzler et al., 2003; Mundschau et al., 2003; Rainis et al., 2003; Xu et al., 2003). In these reports, the mutations have not been detected either in AMKL of non-DS patients or in other types of leukemias in DS patients, indicating that *GATA1* mutations are specific to TL, MDS and AMKL in DS patients. The mutations include a variety of abnormalities, such as nonsense/missense point mutations, deletions, insertions, or splice site mutations, which are so diverse as to be clone-specific markers. However, most of these abnormalities are clustered within exon 2 or less commonly in exon 3 (Fig. 5), resulting in loss of the first initiation codon (Met1) or disruption of the normal reading frame and introduction of a premature termination codon. Since *GATA1* gene is located on the X chromosome, when the allele harboring mutated *GATA1* is active, the other allele with wild-type *GATA1* is inactivated by methylation in female cells. Therefore, only the mutant *GATA1* is expressed in both male and female patients. The mutated *GATA1* gene invariably fails to produce full-length GATA1 and generates only the GATA1s isoform lacking N-terminal transcriptional activation domain using an alternative downstream initiator codon Met84 on exon 3 (Fig. 5). The other mutation, that is, splice site mutation that occurs in the boundary between exon 2 and intron 2 disrupts mRNA splicing and generates only shorter splice variant mRNA (GATA1s mRNA), in which exon 2 is skipped, and, consequently, only short isoform of GATA1, equivalent to GATA1s, is produced (Rainis et al., 2003) (Fig. 5).

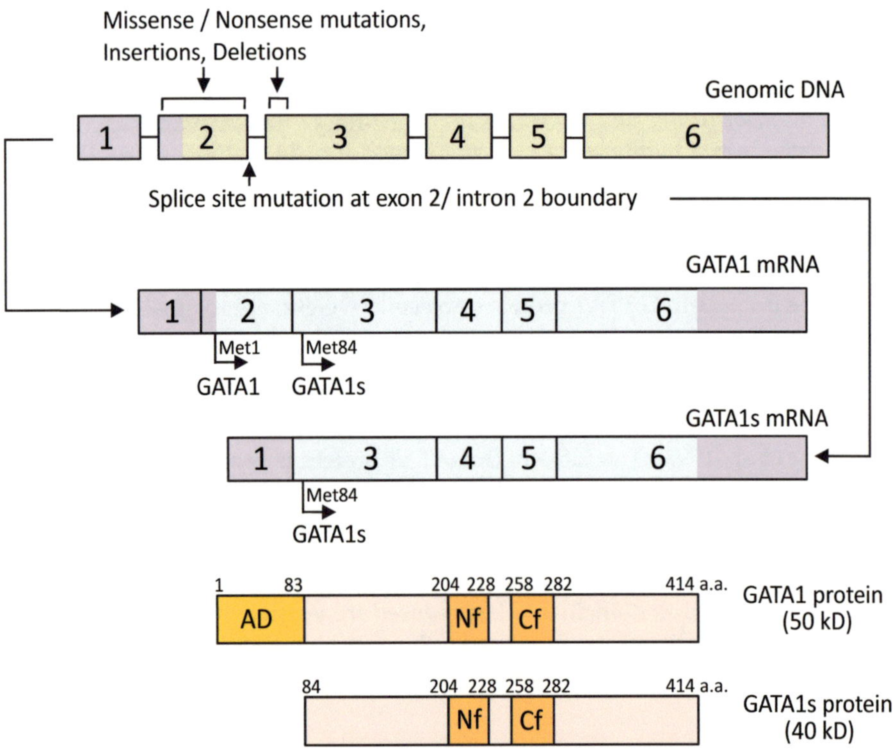

Fig. 5. Mutations of the *GATA1* gene in TL and AMKL-DS. Genomic DNA encoding *GATA1* consists of 6 exons (depicted as boxes and numbered from 1 to 6). The area colored in purple are 5′ and 3′ non-coding regions. Physiologically, normal full-length GATA1 protein is produced by translation from Met1 on exon 2, whereas GATA1s protein from Met84 on exon 3 of full GATA1 mRNA by alternative splicing. Most *GATA1* mutations occur on exon 2 or at exon2/intron2 boundary and all result in the production of only GATA1s, but the former by alternative splicing using downstream initiation codon Met84 whereas the latter by producing GATA1s mRNA and translation from it. Abbreviations: AD, transactivation domain; Nf, N-terminal zinc finger; Cf, C-terminal zinc finger; a.a., amino acid.

GATA1 mutations are not detected at the stage of remission in either TL or AMKL-DS (Rainis et al., 2003; Ahmed et al., 2004), indicating that the mutations are acquired somatic events. Accumulated data suggest that *GATA1* mutations occur in utero: 1) since TL is a disorder of neonates and almost certainly arises in utero, *GATA1* mutations that are present in almost all cases of TL should also occur in utero; 2) exactly the same mutations have been identified in the blasts of AMKL-DS in identical twins (Rainis et al., 2003), indicating that abnormal cells with *GATA1* mutations arose in one of the twins during the fetal stage and transferred to the other twin via anastomosing blood vessels in the placenta; 3) the same *GATA1* mutations have been detected in the neonatal blood spots of patients with AMKL-DS, who did not have clinically overt antecedent TL (Ahmed et al., 2004); 4) *GATA1* mutations have been detected in neonatal blood spots from 2 of 21 otherwise healthy DS children but not from non-DS cord blood samples (Ahmed et al., 2004); and 5) *GATA1* mutations have been detected in genomic DNA from 2 of 9 fetal liver and 2 of 5 infantile bone marrow autopsy specimens from patients with DS (Taub et al., 2004). Thus, *GATA1* mutations appear to occur in utero, if not in all cases, at relatively high frequency and specifically in patients with DS.

Although TL and AMKL-DS are typically disorders consisting of monoclonal population of cells carrying a single type of *GATA1* mutation, there have been reports of cases of TL and AMKL-DS with multiple independent clones with different *GATA1* mutations in single patients (Ahmed et al., 2004; Groet et al., 2005; Miyauchi et al., 2010). In one of four AMKL-DS patients with multiple *GATA1* mutations, neonatal blood spot showed 3 independent mutations but only one of these was present in AMKL-DS blasts (Ahmed et al., 2004), indicating that AMKL-DS had evolved from one of these oligoclonal cells with different *GATA1* mutations that had occurred in utero. Similarly, evolution of AMKL-DS from one of the oligoclonal populations of TL blasts with different chromosomal abnormalities after regression of TL has been demonstrated (Kitoh et al., 2009). While identical mutations between the blasts in TL and AMKL-DS that occurred later in the same patient have been reported by several investigators (Wechsler et al., 2002; Hitzler et al., 2003; Rainis et al., 2003; Shimada et al., 2004), different mutations between the blasts of TL and subsequent AMKL in the same patient have also been reported (Xu et al., 2006b; Kanegane et al., 2007). In the patient of Xu et al., however, although predominant clones of TL and AMKL-DS were different, a minor clone of TL with *GATA1* mutation identical to that of AMKL-DS was present. Taken together, it appears highly likely that AMKL-DS evolves from a minor clone (or multiple clones in some cases) of TL blasts that have persisted after regression, or from one or multiple silent clones of cells with *GATA1* mutations that have not expanded to develop into clinically detectable TL but survived persistently in the body, possibly in the bone marrow.

4.3 The role of GATA1 and GATA1s in TL and AMKL-DS

Since high expression of GATA1s and abrogation of full-length GATA1 is the invariable result of the *GATA1* gene mutations, increased GATA1s and/or loss of full-length GATA1 protein must play a crucial role in leukemogenesis in both TL and AMKL-DS, possibly through altered interaction with their partner proteins. Since GATA1s has a reduced transactivation potential due to the lack of an N-terminal activation domain but can bind DNA and interact with the cofactor FOG1 via zinc finger domains, its role as a dominant negative protein, which fails to activate or repress the function of proteins that are normally regulated by GATA1, has been proposed (Gurbuxani et al., 2004). Alternatively, since normal GATA1 protein binds to RUNX1, which is an important megakaryopoietic regulator encoded by the *RUNX1* gene that resides on chromosome 21, and the binding site has been shown to be located at the N- and C-terminal portions of GATA1 (Elagib et al., 2003), GATA1s lacking an N-terminus may cause abnormal growth and/or differentiation of neoplastic cells involving the megakaryocytic lineage through defective biding to RUNX1. However, the site on GATA1 that binds to RUNX1 is controversial; it has been shown that GATA1 interacts with RUNX1 through zinc fingers, but not the N-terminal portion (Waltzer et al., 2003), and that GATA1s of all patient samples examined bound to RUNX1 through zinc finger domains (Xu et al., 2006a). The role of RUNX1 in leukemogenesis of DS-related leukemias needs to be further determined. We have recently shown that the expression level of GATA1s decreases during the process of growth factor-induced differentiation of TL blasts *in vitro*, indicating that GATA1s may act as a repressor of the GATA1-related proteins that induce differentiation and that the protein level of GATA1s changes depending on the cellular circumferential conditions and may be a key factor that influences the growth and differentiation of TL blasts (Miyauchi et al., 2010). Consistent with this finding, it has been described that expression of GATA1s is decreased *in vivo* in murine mature megakaryocytes carrying a *GATA1* mutation that results in the production of GATA1s equivalent to the protein products of *GATA1* mutations in DS-related leukemias (Majewski et al., 2006). Kanezaki et al. (2010) showed that protein levels of GATA1s in TL blasts differ depending on the sites of mutations and its quantitative differences are significantly associated with patient prognosis and the risk of developing AMKL-DS. These data suggest that protein levels of GATA1s may also be important in the biology of DS-related leukemic cells.

Experiments using mouse models with various *GATA1* gene alterations have shown that the presence of full-length GATA1 is crucial in fetal development, particularly for megakaryocyte and erythroid lineages. Complete absence of GATA1 in male mice (GATA1 null mice) results in embryonic lethality due to severe anemia (Fujiwara et al., 1996). Reduced expression of GATA1 in GATA1.05 mice, in which GATA1 expression is reduced to less than 5% of the normal level, also causes embryonic lethality in male hemizygous and female homozygous mice, whereas female heterozygous mice survive the fetal stage but develop hematological abnormalities similar to MDS and die prematurely (Takahashi et al., 1997; Takahashi et al., 1998). Another mouse strain (lineage-selective GATA1 knock-out mouse), in which GATA1 expression is virtually absent from megakaryocytes, exhibits marked thrombocytopenia and morphologically abnormal megakaryocytes with impaired cytoplasmic maturation proliferate and accumulate in the spleen and bone marrow (Shivdasani et al., 1997). Abnormal proliferation of megakaryocyte/erythroid progenitors in GATA1-deficient murine embryonic stem cell-derived hematopoietic cultures has also been described (Stachura et al., 2006). Thus, loss of normal full-length GATA1 might also play an important role in leukemogenesis of TL and AMKL-DS. However, the extent to which the leukemic phenotype is due to the loss of full-length GATA1 versus high expression of GATA1s remains to be explored.

5. Multistep model of myeloid leukemogenesis in children with DS

Based upon the data described above, a multistep model of leukemogenesis of myeloid leukemias in children with DS has been proposed (Ahmed et al., 2004; Gurbuxani et al., 2004; Cantor, 2005; Hitzler & Zipursky, 2005; Hitzler, 2007; Roy et al., 2009; Zwaan et al., 2010) (Fig. 6). TL and AMKL-DS are disorders closely associated with DS, and although they rarely occur in phenotypically normal patients with trisomy 21 mosaicism, trisomy 21 is always present in all leukemic cells of such patients, indicating that trisomy 21 must be the prerequisite of these disorders. Several mouse models of DS have been developed, which can be used to explore the important dose-dependent genes that are involved in DS-specific disorders and study the pathology of model mice in comparison with human DS patients. These model mice include Ts65DN, Ts1Cje (Carmichael et al., 2009) and Tc1 (Alford et al., 2010) mouse strains, that are trisomic for 143, 94 and 269 gene orthologues, respectively, of 324 recognized genes on human chromosome 21, with the Tc1 strain representing the most complete model of human DS generated to date. These mice all show macrocytic anemia and some of these mouse strains show increased numbers of megakaryocytic and erythroid precursors in the adult spleen and develop myeloproliferative disorder in adults. However, none of these mouse strains develop TL and AMKL, indicating that additional genetic abnormalities are required to cause leukemia. In humans as well, trisomy 21 itself has been shown to disturb fetal liver, but not bone marrow, hematopoiesis, enhance production of megakaryocyte/erythroid progenitors (MEPs), which may be susceptible to acquisition of other genetic abnormalities, and predispose these cells to DS-related leukemias (Chou et al., 2008; De Vita et al., 2008; Tunstall-Pedoe et al., 2008). These data support the model that the genes on chromosome 21 play essential roles in the development of these disorders and trisomy 21 is the first step of myeloid leukemogenesis in DS.

The genes *RUNX1* (alternatively called *AML1*), *BACH1*, *ETS2* and *ERG*, all of which are located on chromosome 21 and are associated with megakaryopoiesis, have been suggested to be the candidate genes involved in leukemogenesis of TL and AMKL-DS (Ahmed et al., 2004; Gurbuxani et al., 2004; Cantor, 2005; Hitzler & Zipursky, 2005; Osato & Ito, 2005; Hitzler, 2007; Roy et al., 2009; Zwaan et al., 2010). Translocations and point mutations of *RUNX1*, leading to loss of function or haploinsufficiency (namely, reduced expression) of RUNX1, have been detected in a variety of human leukemias and are thought to be involved in leukemogenesis (Yamashita et al., 2005). Alternatively, increased dosage of expression of these genes due to trisomy 21 has also been suggested to be another mechanism of leukemogenesis (Yanagida et al., 2005). However, expression levels of RUNX1 are not necessarily increased in all tissues in patients with DS or DS model mice (Osato & Ito, 2005); therefore, the above theory regarding RUNX1 requires further verification. ERG has been shown to be expressed in AMKL-DS, strongly cooperate with GATA1s and immortalize megakaryocytic progenitors (Salek-Ardakani et al., 2009), indicating that ERG in trisomy 21 may play a role in the development of DS-related leukemias. It has been shown recently that miR-125b-2, a microRNA (miRNA) that is located on chromosome 21, is upregulated in the samples of patients with TL and AMKL-DS and that its overexpression stimulates proliferation and self-renewal of megakaryocytic progenitors and MEPs and accentuates proproliferative effects of GATA1s on MEPs in murine fetal liver, indicating that miRNAs related to chromosome 21 might also participate in leukemogenesis in patients with DS (Klusmann et al., 2010). The role of the genes or miRNAs on chromosome 21 in DS-related leukemogenesis would be the major concerns in future studies.

The second step is most likely the acquisition of *GATA1* mutations in hematopoietic progenitor cells (Fig. 6), since it has been demonstrated that 1) *GATA1* mutations are present exclusively in the blasts of TL and AMKL-DS in nearly all patients; 2) these are acquired somatic mutations; and 3) these mutations occur in utero. Furthermore, it has been reported that a germline splicing mutation of *GATA1*, leading to synthesis of only GATA1s, caused anemia and neutropenia but not leukemia in seven affected males from two generations of a family, indicating that a *GATA1* mutation alone may cause hematological abnormalities but requires trisomy 21 to cause TL or AMKL (Hollanda et al., 2006). However, it is of note that N-terminally truncated *GATA1* mutant in a non-DS-model mouse caused massive accumulation of megakaryocytes in the fetal liver that spontaneously resolved after birth, similar to TL in humans, indicating that a *GATA1* mutation alone may cause TL-like megakaryocytic hyperproliferation in mice (Shimizu et al., 2009).

The target cells of *GATA1* mutations are likely to be embryonic or fetal primitive hematopoietic progenitor cells with multilineage differentiation potential. With the acquisition of *GATA1* mutations, these cells would give rise to oligoclonal or monoclonal populations of neoplastic cells in the fetal liver (Fig. 6). The large clone(s) may develop into TL and cause hepatic fibrosis and dysfunction through the production of collagen-stimulating cytokines or infiltrate into the tissue, causing cardiac failure or hydrops fetalis. *GATA1* mutations in cooperation with trisomy 21 may cause TL but they should be insufficient to immortalize the blasts, leading to spontaneous remission before or after birth through unknown mechanism(s).

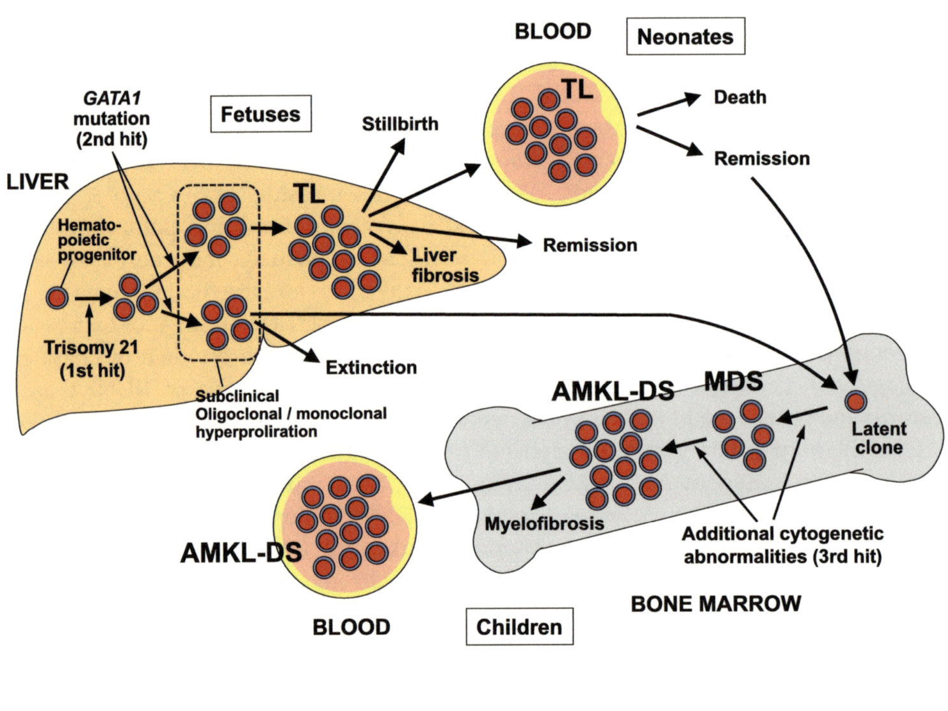

Fig. 6. Multistep model of myeloid leukemogenesis in young children with DS.

It is plausible that minor clones of residual TL blasts or clinically silent neoplastic hematopoietic progenitor cells that have obtained *GATA1* mutations but have not caused TL could survive latently during postnatal life and, with the acquisition of additional genetic abnormalities as the third step, would cause AMKL-DS through the stage of MDS in the bone marrow (Fig. 6). Although trisomy 8, altered telomerase activity (Holt et al., 2002), and mutations in several genes, including *TP53* (Malkin et al., 2000; Hirose et al., 2003), *KIT*, *MPL* and *FLT3* (Malinge et al., 2008), have been identified in some patients with AMKL-DS, genetic abnormalities that cause evolution of AMKL-DS from those latent clones of cells with *GATA1* mutations are largely unknown. Several recent studies have shown activating mutations of the Janus kinase 3 (*JAK3)* gene, which encodes for a non-receptor tyrosine kinase, in some patients with TL and AMKL-DS (De Vita et al., 2007; Kiyoi et al., 2007; Klusmann et al., 2007), but these mutations were present in both TL and AMKL-DS and, therefore, are not likely involved in disease progression from TL to AMKL-DS. Concerning the evolution of AMKL-DS, Kanezaki et al. (2010) have recently demonstrated that the expression levels of GATA1s protein are associated with the type of *GATA1* mutations in TL; low expression of GATA1s is caused by mutations introducing premature termination codon (PTC) at the 5′ side of exon 2 or after codon 84 on exon 3 whereas high expression of GATA1 is associated with mutations causing loss of the first methionine, splicing error or introduction of PTC at the 3′ side of exon 2, and that GATA1s low mutations in TL are significantly associated with higher risk of developing AMKL-DS. The mechanism by which AMKL-DS evolves from minor clones of cells with *GATA1* mutations is currently one of the main areas of research in DS-associated leukemias.

6. Conclusion

Young children with DS are predisposed to unusual leukemias of myeloid origin, namely, TL and AMKL-DS. In contrast to the transient nature of the former, which places it in a category of preleukemia or "unusual" leukemia, the latter is an authentic leukemia leading to a lethal outcome unless treated. Nevertheless, these disorders are closely linked to each other by many common cellular morphological as well as cytogenetic features, including trisomy 21 and *GATA1* gene mutations, and share a distinct pathogenetic basis. Recent investigations have demonstrated much of molecular basis of these disorders and contributed to the proposal of an attractive model of a stepwise leukemogenic process of these disorders. This new model is expected to suggest many directions for future studies on not only DS-related leukemias but also pediatric leukemias in general.

7. References

Ahmed, M.; Sternberg, A.; Hall, G.; Thomas, A.; Smith, O., et al. (2004) Natural history of *GATA1* mutations in Down syndrome. *Blood*, Vol.103, No.7, (Apr 2004), pp.2480-2489, ISSN 0006-4971

Al-Kasim, F.; Doyle, J. J.; Massey, G. V.; Weinstein, H. J.; Zipursky, A., et al. (2002) Incidence and treatment of potentially lethal diseases in transient leukemia of Down syndrome: Pediatric Oncology Group Study. *J Pediatr Hematol Oncol*, Vol.24, No.1, (Jan 2002), pp.9-13, ISSN 1077-4114

Alford, K. A.; Slender, A.; Vanes, L.; Li, Z.; Fisher, E. M., et al. (2010) Perturbed hematopoiesis in the Tc1 mouse model of Down syndrome. *Blood*, Vol.115, No.14, (Apr 2010), pp.2928- 2937, ISSN 1528-0020

Arai, H.; Ishida, A.; Nakajima, W.; Nishinomiya, F.; Yamazoe, A., et al. (1999) Immunohistochemical study on transforming growth factor-beta1 expression in liver fibrosis of Down's syndrome with transient abnormal myelopoiesis. *Hum Pathol*, Vol.30, No.4, (Apr 1999), pp.474-476, ISSN

Becroft, D. M. (1993) Fetal megakaryocytic dyshemopoiesis in Down syndrome: association with hepatic and pancreatic fibrosis. *Pediatr Pathol,* Vol.13, No.6, (Nov-Dec 1993), pp.811-820, ISSN 0277-0938

Becroft, D. M. & Zwi, L. J. (1990) Perinatal visceral fibrosis accompanying the megakaryoblastic leukemoid reaction of Down syndrome. *Pediatric Pathology,* Vol.10, No.3, (n.d. 1990), pp.397-406, ISSN 0277-0938

Bessho, F.; Hayashi, Y. & Ohga, K. (1988) Ultrastructural studies of peripheral blood of neonates with Down's syndrome and transient abnormal myelopoiesis. *Am J Clin Pathol,* Vol.89, No.5, (May 1988), pp.627-633, ISSN 0002-9173

Breton-Gorius, J.; Bizet, M.; Reyes, F.; Dupuy, E.; Mear, C., et al. (1982) Myelofibrosis and acute megakaryoblastic leukemia in a child: topographic relationship between fibroblasts and megakaryocytes with an α-granule defect. *Leuk Res,* Vol.6, No.1, (n.d. 1982), pp.97-110, ISSN 0145-2126

Brodeur, G. M.; Dahl, G. V.; Williams, D. L.; Tipton, R. E. & Kalwinsky, D. K. (1980) Transient leukemoid reaction and trisomy 21 mosaicism in a phenotypically normal newborn. *Blood,* Vol.55, No.4, (Apr 1980), pp.691-693, ISSN 0006-4971

Calligaris, R.; Bottardi, S.; Cogoi, S.; Apezteguia, I. & Santoro, C. (1995) Alternative translation initiation site usage results in two functionally distinct forms of the GATA-1 transcription factor. *Proc Natl Acad Sci U S A,* Vol.92, No.25, (Dec 1995), pp.11598-11602, ISSN 0027-8424

Cantor, A. B. (2005) GATA transcription factors in hematologic disease. *Int J Hematol,* Vol.81, No.5, (Jun 2005), pp.378-384, ISSN 0925-5710

Carmichael, C. L.; Majewski, I. J.; Alexander, W. S.; Metcalf, D.; Hilton, D. J., et al. (2009) Hematopoietic defects in the Ts1Cje mouse model of Down syndrome. *Blood,* Vol.113, No.9, (Feb 2009), pp.1929-1937, ISSN 1528-0020

Chou, S. T.; Opalinska, J. B.; Yao, Y.; Fernandes, M. A.; Kalota, A., et al. (2008) Trisomy 21 enhances human fetal erythro-megakaryocytic development. *Blood,* Vol.112, No.12, (Dec 2008), pp.4503-4506, ISSN 1528-0020

Coulombel, L.; Derycke, M.; Villeval, J. L.; Leonard, C.; Breton-Gorius, J., et al. (1987) Characterization of the blast cell population in two neonates with Down's syndrome and transient myeloproliferative disorder. *Br J Haematol,* Vol.66, No.1, (May 1987), pp.69-76, ISSN 0007-1048

De Vita, S.; Devoy, A.; Groet, J.; Kruslin, B.; Kuzmic-Prusac, I., et al. (2008) Megakaryocyte hyperproliferation without *GATA1* mutation in foetal liver of a case of Down syndrome with hydrops foetalis. *Br J Haematol,* Vol.143, No.2, (Oct 2008), pp.300-303, ISSN 1365-2141

De Vita, S.; Mulligan, C.; McElwaine, S.; Dagna-Bricarelli, F.; Spinelli, M., et al. (2007) Loss-of-function *JAK3* mutations in TMD and AMKL of Down syndrome. *Br J Haematol,* Vol.137, No.4, (May 2007), pp.337-341, ISSN 0007-1048

Dormann, S.; Kruger, M.; Hentschel, R.; Rasenack, R.; Strahm, B., et al. (2004) Life-threatening complications of transient abnormal myelopoiesis in neonates with Down syndrome. *Eur J Pediatr,* Vol.163, No.7, (Jul 2004), pp.374-377, ISSN 0340-6199

Eguchi, M.; Ozawa, T.; Sakakibara, H.; Sugita, K.; Iwama, Y., et al. (1992) Ultrastructural and ultracytochemical differences between megakaryoblastic leukemia in children and adults. Analysis of 49 patients. *Cancer,* Vol.70, No.2, (Jul 1992), pp.451-458, ISSN 0008-543X

Eguchi, M.; Sakaibara, H.; Suda, J.; Ozawa, T.; Hayashi, Y., et al. (1989) Ultrastructural and ultracytochemical differences between transient myeloproliferative disorder and megakaryoblastic leukaemia in Down's syndrome. *Br J Haematol*, Vol.73, No.3, (Nov 1989), pp.315-322, ISSN 0007-1048

Elagib, K. E.; Racke, F. K.; Mogass, M.; Khetawat, R.; Delehanty, L. L., et al. (2003) RUNX1 and GATA-1 coexpression and cooperation in megakaryocytic differentiation. *Blood*, Vol.101, No.11, (Jun 2003), pp.4333-4341, ISSN 0006-4971

Foucar, K.; Friedman, K.; Llewellyn, A.; McConnell, T.; Aisenbrey, G., et al. (1992) Prenatal diagnosis of transient myeloproliferative disorder via percutaneous umbilical blood sampling. Report of two cases in fetuses affected by Down's syndrome. *Am J Clin Pathol*, Vol.97, No.4, (Apr 1992), pp.584-590, ISSN 0002-9173

Fujiwara, Y.; Browne, C. P.; Cunniff, K.; Goff, S. C. & Orkin, S. H. (1996) Arrested development of embryonic red cell precursors in mouse embryos lacking transcription factor GATA-1. *Proc Natl Acad Sci U S A*, Vol.93, No.22, (Oct 1996), pp.12355-12358, ISSN 0027- 8424

Gamis, A. S. & Hilden, J. M. (2002) Transient myeloproliferative disorder, a disorder with too few data and many unanswered questions: does it contain an important piece of the puzzle to understanding hematopoiesis and acute myelogenous leukemia? *J Pediatr Hematol Oncol*, Vol.24, No.1, (Jan 2002), pp.2-5, ISSN 1077-4114

Gray, E. S.; Balch, N. J.; Kohler, H.; Thompson, W. D. & Simpson, J. G. (1986) Congenital leukaemia: an unusual cause of stillbirth. *Arch Dis Child*, Vol.61, No.10, (Oct 1986), pp.1001-1006, ISSN 1468-2044

Greene, M. E.; Mundschau, G.; Wechsler, J.; McDevitt, M.; Gamis, A., et al. (2003) Mutations in GATA1 in both transient myeloproliferative disorder and acute megakaryoblastic leukemia of Down syndrome. *Blood Cells Mol Dis*, Vol.31, No.3, (Nov-Dec 2003), pp.351-356, ISSN 1079-9796

Groet, J.; McElwaine, S.; Spinelli, M.; Rinaldi, A.; Burtscher, I., et al. (2003) Acquired mutations in *GATA1* in neonates with Down's syndrome with transient myeloid disorder. *Lancet*, Vol.361, No.9369, (May 2003), pp.1617-1620, ISSN 0140-6736

Groet, J.; Mulligan, C.; Spinelli, M.; Serra, A.; McElwaine, S., et al. (2005) Independent clones at separable stages of differentiation, bearing different *GATA1* mutations, in the same TMD patient with Down syndrome. *Blood*, Vol.106, No.5, (Sep 2005), pp.1887-1888, ISSN 0006-4971

Gurbuxani, S.; Vyas, P. & Crispino, J. D. (2004) Recent insights into the mechanisms of myeloid leukemogenesis in Down syndrome. *Blood*, Vol.103, No.2, (Jan 2004), pp.399-406, ISSN 0006-4971

Hayashi, Y.; Eguchi, M.; Sugita, K.; Nakazawa, S.; Sato, T., et al. (1988) Cytogenetic findings and clinical features in acute leukemia and transient myeloproliferative disorder in Down's syndrome. *Blood*, Vol.72, No.1, (Jul 1988), pp.15-23, ISSN 0006-4971

Heald, B.; Hilden, J. M.; Zbuk, K.; Norton, A.; Vyas, P., et al. (2007) Severe TMD/AMKL with *GATA1* mutation in a stillborn fetus with Down syndrome. *Nat Clin Pract Oncol*, Vol.4, No.7, (Jul 2007), pp.433-438, ISSN 1743-4262

Hirose, Y.; Kudo, K.; Kiyoi, H.; Hayashi, Y.; Naoe, T., et al. (2003) Comprehensive analysis of gene alterations in acute megakaryoblastic leukemia of Down's syndrome. *Leukemia*, Vol.17, No.11, (Nov 2003), pp.2250-2252, ISSN 0887-6924

Hitzler, J. K. (2007) Acute megakaryoblastic leukemia in Down syndrome. *Pediatr Blood Cancer*, Vol.49, No.7 Suppl, (Dec 2007), pp.1066-1069, ISSN 1545-5009

Hitzler, J. K.; Cheung, J.; Li, Y.; Scherer, S. W. & Zipursky, A. (2003) GATA1 mutations in transient leukemia and acute megakaryoblastic leukemia of Down syndrome. *Blood*, Vol.101, No.11, (Jun 2003), pp.4301-4304, ISSN 0006-4971

Hitzler, J. K. & Zipursky, A. (2005) Origins of leukaemia in children with Down syndrome. *Nat Rev Cancer*, Vol.5, No.1, (Jan 2005), pp.11-20, ISSN 1474-175X

Hollanda, L. M.; Lima, C. S.; Cunha, A. F.; Albuquerque, D. M.; Vassallo, J., et al. (2006) An inherited mutation leading to production of only the short isoform of GATA-1 is associated with impaired erythropoiesis. *Nat Genet*, Vol.38, No.7, (Jul 2006), pp.807-812, ISSN 1061-4036

Holt, S. E.; Brown, E. J. & Zipursky, A. (2002) Telomerase and the benign and malignant megakaryoblastic leukemias of Down syndrome. *J Pediatr Hematol Oncol*, Vol.24, No.1, (Jan 2002), pp.14-17, ISSN 1077-4114

Ishigaki, H.; Miyauchi, J.; Yokoe, A.; Nakayama, M.; Yanagi, T., et al. (2011) Expression of megakaryocytic and myeloid markers in blasts of transient abnormal myelopoiesis in a stillbirth with Down syndrome: report of histopathological findings of an autopsy case. *Hum Pathol*, Vol.42, No.1, (Jan 2011), pp.141-145, ISSN 1532-8392

Kalousek, D. K. & Chan, K. W. (1987) Transient myeloproliferative disorder in chromosomally normal newborn infant. *Med Pediatr Oncol*, Vol.15, No.1, (n.d. 1987), pp.38-41, ISSN 0098-1532

Kanegane, H.; Watanabe, S.; Nomura, K.; Xu, G.; Ito, E., et al. (2007) Distinct clones are associated with the development of transient myeloproliferative disorder and acute megakaryocytic leukemia in a patient with Down syndrome. *Int J Hematol*, Vol.86, No.3, (Oct 2007), pp.250-252, ISSN 0925-5710

Kanezaki, R.; Toki, T.; Terui, K.; Xu, G.; Wang, R., et al. (2010) Down syndrome and *GATA1* mutations in transient abnormal myeloproliferative disorder: mutation classes correlate with progression to myeloid leukemia. *Blood*, Vol.116, No.22, (Nov 2010), pp.4631-4638, ISSN 1528-0020

Kitoh, T.; Taki, T.; Hayashi, Y.; Nakamura, K.; Irino, T., et al. (2009) Transient abnormal myelopoiesis in a Down syndrome newborn followed by acute myeloid leukemia: identification of the same chromosomal abnormality in both stages. *Cancer Genet Cytogenet*, Vol.188, No.2, (Jan 2009), pp.99-102, ISSN 1873-4456

Kiyoi, H.; Yamaji, S.; Kojima, S. & Naoe, T. (2007) JAK3 mutations occur in acute megakaryoblastic leukemia both in Down syndrome children and non-Down syndrome adults. *Leukemia*, Vol.21, No.3, (Mar 2007), pp.574-576, ISSN 0887-6924

Klusmann, J. H.; Creutzig, U.; Zimmermann, M.; Dworzak, M.; Jorch, N., et al. (2008) Treatment and prognostic impact of transient leukemia in neonates with Down syndrome. *Blood*, Vol.111, No.6, (Mar 2008), pp.2991-2998, ISSN 0006-4971

Klusmann, J. H.; Li, Z.; Bohmer, K.; Maroz, A.; Koch, M. L., et al. (2010) miR-125b-2 is a potential oncomiR on human chromosome 21 in megakaryoblastic leukemia. *Genes Dev*, Vol.24, No.5, (Mar 2010), pp.478-490, ISSN 1549-5477

Klusmann, J. H.; Reinhardt, D.; Hasle, H.; Kaspers, G. J.; Creutzig, U., et al. (2007) Janus kinase mutations in the development of acute megakaryoblastic leukemia in children with and without Down's syndrome. *Leukemia*, Vol.21, No.7, (Jul 2007), pp.1584-1587, ISSN 0887-6924

Kurahashi, H.; Hara, J.; Yumura-Yagi, K.; Murayama, N.; Inoue, M., et al. (1991) Monoclonal nature of transient abnormal myelopoiesis in Down's syndrome. *Blood*, Vol.77, No.6, (Mar 1991), pp.1161-1163, ISSN 0006-4971

Langebrake, C.; Creutzig, U. & Reinhardt, D. (2005) Immunophenotype of Down syndrome acute myeloid leukemia and transient myeloproliferative disease differs significantly from other diseases with morphologically identical or similar blasts. *Klin Padiatr*, Vol.217, No.3, (May-Jun 2005), pp.126-134, ISSN 0300-8630

Li, Z.; Godinho, F. J.; Klusmann, J. H.; Garriga-Canut, M.; Yu, C., et al. (2005) Developmental stage-selective effect of somatically mutated leukemogenic transcription factor GATA1. *Nat Genet*, Vol.37, No.6, (Jun 2005), pp.613-619, ISSN 1061-4036

Majewski, I. J.; Metcalf, D.; Mielke, L. A.; Krebs, D. L.; Ellis, S., et al. (2006) A mutation in the translation initiation codon of *Gata-1* disrupts megakaryocyte maturation and causes thrombocytopenia. *Proc Natl Acad Sci U S A*, Vol.103, No.38, (Sep 2006), pp.14146-14151, ISSN 0027-8424

Malinge, S.; Ragu, C.; Della-Valle, V.; Pisani, D.; Constantinescu, S. N., et al. (2008) Activating mutations in human acute megakaryoblastic leukemia. *Blood*, Vol.112, No.10, (Nov 2008), pp.4220-4226, ISSN 1528-0020

Malkin, D.; Brown, E. J. & Zipursky, A. (2000) The role of p53 in megakaryocyte differentiation and the megakaryocytic leukemias of Down syndrome. *Cancer Genet Cytogenet*, Vol.116, No.1, (Jan 2000), pp.1-5, ISSN 0165-4608

Massey, G. V.; Zipursky, A.; Chang, M. N.; Doyle, J. J.; Nasim, S., et al. (2006) A prospective study of the natural history of transient leukemia (TL) in neonates with Down syndrome (DS): Children's Oncology Group (COG) study POG-9481. *Blood*, Vol.107, No.12, (Jun 2006), pp.4606-4613, ISSN 0006-4971

Miyashita, T.; Asada, M.; Fujimoto, J.; Inaba, T.; Takihara, Y., et al. (1991) Clonal analysis of transient myeloproliferative disorder in Down's syndrome. *Leukemia*, Vol.5, No.1, (Jan 1991), pp.56-59, ISSN 0887-6924

Miyauchi, J.; Ito, Y.; Kawano, T.; Tsunematsu, Y. & Shimizu, K. (1992) Unusual diffuse liver fibrosis accompanying transient myeloproliferative disorder in Down's syndrome: a report of four autopsy cases and proposal of a hypothesis. *Blood*, Vol.80, No.6, (Sep 1992), pp.1521-1527, ISSN 0006-4971

Miyauchi, J.; Ito, Y.; Tsukamoto, K.; Takahashi, H.; Ishikura, K., et al. (2010) Blasts in transient leukaemia in neonates with Down syndrome differentiate into basophil/mast-cell and megakaryocyte lineages in vitro in association with down-regulation of truncated form of GATA1. *Br J Haematol*, Vol.148, No.6, (Mar 2010), pp.898-909, ISSN 1365-2141

Mundschau, G.; Gurbuxani, S.; Gamis, A. S.; Greene, M. E.; Arceci, R. J., et al. (2003) Mutagenesis of *GATA1* is an initiating event in Down syndrome leukemogenesis. *Blood*, Vol.101, No.11, (Jun 2003), pp.4298-4300, ISSN 0006-4971

Osato, M. & Ito, Y. (2005) Increased dosage of the *RUNX1/AML1* gene: a third mode of RUNX leukemia? *Crit Rev Eukaryot Gene Expr*, Vol.15, No.3, 2005), pp.217-228, ISSN 1045-4403

Parkin, J. L.; McKenna, R. W. & Brunning, R. D. (1980) Ultrastructural features of basophil and mast cell granulopoiesis in blastic phase Philadelphia chromosome-positive leukemia. *J Natl Cancer Inst*, Vol.65, No.3, (Sep 1980), pp.535-546, ISSN 0027-8874

Rainis, L.; Bercovich, D.; Strehl, S.; Teigler-Schlegel, A.; Stark, B., et al. (2003) Mutations in exon 2 of GATA1 are early events in megakaryocytic malignancies associated with trisomy 21. *Blood*, Vol.102, No.3, (Aug 2003), pp.981-986, ISSN 0006-4971

Roberts, A. B.; Sporn, M. B.; Assoian, R. K.; Smith, J. M.; Roche, N. S., et al. (1986) Transforming growth factor type β: rapid induction of fibrosis and angiogenesis in vivo and stimulation of collagen formation in vitro. *Proc Natl Acad Sci U S A*, Vol.83, No.12, (Jun 1986), pp.4167-4171, ISSN 0027-8424

Robertson, M.; De Jong, G. & Mansvelt, E. (2003) Prenatal diagnosis of congenital leukemia in a fetus at 25 weeks' gestation with Down syndrome: case report and review of the literature. *Ultrasound Obstet Gynecol*, Vol.21, No.5, (May 2003), pp.486-489, ISSN 0960-7692

Roy, A.; Roberts, I.; Norton, A. & Vyas, P. (2009) Acute megakaryoblastic leukaemia (AMKL) and transient myeloproliferative disorder (TMD) in Down syndrome: a multi-step model of myeloid leukaemogenesis. *Br J Haematol*, Vol.147, No.1, (Oct 2009), pp.3-12, ISSN 1365-2141

Ruchelli, E. D.; Uri, A.; Dimmick, J. E.; Bove, K. E.; Huff, D. S., et al. (1991) Severe perinatal liver disease and Down syndrome: an apparent relationship. *Hum Pathol*, Vol.22, No.12, (Dec 1991), pp.1274-1280, ISSN 0046-8177

Salek-Ardakani, S.; Smooha, G.; de Boer, J.; Sebire, N. J.; Morrow, M., et al. (2009) *ERG* is a megakaryocytic oncogene. *Cancer Res*, Vol.69, No.11, (Jun 2009), pp.4665-4673, ISSN 1538-7445

Schwab, M.; Niemeyer, C. & Schwarzer, U. (1998) Down syndrome, transient myeloproliferative disorder, and infantile liver fibrosis. *Med Pediatr Oncol*, Vol.31, No.3, (Sep 1998), pp.159-165, ISSN 0098-1532

Shimada, A.; Xu, G.; Toki, T.; Kimura, H.; Hayashi, Y., et al. (2004) Fetal origin of the *GATA1* mutation in identical twins with transient myeloproliferative disorder and acute megakaryoblastic leukemia accompanying Down syndrome. *Blood*, Vol.103, No.1, (Jan 2004), pp.366, ISSN 0006-4971

Shimizu, R.; Kobayashi, E.; Engel, J. D. & Yamamoto, M. (2009) Induction of hyperproliferative fetal megakaryopoiesis by an N-terminally truncated GATA1 mutant. *Genes Cells*, Vol.14, No.9, (Sep 2009), pp.1119-1131, ISSN 1365-2443

Shiozawa, Y.; Fujita, H.; Fujimura, J.; Suzuki, K.; Sato, H., et al. (2004) A fetal case of transient abnormal myelopoiesis with severe liver failure in Down syndrome: prognostic value of serum markers. *Pediatr Hematol Oncol*, Vol.21, No.3, (Apr-May 2004), pp.273-278, ISSN 0888-0018

Shivdasani, R. A.; Fujiwara, Y.; McDevitt, M. A. & Orkin, S. H. (1997) A lineage-selective knockout establishes the critical role of transcription factor GATA-1 in megakaryocyte growth and platelet development. *EMBO J*, Vol.16, No.13, (Jul 1997), pp.3965-3973, ISSN 0261-4189

Smrcek, J. M.; Baschat, A. A.; Germer, U.; Gloeckner-Hofmann, K. & Gembruch, U. (2001) Fetal hydrops and hepatosplenomegaly in the second half of pregnancy: a sign of myeloproliferative disorder in fetuses with trisomy 21. *Ultrasound Obstet Gynecol*, Vol.17, No.5, (May 2001), pp.403-409, ISSN 0960-7692

Stachura, D. L.; Chou, S. T. & Weiss, M. J. (2006) Early block to erythromegakaryocytic development conferred by loss of transcription factor GATA-1. *Blood*, Vol.107, No.1, (Jan 2006), pp.87-97, ISSN 0006-4971

Suda, J.; Eguchi, M.; Akiyama, Y.; Iwama, Y.; Furukawa, T., et al. (1987) Differentiation of blast cells from a Down's syndrome patient with transient myeloproliferative disorder. *Blood*, Vol.69, No.2, (Feb 1987), pp.508-512, ISSN 0006-4971

Sunami, S.; Fuse, A.; Simizu, B.; Eguchi, M.; Hayashi, Y., et al. (1987) The c-*sis* gene expression in cells from a patient with acute megakaryoblastic leukemia and Down's syndrome. *Blood*, Vol.70, No.2, (Aug 1987), pp.368-371, ISSN 0006-4971

Takahashi, S.; Komeno, T.; Suwabe, N.; Yoh, K.; Nakajima, O., et al. (1998) Role of GATA-1 in proliferation and differentiation of definitive erythroid and megakaryocytic cells in vivo. *Blood*, Vol.92, No.2, (Jul 1998), pp.434-442, ISSN 0006-4971

Takahashi, S.; Onodera, K.; Motohashi, H.; Suwabe, N.; Hayashi, N., et al. (1997) Arrest in primitive erythroid cell development caused by promoter-specific disruption of the GATA-1 gene. *J Biol Chem*, Vol.272, No.19, (May 1997), pp.12611-12615, ISSN 0021-9258

Taub, J. W.; Mundschau, G.; Ge, Y.; Poulik, J. M.; Qureshi, F., et al. (2004) Prenatal origin of GATA1 mutations may be an initiating step in the development of megakaryocytic leukemia in Down syndrome. *Blood*, Vol.104, No.5, (Sep 2004), pp.1588-1589, ISSN 0006-4971

Terui, T.; Niitsu, Y.; Mahara, K.; Fujisaki, Y.; Urushizaki, Y., et al. (1990) The production of transforming growth factor-β in acute megakaryoblastic leukemia and its possible implications in myelofibrosis. *Blood*, Vol.75, No.7, (Apr 1990), pp.1540-1548, ISSN 0006-4971

Tsang, A. P.; Visvader, J. E.; Turner, C. A.; Fujiwara, Y.; Yu, C., et al. (1997) FOG, a multitype zinc finger protein, acts as a cofactor for transcription factor GATA-1 in erythroid and megakaryocytic differentiation. *Cell*, Vol.90, No.1, (Jul 1997), pp.109- 119, ISSN 0092-8674

Tunstall-Pedoe, O.; Roy, A.; Karadimitris, A.; de la Fuente, J.; Fisk, N. M., et al. (2008) Abnormalities in the myeloid progenitor compartment in Down syndrome fetal liver precede acquisition of *GATA1* mutations. *Blood*, Vol.112, No.12, (Dec 2008), pp.4507-4511, ISSN 1528-0020

Waltzer, L.; Ferjoux, G.; Bataille, L. & Haenlin, M. (2003) Cooperation between the GATA and RUNX factors Serpent and Lozenge during Drosophila hematopoiesis. *EMBO J*, Vol.22, No.24, (Dec 2003), pp.6516-6525, ISSN 0261-4189

Wechsler, J.; Greene, M.; McDevitt, M. A.; Anastasi, J.; Karp, J. E., et al. (2002) Acquired mutations in *GATA1* in the megakaryoblastic leukemia of Down syndrome. *Nat Genet*, Vol.32, No.1, (Sep 2002), pp.148-152, ISSN 1061-4036

Worth, L. L.; Zipursky, A.; Christensen, H. & Tubergen, D. (1999) Transient leukemia with extreme basophilia in a phenotypically normal infant with blast cells containing a pseudodiploid clone, 46,XY i(21)(q10). *J Pediatr Hematol Oncol*, Vol.21, No.1, (Jan-Feb 1999), pp.63-66, ISSN 1077-4114

Xu, G.; Kanezaki, R.; Toki, T.; Watanabe, S.; Takahashi, Y., et al. (2006a) Physical association of the patient-specific *GATA1* mutants with RUNX1 in acute megakaryoblastic leukemia accompanying Down syndrome. *Leukemia*, Vol.20, No.6, (Jun 2006), pp.1002-1008, ISSN 0887-6924

Xu, G.; Kato, K.; Toki, T.; Takahashi, Y.; Terui, K., et al. (2006b) Development of acute megakaryoblastic leukemia from a minor clone in a Down syndrome patient with clinically overt transient myeloproliferative disorder. *J Pediatr Hematol Oncol*, Vol.28, No.10, (Oct 2006), pp.696-698, ISSN 1077-4114

Xu, G.; Nagano, M.; Kanezaki, R.; Toki, T.; Hayashi, Y., et al. (2003) Frequent mutations in the *GATA-1* gene in the transient myeloproliferative disorder of Down syndrome. *Blood*, Vol.102, No.8, (Oct 2003), pp.2960-2968, ISSN 0006-4971

Yagihashi, N.; Watanabe, K. & Yagihashi, S. (1995) Transient abnormal myelopoiesis accompanied by hepatic fibrosis in two infants with Down syndrome. *J Clin Pathol*, Vol.48, No.10, (Oct 1995), pp.973-975, ISSN 0021-9746

Yamashita, N.; Osato, M.; Huang, L.; Yanagida, M.; Kogan, S. C., et al. (2005) Haploinsufficiency of *Runx1/AML1* promotes myeloid features and leukaemogenesis in BXH2 mice. *Br J Haematol*, Vol.131, No.4, (Nov 2005), pp.495-507, ISSN 0007-1048

Yanagida, M.; Osato, M.; Yamashita, N.; Liqun, H.; Jacob, B., et al. (2005) Increased dosage of *Runx1/AML1* acts as a positive modulator of myeloid leukemogenesis in BXH2 mice. *Oncogene*, Vol.24, No.28, (Jun 2005), pp.4477-4485, ISSN 0950-9232

Yumura-Yagi, K.; Hara, J.; Kurahashi, H.; Nishiura, T.; Kaneyama, Y., et al. (1992) Mixed phenotype of blasts in acute megakaryocytic leukaemia and transient abnormal myelopoiesis in Down's syndrome. *Br J Haematol*, Vol.81, No.4, (Aug 1992), pp.520-525, ISSN 0007-1048

Zerres, K.; Schwanitz, G.; Niesen, M.; Gembruch, U.; Hansmann, M., et al. (1990) Prenatal diagnosis of acute non-lymphoblastic leukaemia in Down syndrome. *Lancet*, Vol.335, No.8681, (Jan 1990), pp.117, ISSN 0140-6736

Zipursky, A. (2003) Transient leukaemia--a benign form of leukaemia in newborn infants with trisomy 21. *Br J Haematol*, Vol.120, No.6, (Mar 2003), pp.930-938, ISSN 0007-1048

Zipursky, A.; Brown, E.; Christensen, H.; Sutherland, R. & Doyle, J. (1997) Leukemia and/or myeloproliferative syndrome in neonates with Down syndrome. *Semin Perinatol*, Vol.21, No.1, (Feb 1997), pp.97-101, ISSN 0146-0005

Zipursky, A.; Brown, E. J.; Christensen, H. & Doyle, J. (1999) Transient myeloproliferative disorder (transient leukemia) and hematologic manifestations of Down syndrome. *Clin Lab Med*, Vol.19, No.1, (Mar 1999), pp.157-167, vii, ISSN 0272-2712

Zipursky, A.; Rose, T.; Skidmore, M.; Thorner, P. & Doyle, J. (1996) Hydrops fetalis and neonatal leukemia in Down syndrome. *Pediatr Hematol Oncol*, Vol.13, No.1, (Jan-Feb 1996), pp.81-87, ISSN 0888-0018

Zipursky, A.; Thorner, P.; De Harven, E.; Christensen, H. & Doyle, J. (1994) Myelodysplasia and acute megakaryoblastic leukemia in Down's syndrome. *Leuk Res*, Vol.18, No.3, (Mar 1994), pp.163-171, ISSN 0145-2126

Zwaan, C. M.; Reinhardt, D.; Hitzler, J. & Vyas, P. (2010) Acute leukemias in children with Down syndrome. *Hematol Oncol Clin North Am*, Vol.24, No.1, (Feb 2010), pp.19-34, ISSN 1558-1977

Part 4

Prenatal Diagnosis and Genetic Counselling

8

Innovations in Down Syndrome Screening

Wendy Koster[1,2], Annemieke de Vries[1],
Gerard Visser[2] and Peter Schielen[1]
[1]*National Institute for Public Health and the Environment*
[2]*Department of Obstetrics, University Medical Centre Utrecht*
The Netherlands

1. Introduction

Down syndrome (DS) is the most common chromosomal abnormality, with an incidence of approximately 1 per 500 to 800 live births (Egan et al., 2004). DS is associated with an impairment of cognitive ability and physical growth, and a particular set of facial characteristics. Moreover, about 50% of all people with DS suffer from a congenital heart defect and DS patients are more prone to develop serious illnesses such as Alzheimer's disease, leukaemia and epilepsy. These factors all contribute to a shorter life expectancy.
For decades, people developed methods to prenatally diagnose DS. In this chapter an overview is given of non-invasive screening methods for DS. The research described in this chapter was performed at the Dutch National Institute for Public Health and the Environment (RIVM). The RIVM acts as the reference laboratory for DS screening in the Netherlands and processes over 10,000 first-trimester combined tests per year. The RIVM therefore possesses an extensive collection of sera of pregnant women carrying a foetus with DS and other congenital abnormalities. For our scientific studies, serum samples from this large database were used. The aim of our research was to identify new biochemical screening markers using proteomics techniques to improve the performance of the current DS screening.

2. Down syndrome screening

2.1 A historical perspective of Down syndrome

An accurate phenotypic description of Down syndrome (DS) was published by John Langdon Down in 1866 (Down, 1866). Following descriptions of Esquirol and Séguin (Esquirol, 1838, Séguin, 1846), who wrote about phenotypic differences between mentally retarded humans, Down was the first to make the distinction between the phenotype which is now called DS and other disorders. He made this distinction based on an ethnic classification in which he discerned four types; the Ethiopian type, the Malay type, the American type and the Mongolian type (Down, 1866). Down noticed that the 'mongolism' occurred in more that 10% of all mentally retarded children and that it was always congenital.
At the end of the 19th century, the principle of inheritance was explained by the discovery of chromosomes in living organisms. In 1909, Morgan and colleagues began to study the

chromosomes of *Drosophila* (fruit flies), which were very suitable for genetic studies because they bred quickly and only have four chromosomes. During their experiments it was, among others, discovered that occasionally *Drosophila* possessed three sex chromosomes instead of two showing a pattern of XXY or XYY, an abnormality which they called 'trisomy' (Morgan et al., 1925, Morgan et al., 1915). Since this trisomy occurred when two copies of a chromosome failed to disjoin properly, it was described as non-disjunction.
Somewhat later, in the 1930s, two researchers independently linked non-disjunction to DS. Waardenburg stated that, due to the extended clinical features of humans with DS, the syndrome might very well be caused by something as complicated as a chromosomal disorder (Waardenburg, 1932). Bleyer proposed that DS occurs with fertilization or has already occurred before, during the period of maturation of the ovum or spermatozoon (Bleyer, 1934). Therefore, he thought that a chromosomal abnormality such as non-disjunction was most likely to cause DS.
Finally, in 1959, a few years after it had been established that human tissues normally contain 46 chromosomes, Lejeune and Jacobs independently discovered the presence of an extra chromosome in children with DS (Jacobs et al., 1959, Lejeune et al., 1959). Lejeune suggested, principally based on the *Drosophila* research, that the presence of an extra chromosome could well be explained in terms of non-disjunction. As individual chromosomes were identified, it appeared that the extra chromosome in DS was always the 21st chromosome. Therefore, DS was since then referred to as trisomy 21.

2.2 Prenatal screening for Down syndrome

The discovery of a trisomy of chromosome 21 as the underlying cause for DS and the possibility to perform a chromosome analysis on amniotic fluid allowed for the prenatal diagnosis of DS (Valenti et al., 1968).
In 1966 the first chromosome analysis of amniotic fluid was performed (Steele and Breg, 1966). This development allowed for the prenatal detection of DS, which was first achieved in 1968 (Valenti et al., 1968). The relationship between the risk of having a child with DS and advanced maternal age had been known for a long time (Penrose, 1933, Shuttleworth, 1909). A statistical estimation of this relationship is shown in figure 1. Because of an increased risk of DS, in many countries women above a certain age (usually above 35-38 years) were offered prenatal diagnosis by means of amniocentesis.
In 1972 it was discovered that very high levels of alpha fetoprotein (AFP) were present in the amniotic fluid of women carrying a child with a neural tube defect (NTD) (Brock and Sutcliffe, 1972). Two years later the association between high AFP levels and NTD was also seen in second trimester maternal serum samples (Brock et al., 1974, Wald et al., 1974), allowing for a non-invasive screening method for NTD (Wald et al., 1977). Again a few years later, in 1984, it was found that, in contrast to the elevated AFP levels in NTD pregnancies, decreased maternal serum levels of AFP in the second trimester of pregnancy could be linked to DS (Cuckle et al., 1984, Merkatz et al., 1984). This meant that prenatal screening for NTD could be extended with the screening for DS. This way, women of advanced maternal age could now be offered a screening test before opting for an invasive amniocentesis that bears a certain risk of miscarriage (Eddleman et al., 2006, Odibo et al., 2008).
The discovery of AFP as a second trimester screening marker for DS triggered researchers to look for other potential screening markers to even further improve the prenatal detection by screening. In 1987, two new screening markers were presented. Maternal serum levels of

human chorion gonadotropin (hCG) were shown to be, on average, higher in DS pregnancies (Bogart et al., 1987) while levels of unconjugated estriol (uE_3) were mostly decreased in DS (Canick et al., 1988). A year later, Wald and colleagues reported on a new method of screening using the three biochemical markers (AFP, hCG and uE_3) together with maternal age as parameters in a single test (Wald et al., 1988). This test became known as the 'triple test'. With the triple test 60% of all DS cases could be prenatally detected at a 5% false positive rate (FPR) (Wald et al., 1988), which was a significant improvement compared to the detection of the previous screening method based on maternal age and AFP only (Cuckle et al., 1984). The triple test became increasingly popular as a screening test for DS and started to be carried out routinely in several countries. The most optimal cut-off risk for the screening was calculated to be 1 in 250 (Baumgarten, 1985). During the early 1990s, the triple test was adjusted by the replacement of hCG with the free beta subunit of hCG (fβ-hCG) (Macri et al., 1990, Ryall et al., 1992). Moreover, in 1996, inhibin-A was found to contribute to the current triple test (Wald et al., 1996) and with the addition of inhibin-A the 'quadruple test' was conceived.

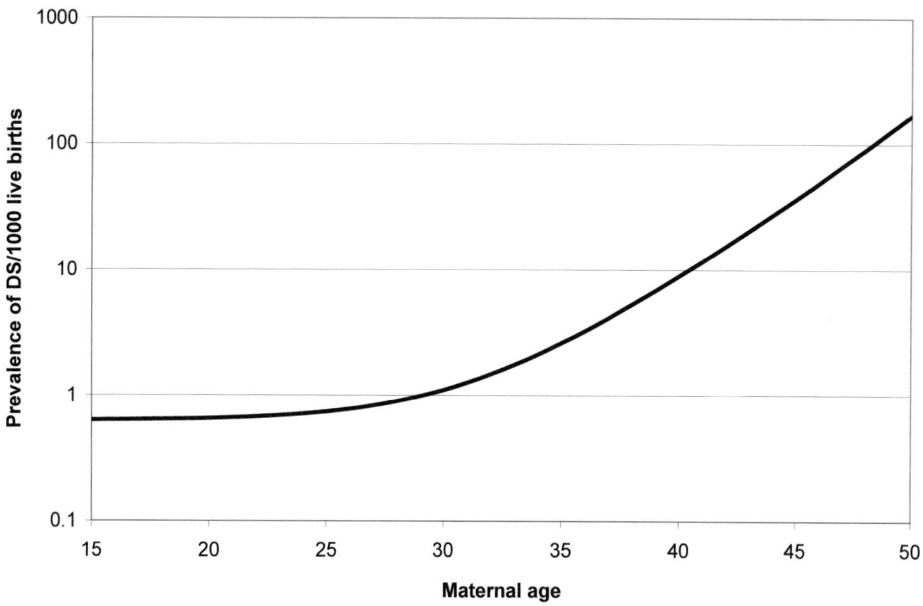

Fig. 1. The relationship between maternal age and the risk of having a child with Down syndrome based on data from Cuckle *et al.* (Cuckle et al., 1987).

In the meantime the focus of prenatal screening for DS shifted more towards the first trimester of pregnancy. This development was in part due to the applicability of chorionic villus sampling, a technique that allows for karyotyping already in the first trimester. Thus, it became possible to detect DS earlier in pregnancy, what subsequently allowed for earlier termination of pregnancy. On the other hand, first trimester screening would not include screening for NTD. However, advanced ultrasound techniques were developed promising high detection rates for NTD in the second trimester.

Except for fβ-hCG (Spencer et al., 1992), the parameters in the current triple test did not perform well in the distinction between DS and euploid pregnancies in the first trimester.

So, to come up with a proper test, new first trimester screening markers were necessary. In 1991, it was found that maternal serum pregnancy associated plasma protein-A (PAPP-A) was reduced about 50% in DS pregnancies (Brambati et al., 1993). Besides PAPP-A, more potential markers were studied (e.g. SP1 (Kornman et al., 1998) and CA125 (Van Lith et al., 1993)), but none of those turned out to be worth adding to the screening test. The search for DS screening markers was not limited to biochemical markers; an enlarged nuchal translucency (NT) on a first trimester ultrasound scan also turned out to be predictive for DS (Nicolaides et al., 1992, Pandya et al., 1994). Combining these three screening markers (fβ-hCG, PAPP-A and NT) with maternal age, using a risk calculation method similar to that of the triple test, originated the 'first trimester combined test' (Wald and Hackshaw, 1997). Over the years, numerous studies have been published showing that with the first trimester combined test approximately 85-90% of all DS cases could be detected at a 5% FPR (Jaques et al., 2007, Nicolaides et al., 2005, Spencer and Nicolaides, 2003, Valinen et al., 2007, Wojdemann et al., 2005).

Under strict guidelines issued by the Dutch Centre for Population Research the first-trimester screening policy for DS was fully implemented in the Netherlands as of January 1, 2007. Since then, all pregnant women are offered such prenatal screening for DS, but the uptake of the test is only 23% (Schielen et al., 2008), which is rather low as compared to other countries. The detection rate (DR) of DS screening in the Netherlands is currently 76% (Wortelboer et al., 2009a).

3. Proteomics techniques to identify new screening markers for Down syndrome

The development of methods for DS screening has so far mainly been based on coincidences. The screening really is a spin-off of the neural tube defect (NTD) screening, and the most effective markers were discovered by fishing expeditions, not by thorough analysis of the causal relationship of genes on chromosome 21 and foetal or placental proteins that are likely to cause an excess or shortage in maternal serum as a result.

A proteome is the entire complement of proteins including the modifications made to a particular set of proteins, produced by an organism or system. Proteomics is the field of research that aims at examination of the proteome in a certain tissue, cell type or body fluid at a certain time point. A plethora of emerging methodological tools allows for the study of proteins, e.g. their quantity, cellular location and post-translational modifications. Understanding the proteome, the structure and function of each protein, and the complexities of protein-interactions during a DS pregnancy may help in the search for additional biomarkers for current first-trimester DS screening.

Our proteomics research consists of three phases (figure 2): i) the discovery of new biomarkers for first-trimester DS screening, ii) the feasibility and validation of proteomics techniques to analyze multiple markers simultaneously, iii) the implementation of a cost-effective assay for large-scale screening programmes.

The presence of an extra chromosome in DS not only leads to anomalies of the foetus, but also of the placenta. In human trophoblast cells, the excess of oxygen radicals produced during oxygen metabolism are eliminated by natural antioxidants and superoxide dismutase (SOD). The gene responsible for this reaction is Zn-SOD and is encoded by chromosome 21. SOD expression and protein levels and activity are significantly higher (about 50%) in trophoblast cells from DS placentas (Pidoux et al., 2004). Over-expression of

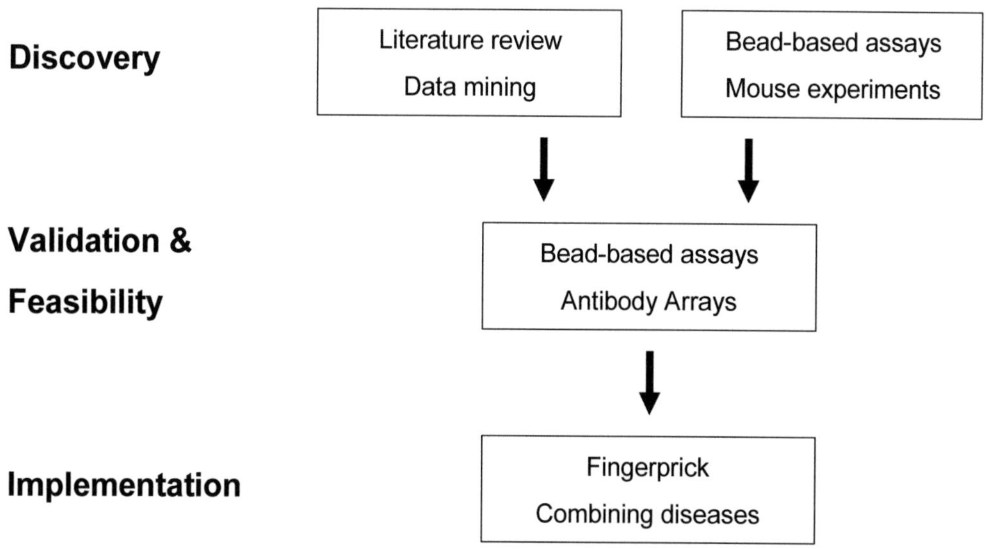

Fig. 2. Three phases of proteomics research for DS screening described in this chapter.

SOD hampers normal trophoblast formation; DS trophoblast cells cannot fully compensate for the reduced oxidative stress resulting in placental abnormalities. DS placentas show signs of impaired differentiation, aggregation and fusion of their trophoblast cells. This could lead to undervascularisation, hypotrophy and cell apoptosis of the placenta already in the first trimester of pregnancy (Koster et al., 2010a). As a result of these pathological changes deregulation and/or differential expression occurs for proteins, e.g. cytokines and growth factors, involved in implantation and placental development (Bromage et al., 2000, Vesce et al., 2002). This may cause an increased or decreased placental expression of biological markers (hormones and proteins). PAPP-A and fβ-hCG, currently used as DS screening markers in the first-trimester combined test, are such markers. PAPP-A is a protein which is thought to be an important regulator of IGF bioavailability and cell growth (Giudice et al., 2002) and fβ-hCG is a subunit of total hCG, which is the most important hormone involved in early pregnancy and provides for the maintenance of the corpus luteum and of pregnancy (Stenman et al., 2006). Based on this knowledge the differential expression of other placenta derived proteins, given that it is traceable in maternal blood, could be used in the search for new screening markers.

In the discovery phase of our research, an extensive review of the literature was carried out to study normal placental development and function during early pregnancy (Koster et al., 2010a). Using this knowledge, candidate biomarkers were proposed which may be useful in screening for DS. Current screening markers for DS indeed mainly originate from the placenta, but can also be traced to the foetal liver, e.g. alpha-fetoprotein (AFP). It is therefore hypothesized that new screening markers may also originate from these tissues. However, a prerequisite of a good screening marker is that concentrations of a protein are detectable in maternal serum. The amount of information on genes and proteins in public databases is increasing rapidly, which allows for a bioinformatics approach that involves automated collection and combination of information from biological databases, known as data mining. A bioinformatics approach was developed to use data from the literature on genes and protein expression and data-textmining tools. This way, a list of 49 potential DS screening markers was generated (Pennings et al., 2009). The list included three biomarkers that are already used for DS screening (AFP, fβ-hCG and PAPP-A) and several others, among which proteins that have been examined as potential biomarkers before. Furthermore, there was a large overlap between the proposed screening markers based on the literature review and the data mining (table 1).

Biomarker discovery research within our proteomics project also included the use of mouse-models for biomarker identification (Pennings et al, 2011). Breeding healthy female mice and male transgenic mice with DS (type Ts(16C-tel)1Cje; The Jackson Laboratory, Bar Harbor, ME, USA) produces healthy females pregnant with, on average, 50% DS embryos. Blood was drawn from the pregnant mice during the first trimester, for the identification of potential screening markers in maternal serum. Then, the pregnancy was terminated and the placenta and foetal organs were collected. Gene profiles were analyzed using a whole genome microarray approach to study the difference between DS and unaffected siblings. Genes that showed over- or underexpression in the placentas of DS foetuses were C2cd2, Dyrk1a, Ifnar2, Morc3, Sfrs15, Sod1, Tmprss2, Fgfbp3. Ongoing research focuses on the serum detectability of these gene products, and their potential as a biomarker for DS screening in human serum.

We continued our search for potential screening markers by examining the proteins that have been suggested as first-trimester screening markers for aneuploidies in international studies. One of those markers is placental protein 13 (PP13) which plays an important role in the implantation and modelling of foetal-maternal blood spaces between placenta and endometrium. PP13 is produced by the placenta, which is hampered in trisomic pregnancies, and was found to be decreased in DS pregnancies and, to greater extent, in trisomy 18 and 13 pregnancies (Akolekar et al., 2010, Koster et al., 2009b). Serum concentrations of a disintegrin and metalloprotease 12 (ADAM12) and placental growth factor (PlGF) are also decreased in DS pregnancies (Wortelboer et al., 2009b, Zaragoza et al., 2009). Total hCG (thCG), which is a screening marker for DS in the second trimester of pregnancy, is increased in maternal serum from first-trimester DS pregnancies (Hallahan et al., 2000). However, when these four markers were added to the current first-trimester combined test algorithm the DR increased by only 3% (table 2a) (Koster et al., 2010d).

These studies show that the predictive power of maternal serum markers is not constant during the first trimester. For three markers (PAPP-A, ADAM12 and PP13) the difference between DS and unaffected pregnancies is more distinct early in the first trimester (before 11 weeks), while for the remaining markers (fβ-hCG, thCG and PlGF) the difference is more pronounced later on (after 11 weeks) (Kuc et al., 2010). Based on this knowledge, it would be useful to draw two separate blood samples (a so-called two-sample combined test) to increase the DR of first-trimester screening to almost 90% at a 5% FPR, which is obviously a tremendous improvement compared to the DR of the current screening program (table 2b). On the other hand, adding new markers to the screening test and taking an extra blood sample bears extra costs and complicates the logistic process of first-trimester screening. A cost-effectiveness analysis is therefore necessary to evaluate the potential of such a two-sample first-trimester screening setting.

A more experimental proteomics approach was carried out by analyzing 90 different proteins from a pre-existing non-pregnancy-specific bead-based multiplexed immunoassay. By comparing the protein concentrations in a small cohort of DS and control sera, seven

Marker	Description	Function	Potential
ADAM12	ADAM metallopeptidase domain 12	* Involved in proteolysis, adhesion, fusion and intracellular signalling * Interacts with IGF binding proteins	biomarker
EGF	Epidermal growth factor (β-urogastrone)	* Promotes differentiation and prevents apoptosis in trophoblasts * Involved in trophoblast invasion and proliferation	examined
hCG	Chorionic gonadotropin	* Glycoprotein hormone that consists of a common α subunit and a unique β subunit * Stimulates the ovaries to synthesize steroids to maintain pregnancy * Involved in trophoblast differentiation and cell aggregation	in use
hPL	Chorionic somatomammotropin hormone 1 (placental lactogen)	* Member of the somatotropin/prolactin family that is expressed mainly in the placenta * Plays an important role in growth control	biomarker
IGF-1	Insulin-like growth factor 1	* Regulates placental growth and transport, trophoblast invasion and placental angiogenesis	examined
IGF-2	Insulin-like growth factor 2	* Has large effects on cell proliferation and differentiation	examined
IGFBP-1	Insulin-like growth factor binding protein 1	* Bind both IGF I and II * Restrict trophoblast invasion	examined
IGFBP-2	Insulin-like growth factor binding protein 2	* Stimulate trophoblast cell migration and invasion	examined
IGFBP-3	Insulin-like growth factor binding protein 3	* Regulate IGF bioavailability and cell growth	examined
IGFBP-4	Insulin-like growth factor binding protein 4		unknown
IGFBP-5	Insulin-like growth factor binding protein 5		unknown
IGFBP-6	Insulin-like growth factor binding protein 6		unknown
IGFBP-7	Insulin-like growth factor binding protein 7		unknown
Leptin	Leptin	* Involved in angiogenesis, growth and immunomodulation * Regulation of foetal and uterine metabolism	examined
MMP-2	Matrix metallopeptidase 2 (gelatinase A)	* Involved in extracellular matrix degeneration in embryonic development, reproduction and tissue remodelling * Play a role in endometrial menstrual breakdown, regulation of vascularization and the inflammatory response	unknown
MMP-9	Matrix metallopeptidase 9 (gelatinase B)	* Regulate several growth factors and cytokines	unknown
PAPP-A	Pregnancy-associated plasma protein A	* Cleaves IGFBPs * Important regulator of IGF bioavailability and cell growth	in use
PGH	Placenta-specific growth hormone	* Member of the somatotropin/prolactin family that is expressed mainly in the placenta * Plays an important role in growth control. * Has a key role in the control of IGF-1 levels	biomarker
PLGF	Placental growth factor	* Mainly involved in angiogenesis * Has an autocrine function in regulating trophoblast function	biomarker
SOD-1	Superoxide dismutase 1	* Binds copper and zinc ions * Responsible for catalyzing free superoxide radicals	examined
TGF-β	Transforming growth factor β 1	* Inhibits cytotrophoblast migration * Decreases trophoblast proliferation * Increases formation of placental giant cells * Regulates many other growth factors	unknown
TIMP-1	Tissue inhibitor of matrix metallopeptidase 1	* Natural inhibitors of MMPs * Promote cell proliferation * Anti-apoptotic function * Suppress endothelial proliferation	unknown
TIMP-2	Tissue inhibitor of matrix metallopeptidase 2	* Maintain tissue homeostasis	unknown
TIMP-3	Tissue inhibitor of matrix metallopeptidase 3	* Regulate platelet aggregation and recruitment	unknown
TIMP-4	Tissue inhibitor of matrix metallopeptidase 4	* Play a role in hormonal regulation and endometrial tissue remodelling	unknown
VEGF	Vascular endothelial growth factor	* Mediates vascular permeability * Induces angiogenesis, vasculogenesis and endothelial cell proliferation	examined

Table 1. Early biomarkers involved in placental development according to a literature study and data-mining. Potential for DS screening is indicated as follows: In use, currently widely used in DS screening; Biomarker, studies showed overall significant concentrations; Examined, examined as biomarker but not significant or inconclusive overall results.

A One-sample test (8-13 wks)	DR at FPR 5%	3%	1%
PAPP-A & fβ-hCG	*77*	*71*	*59*
+ ADAM12	77	72	60
+ thCG	77	71	60
+ PP13	77	71	60
+ PIGF	78	73	61
+ ADAM12, thCG, PP13 & PIGF	**80**	**74**	**63**
+ ADAM12, thCG & PIGF	79	74	62
+ ADAM12 & PIGF	79	73	62

B Two-sample test 1st (8-10 wks)	2nd (11-13 wks)	DR at FPR 5%	3%	1%
PAPP-A	*fβ-hCG*	*83*	*79*	*68*
+ ADAM12		84	80	69
	+ thCG	85	80	70
+ PP13		84	79	69
	+ PIGF	85	80	69
+ ADAM12 & PP13	**+ thCG & PIGF**	**89**	**85**	**75**
+ ADAM12	+ thCG & PLGF	88	84	74
+ ADAM12	+ PIGF	85	81	70

Table 2. Modeled detection rates (DR) at given false positive rates (FPR) for NT at 11-13 weeks and several serum marker combinations in a one-sample (A) or two-sample test (B). Models containing all markers are displayed in bold.

potential screening markers were identified (Koster et al., 2009a): alpha fetoprotein (AFP), epidermal growth factor (EGF), extracellular rage binding protein (EN-RAGE), eotaxin, haptoglobin (HP), insulin (INS) and lipoprotein A (LPA). None of the identified proteins is linked to genes located on chromosome 21. However, some of the markers are known to be highly expressed in the placenta or foetal liver and were also proposed in the candidate biomarker lists from the previously described discovery studies. Unfortunately, none of the seven identified single markers showed significant differences between cases and controls. It might be that biomarkers with large distinctive power were not present on the immunoassay or, alternatively, that fold changes are inherently not high in maternal blood. Interestingly, the addition of the whole panel of seven biomarkers to the current screening test provided a significant improvement of the detection rate for DS.

Despite these promising results, it is obvious that test performance is always better when a screening test is applied to the same cases from which the markers are derived and therefore application of the proposed markers on a different cohort of cases is essential to establish the

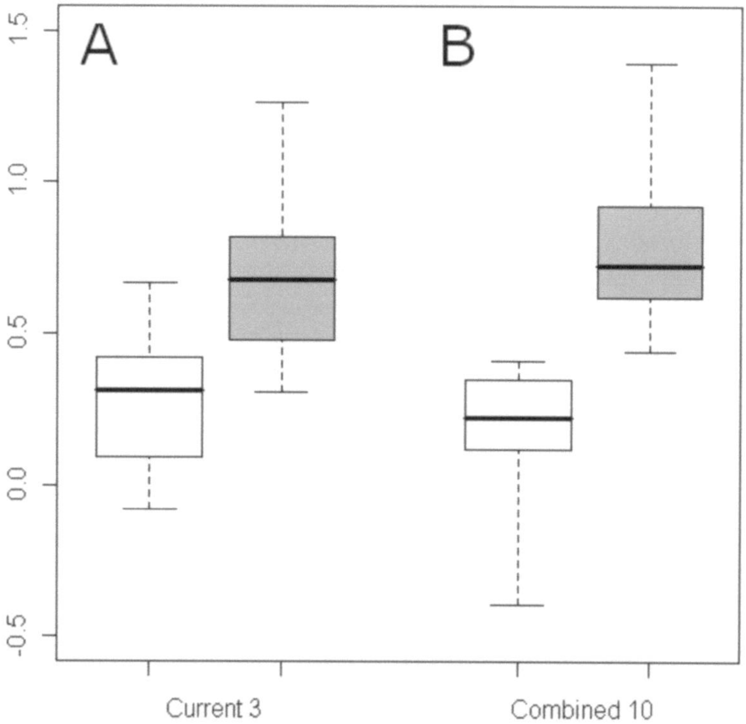

Fig. 2. Boxplots showing the distinction between Down syndrome cases (grey) and the controls (white) by plotting the median, quartiles and minimum/maximum values. (A) Difference between cases and controls when the three current screening markers (PAPP-A, fβ-hCG and NT) are used, (B) Difference between cases and controls when the current three screening markers are combined with the seven newly identified potential biomarkers (AFP, EGF, EN-RAGE, Eotaxin, HP, INS and LPA). Values along the vertical axis indicate prediction scores expressed as arbitrary units.

true diagnostic accuracy of the immunoassay. This was done in a subsequent validation study in which 34 DS cases and matching controls were included to confirm the predictive value of the seven markers found in the discovery study. EGF and EN-RAGE were confirmed to be potential screening markers for DS and improved the DR of the current first-trimester combined test with approximately 6% (table 3) (Koster et al., 2010b). This may seem rather disappointing considering the initial identification of seven potential markers. On the other hand, the finding that two markers again improved the DS screening performance in an independent study is highly encouraging. Clearly, large scale validation experiments need to be performed to provide sufficient evidence for potential markers before they can be implemented in a screening test.

4. Screening for Down syndrome using cell-free foetal DNA/RNA in maternal blood

Currently, not only knowledge to do in-depth evaluations based on proteomic techniques is available, but more and more research focuses on the genomic detection of DS in maternal

markers in the model	DR at a 5% FPR			
	discovery fit + discovery data	discovery fit + validation data	validation fit + discovery data	validation fit + validation data
current screening (PAPP-A, fβ-hCG, NT)	56.2	65.2	39.7	64.0
PAPP-A+ fβ-hCG	38.9	57.1	32.7	57.6
current+AFP	**58.9**	64.1	**40.6**	64.0
current+EGF	**62.6**	**67.1**	**51.7**	**68.0**
current+EN-RAGE	**58.7**	**68.4**	**47.7**	**68.1**
current+Eotaxin	**61.1**	55.8	**40.7**	63.8
current+Haptoglobin	**61.8**	62.3	36.1	**64.2**
current+Insulin	**59.7**	65.2	37.4	63.7
current+LPA	**61.0**	65.0	**51.6**	63.4
10 markers (current + 7 new)	**82.5**	42.4	**59.2**	**71.5**
current+EGF+EN-RAGE	**62.1**	**70.1**	**53.8**	**71.4**

Table 3. Modeled detection rates (DR) at a given 5% false positive rate (FPR) for several marker combinations. Models were fitted based on the data of the discovery study or based on the validation study and tested on both datasets. DRs displayed in bold indicate an improvement compared to the current screening model.

blood. We feel therefore that we should devote a paragraph on the potential value of this technique and its possible role within the screening process. One line of research concerning DS screening tries to put high-end sequencing quantification techniques for DNA and RNA into use to quantify foetal DNA or RNA, either in nuclei of foetal cells or free-floating in maternal serum (Lo, 2000). Non-invasive foetal genotyping became feasible when, foetal DNA was found to constitute approximately 10% of the DNA circulating in the mother's plasma (Lo et al., 1998). However, determination of the maternally inherited alleles was a considerable challenge because the foetal contribution to the plasma DNA can only result in subtle shifts to the total allelic balance, rather than providing a novel allele.

Currently, the most promising technique is so-called massive parallel genomic sequencing. This technique can identify and quantify many DNA fragments in a relatively short time span (Chiu et al., 2008, Fan et al., 2008). Recently, a large-scale study in a high risk cohort was conducted to investigate the performance of massive parallel genomic sequencing in terms of detection and false positive rates. In this study, all DS pregnancies could be identified at a 2.1% false positive rate (Chiu et al., 2011). The authors claim that if such a test would be carried out in all women who initially had a high risk pregnancy (based on first trimester screening), only very few women would need a referral for an invasive diagnostic procedure such as amniocentesis. However, it is unclear how the test would perform in a more representative low-risk pregnant population.

With this promising non-invasive technique, it seems possible to provide definite identification of DS. However, there are still limitations to the technique and some reputable experts in the field have expressed doubts concerning these developments (Community Corner Nature Medicine, 2011). This line of research has been going on for over ten years now; the major technical challenges of sequencing foetal DNA from maternal blood may have been largely solved, but now the practical issues raised by applying this technology need to be addressed. For a diagnostic test, a false positive rate of 2.1% is unacceptable, since it would lead to termination of pregnancy in an equal percentage unaffected pregnancies. For a screening test on the other hand, the technique is still too expensive and time-consuming. And furthermore, if this technique keeps evolving it might even become possible to prenatally offer whole genome sequencing, which obviously raises a complex set of social and ethical issues.

So we feel that, although it is likely that, somewhere in the near future, massive parallel genomic sequencing will be used as an intermediate step in the prenatal detection of DS to decrease the number of invasive procedures such as amniocentesis, the technique is still a long way from implementation in a high-throughput screening setting.

5. Future perspectives and ongoing research

The research described in this chapter focuses on the directive search for new markers for DS using the ever expanding knowledge of the human genome and proteome and combines both laboratory techniques and digital evaluation of data (data mining). The current first trimester combined test is based on enzyme-linked immunosorbent assay (ELISA) methods, which is widely used for quantitative protein measurements. Recently, two-dimensional gel electrophoresis (2-D), tandem mass spectrometry (MS-MS) and bead-based multiplexed immunoassays have been used to identify several potential biomarkers in amniotic fluid and maternal blood (Busch et al., 2005, Kolialexi et al., 2008, Nagalla et al., 2007, Tsangaris et al., 2006), clearly demonstrating the potential of applying proteomics techniques in the quest for new biomarkers. Bead-based multiplexed immunoassays use color-coded tiny beads in up to 100 distinct sets. Coating each bead set with a specific reagent allows the capture and detection of many specific analytes, such as proteins, from a sample. Next, labeled beads are incubated with serum samples and, subsequently, with a detection antibody labeled with a reporter dye in a bead-based immunoassay. Flow cytometry equipment measures the internal dyes to identify each particle and the reporter dye captured during the assay (Krishhan et al., 2009). Another proteomics technique is the use of Antibody microarrays (Ab-arrays). Ab-arrays are a platform for protein expression profiling. Small amounts of capture antibodies for the selected targets are immobilized or spotted on a very small area on coated glass slides. The high density of the capture antibodies in the spots that is obtained enables high sensitivity (Ekins, 1989). These technologies allow analyzing many unique markers within a single sample, both rapidly and precisely, in a high-throughput setting. In the boost of new development the question arises whether these advanced detection techniques will be available at a reasonable cost, a prerequisite for screening tests. In principle however, Ab-array techniques are calculated to cost within the range of 20-50 Euros per screening.

In recent years, the focus of prenatal screening has expanded. Several studies have been performed to evaluate the potential of prenatal screening for foetal chromosomal abnormalities other than DS, in particular Edwards syndrome (trisomy 18) and Patau syndrome (trisomy 13). With the first-trimester combined test it is possible to detect these trisomies using the same algorithm as for DS screening (Spencer et al., 2000, Tul et al., 1999). In trisomy 18 and 13 pregnancies PAPP-A levels are decreased to a greater extent than in DS and the NT is often very large. However, as opposed to DS, serum concentrations of fβ-hCG are decreased in trisomy 18 and 13 pregnancies. Thus, with a slight adjustment of the DS risk calculation, it would be possible to provide separate risks specifically for trisomy 18 and 13. This would lead to the detection of many trisomy 18 and 13 cases with only 0.2% extra false positives (Koster et al., 2010c).

This spin-off of the current proteomics project may have opened a completely new field of research. Currently, a similar approach has been set up to identify potential screening markers for pregnancy complications such as pre-eclampsia (PE), intrauterine growth restriction and foetal death. PE is a serious complication of pregnancy that affects approximately 1-2% of all pregnant women and it is the leading cause of maternal and perinatal morbidity and mortality (Gaugler-Senden et al., 2006). Because of the serious health consequences of PE, risk assessment for PE is highly recommended. Early identification of women at risk might facilitate better antenatal surveillance, timely intervention and better outcomes.

Especially new proteomic techniques will need only minute amounts of test material; 10-20 micro-litres serum instead of 1-2 ml. Hypothetically, this downscaling opens the possibility to draw small amounts of blood and to replace the relatively laborious venous puncture with a finger prick. Our first studies comparing venous blood with capillary blood (derived from a finger prick), drawn at the same time from pregnant women, indeed show that capillary blood can be reliably used to determine the currently used biomarkers in serum. The laboratory will be able to analyze a combination of approximately ten markers. Based on these developments, it must surely be possible to detect, in the same samples, all parameters of prenatal screening (e.g. irregular blood types and infectious diseases, like HIV and hepatitis) and to identify high risks for foetal (e.g. chromosomal abnormalities) and maternal (e.g. pre-eclampsia) pregnancy complications.

In the next coming years, the outline of such a future prenatal screening is feasible, however; it will probably take some time before these methods can be tested in large cohorts that proof their efficacy as a screening tool, a bare necessity before actual implementation can take place.

6. Conclusion

It is anticipated that the introduction of a new screening method consists of a discovery phase, taking 1-3 years, a validation phase, taking 2-5 years, and an implementation phase, taking 5-7 years. This means that of all of the discoveries presented in this paper, which are clearly done in the realm of the discovery phase, very few will make it to becoming an element of an implemented screening test. While we cannot predict what the prenatal screening test for Down syndrome, other aneuplodies and foetal and maternal health will be in ten years time, we can state that it will not be the first trimester combined test. The past decades have learned sufficiently that the screening tests, while not being volatile, are liable to changes, and this will not stop in the next years. It is safe to say that the future test will use the complete array of proteomics, genomics and ultrasound markers, to provide a continuum of tests, with the sole purpose of improving in general the outcome of pregnancies, including the health perspective of the mother, worldwide.

7. Acknowledgments

This chapter is based on research described in PhD-thesis "Innovations in Down syndrome screening" by M.P.H. Koster, Utrecht University, the Netherlands; 2010. ISBN: 978-90-5335-305-9 [dissertation]. The authors would like to thank everyone who contributed to this research: Idder Belmouden, Bert Elvers, José Ferreira, Gert-Jan Gödeke, Kirsten Heetkamp, Sandra Imholz, Mark Jonker, Gerard Loeber, Jeroen Pennings, Johan Reimerink, Wendy

Rodenburg and Conny van Oostrom at the National Insititute for Public Health and the Environment; Sylwia Kuc, Philip Stoutenbeek and Esther Wortelboer at the Department of Obstetrics of the University Medical Centre Utrecht; Howard Cuckle at Columbia University, New York, USA.

8. References

Akolekar, R., Perez Penco, J. M., Skyfta, E., Rodriguez Calvo, J. & Nicolaides, K. H. 2010. Maternal serum placental protein 13 at eleven to thirteen weeks in chromosomally abnormal pregnancies. *Fetal Diagn Ther,* 27, 72-7.

Baumgarten, A. 1985. AFP screening and Down syndrome. *Lancet,* 1, 751.

Bleyer, A. 1934. Indications that mongoloid imbecility is a gametic mutation of degressive type. *Amer J Dis Child,* 47, 342-348.

Bogart, M. H., Pandian, M. R. & Jones, O. W. 1987. Abnormal maternal serum chorionic gonadotropin levels in pregnancies with fetal chromosome abnormalities. *Prenat Diagn,* 7, 623-30.

Brambati, B., Macintosh, M. C., Teisner, B., Maguiness, S., Shrimanker, K., Lanzani, A., Bonacchi, I., Tului, L., Chard, T. & Grudzinskas, J. G. 1993. Low maternal serum levels of pregnancy associated plasma protein A (PAPP-A) in the first trimester in association with abnormal fetal karyotype. *Br J Obstet Gynaecol,* 100, 324-6.

Brock, D. J., Bolton, A. E. & Scrimgeour, J. B. 1974. Prenatal diagnosis of spina bifida and anencephaly through maternal plasma-alpha-fetoprotein measurement. *Lancet,* 1, 767-9.

Brock, D. J. & Sutcliffe, R. G. 1972. Alpha-fetoprotein in the antenatal diagnosis of anencephaly and spina bifida. *Lancet,* 2, 197-9.

Bromage, S. J., Lang, A. K., Atkinson, I. & Searle, R. F. 2000. Abnormal TGFbeta levels in the amniotic fluid of Down syndrome pregnancies. *Am J Reprod Immunol,* 44, 205-10.

Busch, A., Michel, S., Hoppe, C., Driesch, D., Claussen, U. & Von Eggeling, F. 2005. Proteome analysis of maternal serum samples for trisomy 21 pregnancies using ProteinChip arrays and bioinformatics. *J Histochem Cytochem,* 53, 341-3.

Canick, J. A., Knight, G. J., Palomaki, G. E., Haddow, J. E., Cuckle, H. S. & Wald, N. J. 1988. Low second trimester maternal serum unconjugated oestriol in pregnancies with Down's syndrome. *Br J Obstet Gynaecol,* 95, 330-3.

Chiu, R. W., Akolekar, R., Zheng, Y. W., Leung, T. Y., Sun, H., Chan, K. C., Lun, F. M., Go, A. T., Lau, E. T., To, W. W., Leung, W. C., Tang, R. Y., Au-Yeung, S. K., Lam, H., Kung, Y. Y., Zhang, X., Van Vugt, J. M., Minekawa, R., Tang, M. H., Wang, J., Oudejans, C. B., Lau, T. K., Nicolaides, K. H. & Lo, Y. M. 2011. Non-invasive prenatal assessment of trisomy 21 by multiplexed maternal plasma DNA sequencing: large scale validity study. *Bmj,* 342, c7401.

Chiu, R. W., Chan, K. C., Gao, Y., Lau, V. Y., Zheng, W., Leung, T. Y., Foo, C. H., Xie, B., Tsui, N. B., Lun, F. M., Zee, B. C., Lau, T. K., Cantor, C. R. & Lo, Y. M. 2008. Noninvasive prenatal diagnosis of fetal chromosomal aneuploidy by massively parallel genomic sequencing of DNA in maternal plasma. *Proc Natl Acad Sci U S A,* 105, 20458-63.

Community Corner: Opening the Pandora's box of prenatal genetic testing. *Nat Med,* 17, 250-1.

Cuckle, H. S., Wald, N. J. & Lindenbaum, R. H. 1984. Maternal serum alpha-fetoprotein measurement: a screening test for Down syndrome. *Lancet,* 1, 926-9.

Cuckle, H. S., Wald, N. J. & Thompson, S. G. 1987. Estimating a woman's risk of having a pregnancy associated with Down's syndrome using her age and serum alpha-fetoprotein level. *Br J Obstet Gynaecol,* 94, 387-402.

Down, J. L. 1866. Observations on an ethnic classification of idiots. *Lond Hosp Clin Lect Rep,* 3, 259-262.

Eddleman, K. A., Malone, F. D., Sullivan, L., Dukes, K., Berkowitz, R. L., Kharbutli, Y., Porter, T. F., Luthy, D. A., Comstock, C. H., Saade, G. R., Klugman, S., Dugoff, L., Craigo, S. D., Timor-Tritsch, I. E., Carr, S. R., Wolfe, H. M. & D'alton, M. E. 2006. Pregnancy loss rates after midtrimester amniocentesis. *Obstet Gynecol,* 108, 1067-72.

Egan, J. F., Benn, P. A., Zelop, C. M., Bolnick, A., Gianferrari, E. & Borgida, A. F. 2004. Down syndrome births in the United States from 1989 to 2001. *Am J Obstet Gynecol,* 191, 1044-8.

Ekins, R. P. 1989. Multi-analyte immunoassay. *J Pharm Biomed Anal,* 7, 155-68.

Esquirol, J. E. D. 1838. Des maladies mentales considérées sous les rapports médical, hygiénique et médico-légal. *Paris: JB Baillière.*

Fan, H. C., Blumenfeld, Y. J., Chitkara, U., Hudgins, L. & Quake, S. R. 2008. Noninvasive diagnosis of fetal aneuploidy by shotgun sequencing DNA from maternal blood. *Proc Natl Acad Sci U S A,* 105, 16266-71.

Gaugler-Senden, I. P., Huijssoon, A. G., Visser, W., Steegers, E. A. & De Groot, C. J. 2006. Maternal and perinatal outcome of preeclampsia with an onset before 24 weeks' gestation. Audit in a tertiary referral center. *Eur J Obstet Gynecol Reprod Biol,* 128, 216-21.

Giudice, L. C., Conover, C. A., Bale, L., Faessen, G. H., Ilg, K., Sun, I., Imani, B., Suen, L. F., Irwin, J. C., Christiansen, M., Overgaard, M. T. & Oxvig, C. 2002. Identification and regulation of the IGFBP-4 protease and its physiological inhibitor in human trophoblasts and endometrial stroma: evidence for paracrine regulation of IGF-II bioavailability in the placental bed during human implantation. *J Clin Endocrinol Metab,* 87, 2359-66.

Hallahan, T., Krantz, D., Orlandi, F., Rossi, C., Curcio, P., Macri, S., Larsen, J., Buchanan, P. & Macri, J. 2000. First trimester biochemical screening for Down syndrome: free beta hCG versus intact hCG. *Prenat Diagn,* 20, 785-9;discussion 790-1.

Jacobs, P. A., Baikie, A. G., Court Brown, W. M. & Strong, J. A. 1959. The somatic chromosomes in Mongolism. *Lancet,* 1, 710.

Jaques, A. M., Halliday, J. L., Francis, I., Bonacquisto, L., Forbes, R., Cronin, A. & Sheffield, L. J. 2007. Follow up and evaluation of the Victorian first-trimester combined screening programme for Down syndrome and trisomy 18. *BJOG,* 114, 812-8.

Kolialexi, A., Tsangaris, G. T., Papantoniou, N., Anagnostopoulos, A. K., Vougas, K., Bagiokos, V., Antsaklis, A. & Mavrou, A. 2008. Application of proteomics for the identification of differentially expressed protein markers for Down syndrome in maternal plasma. *Prenat Diagn,* 28, 691-8.

Kornman, L. H., Morssink, L. P., Ten Hoor, K. A., De Wolf, B. T., Kloosterman, M. D., Beekhuis, J. R. & Mantingh, A. 1998. Schwangerschafts protein 1 (SP1) adds little to the age-related detection of fetal Down syndrome in the first trimester of pregnancy. *Prenat Diagn,* 18, 1086-90.

Koster, M. P., Heetkamp, K. M., Pennings, J. L., De Vries, A., Visser, G. H. & Schielen, P. C. 2010a. Down syndrome screening: imagining the screening test of the future. *Expert Rev Mol Diagn,* 10, 445-57.

Koster, M. P., Pennings, J. L., Imholz, S., Rodenburg, W., Visser, G. H., De Vries, A. & Schielen, P. C. 2009a. Bead-based multiplexed immunoassays to identify new biomarkers in maternal serum to improve first trimester Down syndrome screening. *Prenat Diagn,* 29, 857-62.

Koster, M. P., Pennings, J. L., Imholz, S., Rodenburg, W., Visser, G. H., De Vries, A. & Schielen, P. C. 2010b. Proteomics and Down syndrome screening: a validation study. *Prenat Diagn,* 30, 1039-43.

Koster, M. P., Stoutenbeek, P., Visser, G. H. & Schielen, P. C. 2010c. Trisomy 18 and 13 screening: consequences for the Dutch Down syndrome screening programme. *Prenat Diagn,* 30, 287-9.

Koster, M. P., Wortelboer, E. J., Cuckle, H. S., Stoutenbeek, P., Visser, G. H. & Schielen, P. C. 2009b. Placental protein 13 as a first trimester screening marker for aneuploidy. *Prenat Diagn,* 29, 1237-41.

Koster, M. P., Wortelboer, E. J., Stoutenbeek, P., Visser, G. H. & Schielen, P. C. 2010d. Modeling the Down syndrome screening performance using first trimester serum markers. *Ultrasound Obstet Gynecol.*

Krishhan, V. V., Khan, I. H. & Luciw, P. A. 2009. Multiplexed microbead immunoassays by flow cytometry for molecular profiling: Basic concepts and proteomics applications. *Crit Rev Biotechnol,* 29, 29-43.

Kuc, S., Koster, M. P., Visser, G. H. & Schielen, P. C. 2010. Performance of first-trimester serum screening for trisomy 21 before and from 11 + 0 weeks of gestational age in The Netherlands. *Prenat Diagn,* 30, 906-8.

Lejeune, J., Gautier, M. & Turpin, R. 1959. Étude des chromosomes somatiques de neuf enfants mongoliens. *CR Acad Sci,* 248, 1721-1722.

Lo, Y. M. 2000. Fetal DNA in maternal plasma. *Ann N Y Acad Sci,* 906, 141-7.

Lo, Y. M., Tein, M. S., Lau, T. K., Haines, C. J., Leung, T. N., Poon, P. M., Wainscoat, J. S., Johnson, P. J., Chang, A. M. & Hjelm, N. M. 1998. Quantitative analysis of fetal DNA in maternal plasma and serum: implications for noninvasive prenatal diagnosis. *Am J Hum Genet,* 62, 768-75.

Macri, J. N., Kasturi, R. V., Krantz, D. A., Cook, E. J., Moore, N. D., Young, J. A., Romero, K. & Larsen, J. W., Jr. 1990. Maternal serum Down syndrome screening: free beta-protein is a more effective marker than human chorionic gonadotropin. *Am J Obstet Gynecol,* 163, 1248-53.

Merkatz, I. R., Nitowsky, H. M., Macri, J. N. & Johnson, W. E. 1984. An association between low maternal serum alpha-fetoprotein and fetal chromosomal abnormalities. *Am J Obstet Gynecol,* 148, 886-94.

Morgan, T. H., Bridges, C. B. & Sturtevant, A. H. 1925. The genetics of Drosophila. *The Hague: M Nijhoff.*

Morgan, T. H., Sturtevant, A. H., Muller, H. J. & Bridges, C. B. 1915. The mechanism of Mendelian heredity. *London: Constable,* 149-50.

Nagalla, S. R., Canick, J. A., Jacob, T., Schneider, K. A., Reddy, A. P., Thomas, A., Dasari, S., Lu, X., Lapidus, J. A., Lambert-Messerlian, G. M., Gravett, M. G., Roberts, C. T., Jr., Luthy, D., Malone, F. D. & D'alton, M. E. 2007. Proteomic analysis of maternal serum in down syndrome: identification of novel protein biomarkers. *J Proteome Res,* 6, 1245-57.

Nicolaides, K. H., Azar, G., Byrne, D., Mansur, C. & Marks, K. 1992. Fetal nuchal translucency: ultrasound screening for chromosomal defects in first trimester of pregnancy. *BMJ,* 304, 867-9.

Nicolaides, K. H., Spencer, K., Avgidou, K., Faiola, S. & Falcon, O. 2005. Multicenter study of first-trimester screening for trisomy 21 in 75 821 pregnancies: results and estimation of the potential impact of individual risk-orientated two-stage first-trimester screening. *Ultrasound Obstet Gynecol,* 25, 221-6.

Odibo, A. O., Gray, D. L., Dicke, J. M., Stamilio, D. M., Macones, G. A. & Crane, J. P. 2008. Revisiting the fetal loss rate after second-trimester genetic amniocentesis: a single center's 16-year experience. *Obstet Gynecol,* 111, 589-95.

Pandya, P. P., Brizot, M. L., Kuhn, P., Snijders, R. J. & Nicolaides, K. H. 1994. First-trimester fetal nuchal translucency thickness and risk for trisomies. *Obstet Gynecol,* 84, 420-3.

Pennings, J. L., Koster, M. P., Rodenburg, W., Schielen, P. C. & De Vries, A. 2009. Discovery of novel serum biomarkers for prenatal Down syndrome screening by integrative data mining. *PLoS One,* 4, e8010.

Pennings, J.L., Rodenburg, W., Imholz, S., Koster, M.P., van Oostrom, C.T., Breit, T.M., Schielen, P.C. & de Vries, A. Gene expression profiling identifies new liver-derived potential biomarkers for Down syndrome screening. *Plos One* [in press].

Penrose, L. S. 1933. The relative effects of paternal and maternal age in mongolism. *J Genet,* 27, 219.

Pidoux, G., Guibourdenche, J., Frendo, J. L., Gerbaud, P., Conti, M., Luton, D., Muller, F. & Evain-Brion, D. 2004. Impact of trisomy 21 on human trophoblast behaviour and hormonal function. *Placenta,* 25 Suppl A, S79-84.

Ryall, R. G., Staples, A. J., Robertson, E. F. & Pollard, A. C. 1992. Improved performance in a prenatal screening programme for Down's syndrome incorporating serum-free hCG subunit analyses. *Prenat Diagn,* 12, 251-61.

Schielen, P. C., Koster, M. P., Elvers, L. H. & Loeber, J. G. 2008. First trimester combined test screening for Down's syndrome 2004-2006. *RIVM report 230024002/2008.*

Séguin, E. 1846. Le traitement moral, l'hygiène et l'éducation des idiots et des autres enfants arrières. *Paris: JB Baillière.*

Shuttleworth, G. E. 1909. Mongolian imbecility. *Brit Med J,* 2, 661-665.

Spencer, K., Macri, J. N., Aitken, D. A. & Connor, J. M. 1992. Free beta-hCG as first-trimester marker for fetal trisomy. *Lancet,* 339, 1480.

Spencer, K. & Nicolaides, K. H. 2003. Screening for trisomy 21 in twins using first trimester ultrasound and maternal serum biochemistry in a one-stop clinic: a review of three years experience. *BJOG,* 110, 276-80.

Spencer, K., Ong, C., Skentou, H., Liao, A. W. & K, H. N. 2000. Screening for trisomy 13 by fetal nuchal translucency and maternal serum free beta-hCG and PAPP-A at 10-14 weeks of gestation. *Prenat Diagn,* 20, 411-6.

Steele, M. W. & Breg, W. R., Jr. 1966. Chromosome analysis of human amniotic-fluid cells. *Lancet,* 1, 383-5.

Stenman, U. H., Tiitinen, A., Alfthan, H. & Valmu, L. 2006. The classification, functions and clinical use of different isoforms of HCG. *Hum Reprod Update,* 12, 769-84.

Tsangaris, G. T., Karamessinis, P., Kolialexi, A., Garbis, S. D., Antsaklis, A., Mavrou, A. & Fountoulakis, M. 2006. Proteomic analysis of amniotic fluid in pregnancies with Down syndrome. *Proteomics,* 6, 4410-9.

Tul, N., Spencer, K., Noble, P., Chan, C. & Nicolaides, K. 1999. Screening for trisomy 18 by fetal nuchal translucency and maternal serum free beta-hCG and PAPP-A at 10-14 weeks of gestation. *Prenat Diagn,* 19, 1035-42.

Valenti, C., Schutta, E. J. & Kehaty, T. 1968. Prenatal diagnosis of Down's syndrome. *Lancet,* 2, 220.

Valinen, Y., Rapakko, K., Kokkonen, H., Laitinen, P., Tekay, A., Ahola, T. & Ryynanen, M. 2007. Clinical first-trimester routine screening for Down syndrome in singleton pregnancies in northern Finland. *Am J Obstet Gynecol,* 196, 278 e1-5.

Van Lith, J. M., Mantingh, A. & De Bruijn, H. W. 1993. Maternal serum CA 125 levels in pregnancies with chromosomally-normal and -abnormal fetuses. Dutch Working Party on Prenatal Diagnosis. *Prenat Diagn,* 13, 1123-31.

Vesce, F., Scapoli, C., Giovannini, G., Tralli, L., Gotti, G., Valerio, A. & Piffanelli, A. 2002. Cytokine imbalance in pregnancies with fetal chromosomal abnormalities. *Hum Reprod,* 17, 803-8.

Waardenburg, P. J. 1932. Das menschliche Auge und seine Erbanlagen. *The Hague: M Nijhoff.*

Wald, N. J., Brock, D. J. & Bonnar, J. 1974. Prenatal diagnosis of spina bifida and anencephaly by maternal serum-alpha-fetoprotein measurement. A controlled study. *Lancet,* 1, 765-7.

Wald, N. J., Cuckle, H., Brock, J. H., Peto, R., Polani, P. E. & Woodford, F. P. 1977. Maternal serum-alpha-fetoprotein measurement in antenatal screening for anencephaly and spina bifida in early pregnancy. Report of U.K. collaborative study on alpha-fetoprotein in relation to neural-tube defects. *Lancet,* 1, 1323-32.

Wald, N. J., Cuckle, H. S., Densem, J. W., Nanchahal, K., Royston, P., Chard, T., Haddow, J. E., Knight, G. J., Palomaki, G. E. & Canick, J. A. 1988. Maternal serum screening for Down's syndrome in early pregnancy. *BMJ,* 297, 883-7.

Wald, N. J., Densem, J. W., George, L., Muttukrishna, S. & Knight, P. G. 1996. Prenatal screening for Down's syndrome using inhibin-A as a serum marker. *Prenat Diagn,* 16, 143-53.

Wald, N. J. & Hackshaw, A. K. 1997. Combining ultrasound and biochemistry in first-trimester screening for Down's syndrome. *Prenat Diagn,* 17, 821-9.

Wojdemann, K. R., Shalmi, A. C., Christiansen, M., Larsen, S. O., Sundberg, K., Brocks, V., Bang, J., Norgaard-Pedersen, B. & Tabor, A. 2005. Improved first-trimester Down syndrome screening performance by lowering the false-positive rate: a prospective study of 9941 low-risk women. *Ultrasound Obstet Gynecol,* 25, 227-33.

Wortelboer, E. J., Koster, M. P., Stoutenbeek, P., Elvers, L. H., Loeber, J. G., Visser, G. H. & Schielen, P. C. 2009a. First-trimester Down syndrome screening performance in the Dutch population; how to achieve further improvement? *Prenat Diagn,* 29, 588-92.

Wortelboer, E. J., Linskens, I. H., Koster, M. P., Stoutenbeek, P., Cuckle, H., Blankenstein, M. A., Visser, G. H., Van Vugt, J. M. & Schielen, P. C. 2009b. ADAM12s as a first-trimester screening marker of trisomy. *Prenat Diagn,* 29, 866-9.

Zaragoza, E., Akolekar, R., Poon, L. C., Pepes, S. & Nicolaides, K. H. 2009. Maternal serum placental growth factor at 11-13 weeks in chromosomally abnormal pregnancies. *Ultrasound Obstet Gynecol,* 33, 382-6.

9

Early Diagnosis of Congenital Heart Disease in the Neonatal Period

Alfonso Ortigado
Pediatric Cardiology, Guadalajara Hospital, University of Alcala
Spain

1. Introduction

Congenital heart disease (CHD) is present in 40-60% of children with Down syndrome (DS) and it is the principal variable that determines the morbimortality during the first two years of life of these patients.

Advances in fetal echocardiography are providing highly accurate diagnoses of congenital heart disease prior to delivery, making it possible to plan the delivery-room management of these newborns. However, the majority of neonates who have congenital heart disease will not require delivery room resuscitation in excess of routine care.

Although cardiovascular evaluation is a standard component of the diagnostic work-up in patients with Down syndrome, physical examination alone does not predict the presence or absence of congenital heart disease en the neonatl period. The changeover of fetal to neonatal circulation with the decrease in pulmonary vascular resistance (increase in pulmonary blood flow), the increase in systemic vascular resistance (the lower-resistance placenta is excluded from the circulation) and the timing of functional closure of the ductus arteriosus may determine the clinical presentation.

As physical examination alone is not sufficient to identify cardiovascular anomalies in neonates with Down syndrome and the early detection can improve the outcome of congenital heart defects, we need a newborn screening strategy, because failure to recognise these defects early in life can have serious consequences. Echocardiographic examination provides extensive anatomic and hemodynamic information noninvasively, in real time, and at relatively low cost. A routine echocardiography should be performed in this population in the neonatal period.

The aims of this chapter are:

1. Congenital heart disease in Down syndrome.
2. Normal and pathologic transitional circulation.
3. Correlation between cardiac physical examination and echocardiography.
4. Potential benefits of early diagnosis.

2. Congenital heart disease in Down syndrome

The association between DS and CHD has been well established since 1950, when the incidence and type of CHD present in newborns and infants with SD was thoroughly described (Evans, 1950)

In general population, CHD is one of the most common serious congenital anomalies, with an incidence about 1%occurring in up to 2% of liveborn children, and in an even higher percentage of fetuses. Children with DS have an increased incidence of CHD, 40%-60% is the range described in the world literature. The life expectancy of children with DS depends primarily on the risk of mortality in the first year of life and CHD is the major cause of mortality during the postneonatal period with 70% of cases (Weijerman et al, 2008)
Nevertheless, there are several factors that influence to determine the true incidence on CHD. Many forms of CHD are now detected by fetal echocardiography with early prenatal diagnosis of chromosomal abnormalities, and the parents may choose to abort these fetuses. Fetal echocardiography has shown that certain ventricular septal defects, may be detected in utero but have disappeared at the time of birth or within 6-12 months after. Studies using neonatal echocardiography have shown prevalence of muscular ventricular defect as high as 53 per 1000 live births, most babies were asymptomatic and most defects were small with early spontaneous closure rate of 89% within 1 to 10 months. These muscular ventricular defects may result from delayed physiologic development rather than from disease (Roguin et al, 1995). If they are not all included, this leads to the underestimation of the true incidence.
In general population, ventricular septal defects are the most common form of CHD, accounting for approximately 30%, but in DS patients, the endocardial cushion defect, also known as atrioventricular septal defects (AVSD), is the leading type, up to 40%(fig.1), followed in frecuency by ventricular septal defect (fig.2), atrial septal defect, patent ductus arteriosus and tetralogy of Fallot. Recent reports have shown that te distribution of congenital heart disease in children with DS may vary with ethnicity (De Rubens et al, 2003). Atrioventricular septal defects show the most significant sex and ethnic differences with twice as many affected females, and compared with whites, twice as many blacks, and half as many Hispanics (Freeman et al, 2008).

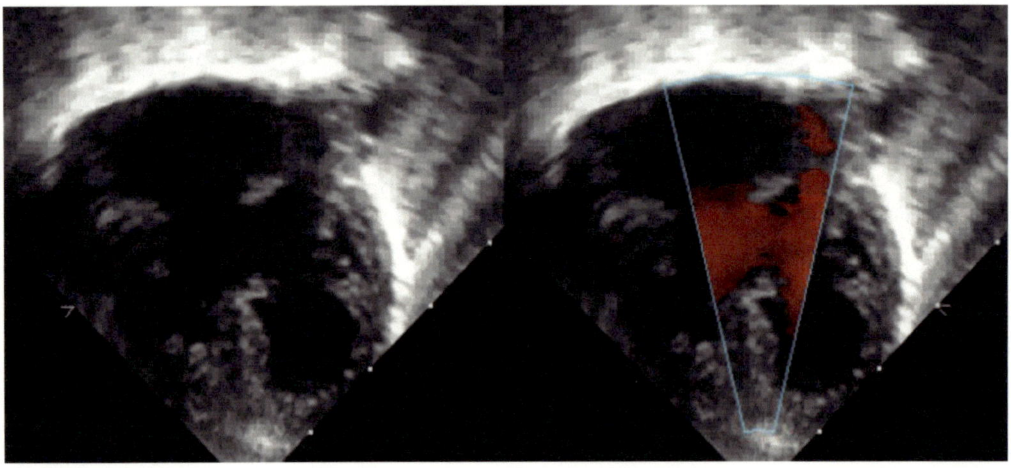

Fig. 1. Echocardiographic s apical four-chamber image demonstrating a complete atrioventricular septal defect (laminar flow without aliasing).

AVSD is caused by abnormal embryologic development of endocardial cushions and the bulboventricular fold. AVSD can be complete (common atrioventricular canal) , partial (atrial septal defect of the ostium primum type or cleft anterior mitral leaflet) or intermediate form. Complete AVSD is characterized by the presence of a common atrioventricular orifice, an interatrial communication and a ventricular septal defect. In partial AVSD, also referred to as primum type atrial septal defect, the superior and inferior bridging leaflets arae connected bya a fibrous continuity in two functionally separate right and left atrioventricular orifices, and are firmly attached to the deficient septal crest, and the interventricualr communication is lacking. The intermediate form is defined as having a "scooped out" interventricular septum with the atrioventricular valves being connected to the top of the septum by fibrous tissue "curtains" and tendinous chordae, consequentelly resulting in a small or absent ventricular septal defect component (Hoohenkerk al, 2010).

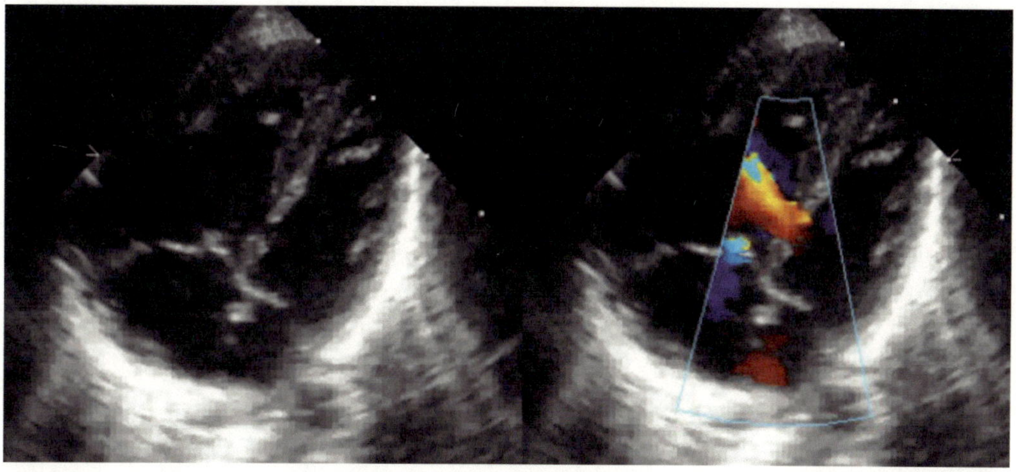

Fig. 2. Echocardiographic apical four-chamber image demonstrating a ventricular septal defect (turbulent flow with aliasing).

Complete AVSD is associated with DS (60-86%) and clinically relevant differences have been identified in children with and without DS. Thus, left-side obstructions and right ventricular dominance, as well as left atrioventricular valve abnormalities such as double orifice valve and single papillary muscle, seem to be more prevalent in children with a normal chromosomal pattern, whereas Rastelli types B and C are more often found in patients with DS. Early progression of pulmonary vascular obstructive disease has been reported especially in patients with AVSD and DS (Lange et al, 2007).

AVSD can be complete (common atrioventricular canal), partial (atrial septal defect of the ostium primum type or cleft anterior mitral leaflet) or intermediate form, it can be isolated or combined with other cardiac anomalies, such as tetralogy of Fallot. Conversely, approximately 80% of all AVSD occur in children with DS.

Left-side obstructive defects such as coarctation of aorte and valvar aortic stenosis are rare, and transposition of the great arteries has not been reported in Down syndrome.

Many chromosomal syndromes are associated with a variety of CHD. Several of theses syndromes show a fixed pattern of CHD, such as 22q11-deletion syndrome, Noonan syndrome, Turner syndrome and Williams syndrome. Down syndrome also shows a fixed patern of CHD, with overrepresentation of septal defects and undrerepresentation of left-side obstructive defects and transposition of the great vessels. This observation, indicates that a locus on chromosome 21 is involved in the development of CHD. Althoug no single gene candidate has yet been identified to be responsible for this phenotype, genes for several matrix-related proteins (alfa-1 and alfa-2 type VI collagen, Down´s Syndrome Cell Adhesion Molecule, integrin beta-2 and alfa-1 XVIII collagen) are located on chromosome 21. Overexpression of type VI collagen has been suggested to play a role in the pathogenesis of atrioventricular septal defects in DS (Vis et al, 2009).

3. Normal and pathologic transitional circulation.

The pulmonary circulation undergoes a near-instantaneous change from its high resistance state in utero to a low resistance circuit after delivery to allow adequate pulmonary perfusion.

Delivery of the fetus from the uterus disrupts the umbilical-placental circulation and the functions of oxygen uptake and carbon dioxide removal are transferred to the lungs. The foramen ovale (fig.3) and the ductus arteriosus (fig.4) have to be closed functionally or anatomically to establish the adult circulation. Physical expansion of the lung, ventilation with oxygen and umbilical cord occlusion produce an increased in pulmonary blood flow and decrease in pulmonary vascular resistance. The pulmonary endothelium plays a crucial role in this adaption, the onset of breathing is associated with an increase in specific mediators such us nitric oxide and prostacyclin (pulmonary vasodilators and inhibitors of smooth muscle cell proliferation), and a decrease of vasoconstrictors (angiotensin and endothelin-1).

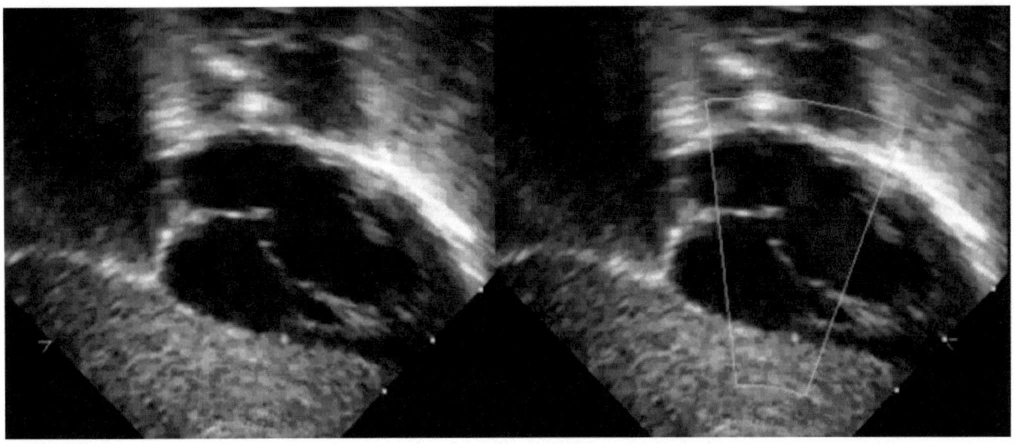

Fig. 3. Echocardiographic subcostal four-chamber image demonstrating a patent foramen ovale .

If pulmonary vascular resistance does not fall normally after birth, pulmonary arterial pressure will not drop to normal postnatal level, and pulmonary blood flow adequate for oxygen needs may not be established. This phenomenon has been named persistent pulmonary hypertension of the newborn (PPHN), and may result from several condition (perinatal asphyxia, meconium aspiration) (Suesaowalak et al, 2010).

A wide variety of cardiac disorders has been reported to cause PPHN and have been grouped into five types based on the physiology of the lesion (Long, 1990):

Group 1. Obstructions to pulmonary venous drainage (obstructed total anomalous pulmonary venous drainage, cor triatriatum, mitral stenosis...)

Group 2. Congenital cardiomyopathies (endocardial fibroelastosis, myocarditis...).

Group 3. Obstructions to left ventricular outflow (aortic atresia, critical aortic stenosis, interrupted aortic arch, coarctation...).

Group 4. Obligatory left-to-right shunts (cerebral arteriovenous malformations, hepatic arteriovenous malformations, complete atrioventricular septal defect...)

Group 5. miscellaneous cardiac disorders (Ebstein anomaly, tricuspid atresia, pulmonary atresia, transposition of the great vessels...)

Children with Down syndrome have an increased risk for developing pulmonary hypertension. The cause of pulmonary hypertension in this population is multifactorial and may be due to both anatomical and physiological alterations in the pulmonary circulation, including the presence of congenital heart disease with persistent left-to-right shunts, chronic upper airway obstruction, or abnormal pulmonary vasculature growth. Although damage to the pulmonary vasculature occurs over time, there also appears to be a subset of Down syndrome patients who develop pulmonary hypertension in the neonatal period. Neonatal DS patients have a greater incidence of persistent pulmonary hypertension of the newborn (PPHN) compared to the general population, and suggests that there may be something intrinsically related to DS that put these patients at increased risk for PPHN (Cua et al, 2007).

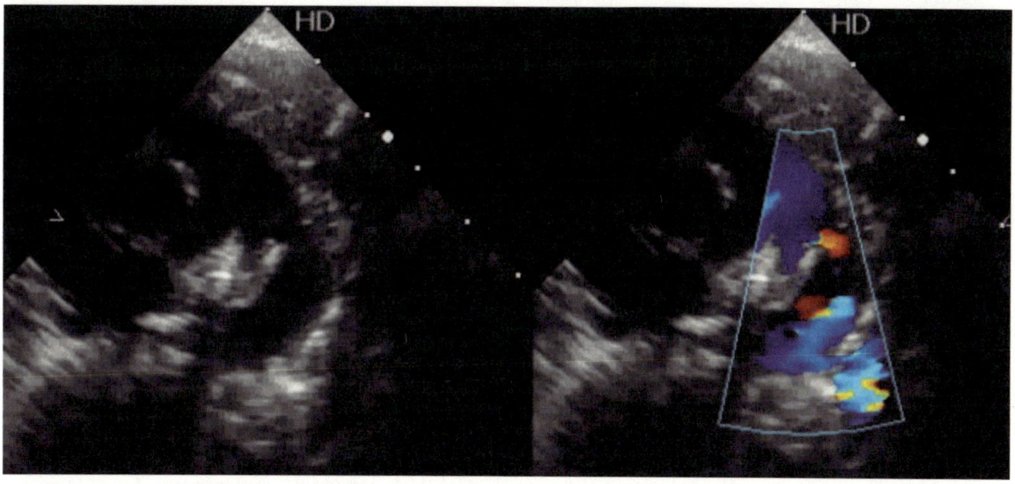

Fig. 4. Echocardiographic parasternal short-axis image demonstrating a patent ductus arteriosus (red flow at the ductus arteriosus and blue flow at both pulmonary arteries).

4. Correlation between cardiac physical examination and echocardiography

4.1 Clinical examination

Although CHD is present at birth, there are often no signs and most babies are asymptomatic. Skilled physical examination, a sensitive and specific screening tool in older children, does not always distinguish between neonates with or without CHD (Griebsch, 2007).

Wren et al. (1999) found no clinical signs in the first weeks in some children with DS, with major cardiac malformations and associated pulmonary hypertension, even in some who progressed to irreversible pulmonary vascular disease.

A normal neonatal examination in children with DS does not therefore exclude a serious CHD. Basic neonatal characteristics, Apgar scores, birth weight and gestational age are not different in children with DS with and without CHD (Weijerman et al, 2010).
The natural history of specific heart defects depends on the transitional circulation in the neonatal period, so the timing of the routine examination is very important. Heart murmurs have a prevalence of between 0.6% and 4.2% in newborns and are mistakenly considered a hallmark of heart disease (Patton, 2006). Transient murmurs due to tricuspid regurgitation (fig.5) and physiological peripheral pulmonic stenosis (fig.6) are the most common innocent murmurs in neonates (Du et al, 1997).

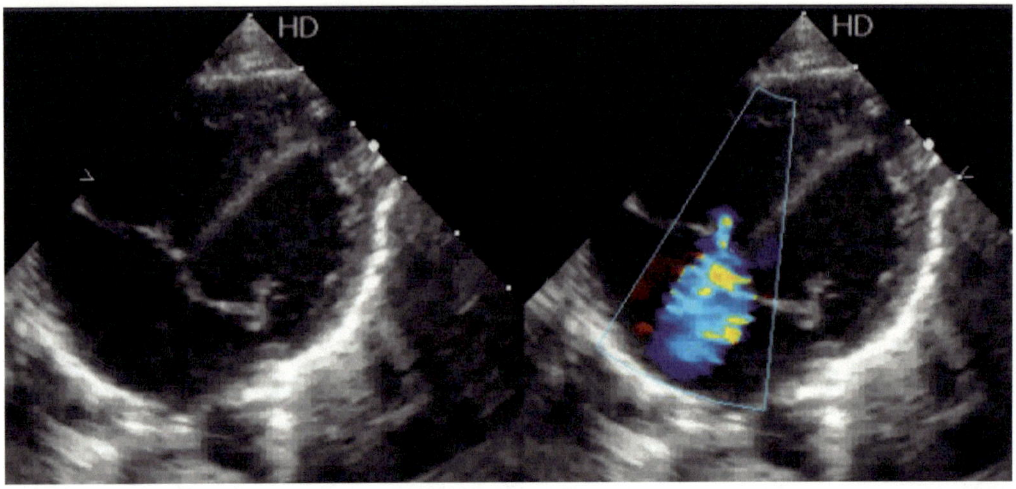

Fig. 5. Echocardiographic apical four-chamber image demonstrating a tricuspid regurgitation (blue jet from right ventricule to right atrium).

Practising pediatricians currently have limited experience in discriminating innocent from pathological murmurs. Detection of a murmur depends on the examiner´s skill and experience, the timing and the frequency of examination, and the conditions under which examination takes place.
Detection of a murmur on routine examination may be a clue to the presence of heart disease and offers the possibility of early, presymptomatic diagnosis. Early referral of all asymptomatic babies with murmurs is recommended for early definitive diagnosis by echocardiography. However, the absence of a murmur does not exclude the presence of potentially serious heart disease (Ainsworth et al, 1999).
Murmurs of atrioventricular septal defect and septal defect, the most common forms of CHD in SD, emerge after the decline in pulmonary resistance and may happen after neonatal discharge.

4.2 Electrocardiography

Electrocardiography (ECG) do not improve the sensitivity of the clinical assessment in the detection of CHD. Atrioventricular septal defects is associated with abnormal ECG (superior QRS axis), but most of the CHD have normal results on ECG (Mackie et al, 2009).

Sensivity and specific of a superior QRS axis to diagnose complete atrioventricular septal defect is 100% and 96.8%, respectively. However, the predictive value of neonatal ECG for other CHD is poor (Dennis et al, 2010).

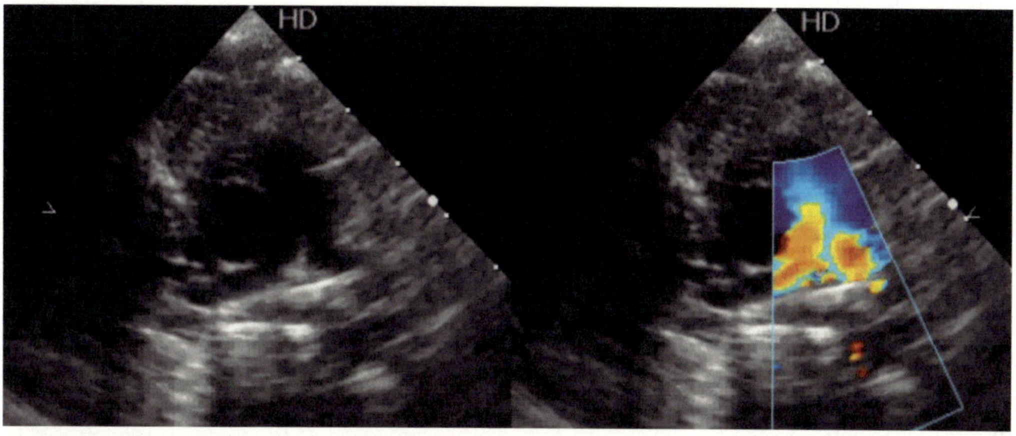

Fig. 6. Echocardiographic parasternal short-axis image demonstrating a physiological peripheral pulmonic stenosis (yellow colour due to aliasing at the origin of both pulmonary arteries).

4.3 Chest radiography

There is no evidence that chest x ray (CXR) is a useful addition for neonatal diagnosis of CHD. CXR alone missed 39% of the cases of complete atrioventricular septal defect, whereas ECG missed only 17%. Combinig CXR, ECG and clinical examination gave little added benefit only 15% missed (Dennis et al, 2010).

In the evolution, but out of neonatal period, radiographic manifestations in infants with left-to-right shunts include cardiomegaly, prominence of the pulmonary vasculature, and dilatation of the central pulmonary arteries. With the severe and longstanding process, pulmonary artery hypertension appears, this shunt flow decreases and reverse, resulting in peripheral prunting of pulmonary vessels. As the pulmonary vascular resistance increases, if the congenital CHD is not corrected, the heart size may decrease (Suesaowalak et al, 2010).

4.4 Pulse oxymetry

Cyanosis in the newborn is difficult to detect at clinically important levels, murmurs may be missed or over diagnosed and femoral pulses are challenging to asses. Together with early discharge and failure to asses infants identified as at risk. The introduction of additional oxymetry screening could achieve better results at the relatively small cost. Pulse oximetry is a symple, non-invasive method of monitoring the pordentage of haemoglobin which is saturated with oxygen. The pulse oximeter consists of a probe attached to the infant´s finger, toe or edge of the foot, which is in turn linked to a computerised display of the porcentage of haemoglobin satured with oxigen and the heart rate. The examination can be performed by a junior doctor, midwife or other health professional. The equipment required is portable and ca be used in the home and hospital. An oximeter identifies hypoxemia and is dependent on a good peripheral circulation and so does not work reliably when a baby has a low blood pressure or is dehydrated, for example. Pulse oximetry may identify babies with cianotic CHD but not defects that only associated with murmurs or delay or absent pulses. Nevertheless, some authors thinks that pulse oximetry is a promising alternative newborn screening strategy (Knowles, 2005; Meberg, 2009), but others not (Reich, 2008. Sendelbach, 2008). Pulse oximetry cannot detect all cases of CHD, and parents should be informed, and hence, a negative test result does not exclude the possibility of heart disease. According to the American Heart Association and American Academy of Pediatrics, the usefulness of oximetry in clinical studies is not well stablished (Class IIb, Level of Evidence C), and future studies are needed to determine whether this practise should become standard of care in the routine assesment of the neonate (Mahle et al, 2009). Therefore, the screening with pulse oximetry should be carried out together with a clinical examination, never alone.

4.5 Echocardiography

Echocardiographic examination provides extensive anatomic and hemodynamic information noninvasively, in real time, and at relatively low cost. Echocardiographic windows are better in the newborn than at any other age because the lungs (impenetrable to ultrasound) do not get in the way as much, and the heart and great vessels are nearer the probe. The echocardiography must be a sistematic study with the standard views (left parasternal, apical, subcostal and suprasternal) and completed with Doppler ultrasound (colour Doppler, pulsed Doppler and continuous wave Doppler). Echocardiography is useful for initial evalution, cardiac defects, level of shunting, degree and directions of shunts, severety of pulmonary arterial hypertension, follow-up of the teatment and ventricular function can be delinaeted systematically. A routine echocardiography should be performed in this population in the neonatal period (AAP´s Committee on Genetics, 2001).

A patient is considered to have an abnormal cardiac physical examination if there is a cardiac murmur and/or cyanosis or an abnormal systemic arterial oxygen saturation, but a newborn without congenital heart disease but with persistent pulmonary hypertension of the newborn (PPHN) may present a cardiac murmur due to transient tricuspid insufficiency of cardiac dysfuntion, and cyanosis due to right-to-left shunting of blood across the patent ductus arteriosus and the foramen ovale. These clinical manifestations may alert the neonatologist and suspect the presence of a congenital heart diasease, but in deed, there is not.

The diagnosis can be confirmed by echocardiography with color Doppler imaging and documenting right-to lef shunting of blood through fetal circulatory pathways (ductus arteriosus and foramen ovale), in the abscence of CHD (fig 7, Fig 8). Contrast echocardiography is performed by rapidly injecting approximately 1ml of saline/blood mixture into a pheriperal vein while capturing a four-chamber view of the heart. The simultaneous appearance of bright echoes from cavitations in the fluid in the right ventricle and left atrium documents right-to-left atrial shunting. Because the right-to-left atrial shunt may be predominately of inferior vena cava, as it is in the normal fetal state, injection of fluid into a vein draining to the inferior vena cava may yield the best results (Fineman, Heymann & Morin, 2001).

Doppler echocardiography allows estimation of pulmonary artery systolic pressure. Because pulmonary artery and right ventricule systolic pressure are nearly equal in the absence of

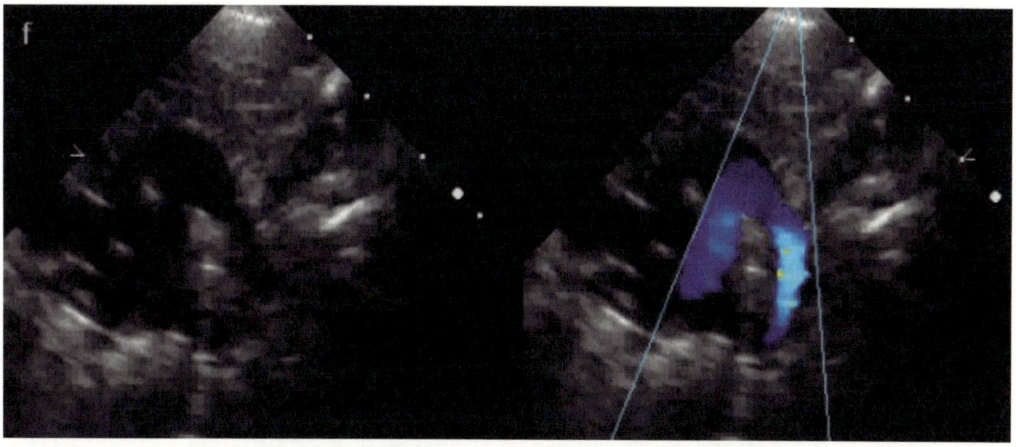

Fig. 7. Echocardiographic parasternal short-axis image demonstrating a patent ductus arteriosus with right-to-left shunt (blue flow).

stenosis of right ventricule outflow tract, pulmonary artery systolic pressure is commonly estimated by techniques that measures right ventricule systolic prresure. In the method most commonly used, the tricuspid regurgitation jet is used to calculate the right ventricular-right atrial pressure gradient (Snider & Serwer, 1990).

Transthoracic echocardiograpy is useful for evaluation of severity of pulmonary arterial hypertension and ventricular function can be delineated systematically. The abnormal motion of the interventricualr septum and the eccentricity index estimate right ventricular pressure overload. The Tei index and the tricuspid annular plane systolic excursion (TAPSE) correlate with right ventricular function (Suesaowalak et al, 2010).

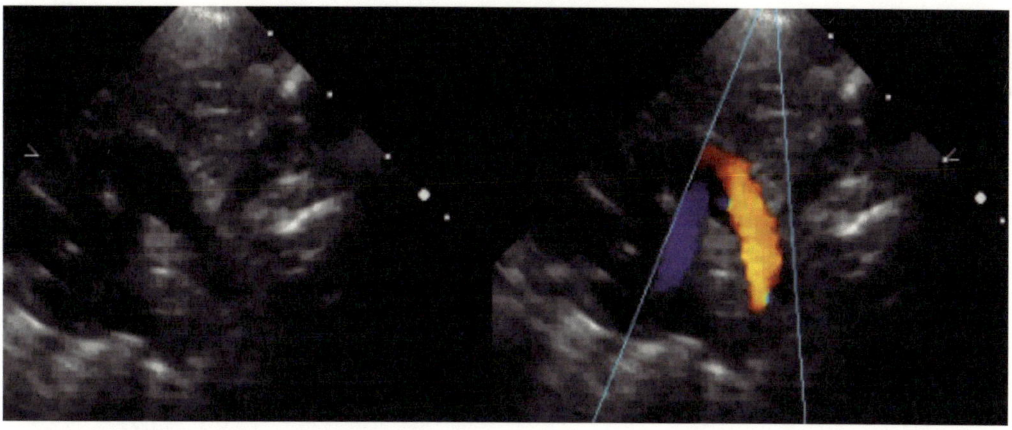

Fig. 8. Echocardiographic parasternal short-axis image demonstrating a patent ductus arteriosus with left-to-right shunt (orange flow).

5. Potencial benefits of early diagnosis.

Because of the high incidence of a significant CHD in children with DS, the early recognition of CHD can lead to the optimal management of the defect and emphasizes the importance of an early echocardiography of neonates with DS.

Early diagnosis of CHD in DS is important firstly because both the parents and the paediatrician need to know the implications of the heart defect. Secondly some major malformations with pulmonary hypertension may show no signs and may progress to irreversible pulmonary vascular disease before the heart defect has been recognised.
When fetal echocardiography was introduced into clinical practise, it become possible to study the spectrum of lesions associated with DS in prenatal life (fig.9) and the early diagnosis is of paramount importance (Paladini et al, 2000).

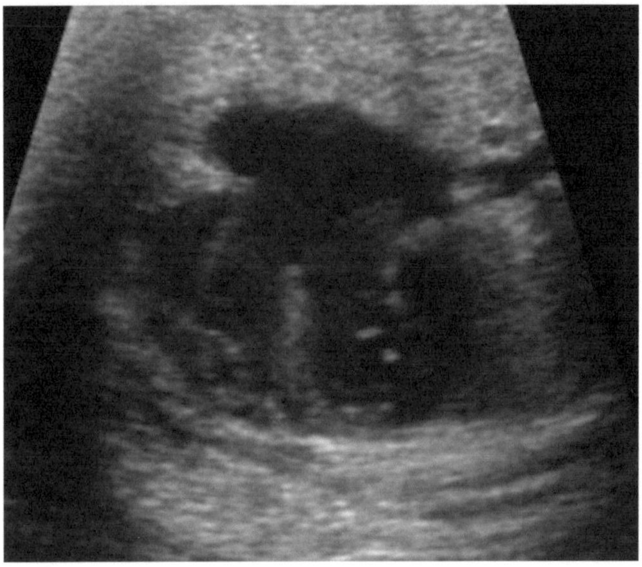

Fig. 9. Fetal echocardiography demonstrating a complete atrioventricular septal defect.

5.1 Pulmonary arterial hypertension

About half of all babies with DS will have CHD, and in around one-third of these this will comprise a complete atrioventricular septal defect with high risk of pulmonary vascular disease due to high pulmonary blood flow.
Among the numerous causes of pulmonary arterial hypertension, left-to-right shunt and chronic upper airway obstruction are frequently encountered in children with DS. Obstructive sleep apnoea is common in children with SD, affecting 30-50% of this patient group compared with 3% of the general paediatric population. This may result from a number of factors, including hypotonic upper airway, adeno-tonsillar hypertrophy, macroglossia, glossoptosis, flattened mid-face and narrow nasopharynx in these patients (Hawkins et al, 2011). This association of CHD in DS with pulmonary arterial hypertension, has led a neonatal screening and, as medical treatment becomes increasingly unsuccessful, early definitive cardiac surgery is usually undertaken at 3-6 months of age (Vohra et al, 2010). Many reports have demonstrated safe and effective repair in infants with atrioventricular septal defects within the first few months of live, and the presence of DS is not a risk factor (Lange et al, 2007).
In the past, infants with complete AVSD were initially palliated with pulmonary artery banding to prevent pulmonary vascular disease, followed by complete repair at a later stage to reduce mortality and morbidity. Better perioperative care and improvements in surgical

and cardiopulmonary bypass techniques, allowed surgeons to successfully perform early repair. Nevertheless, there are situations in which early primary repair is not feasible or is accompanied by unacceptable risk. Reasons include unfavourable intracardiac anatomy (unbalanced ventricular morphology, associated lesions, or both), associated non cardiac malformation (exomphalos), or poor clinical condition (infection, chronic lung disease, renal or liver dysfunction, gastrointestinal or neurological complications). In these situations palliation with pulmonary artery banding followed by late repair is recognized as a viable surgical option (Dhannapuneni et al, 2011).

5.2 Nutrition

Failure to thrive is common in children with congenital heart disease. Infants with CHD are particularly at risk of energy imbalance that can involve deficiencies of specific nutrients, or insufficient total caloric intake. Malnutrition undermines the outcome of corrective surgical operations and postoperative recovery. Most infants with CHD have a normal weight for gestational age at birth but develop nutritional and growth problems in early infancy. Weight tends to be more effected than height; even so, almost half of infants younger than 2 years are stunted (Nydegger and Bines, 2006).

Mechanisms linking CHD to malnutrition may be related either to decreased energy intake and/or to increased energy requirements.

Decreased energy intake are in relation with anorexia and aerly satiety of these patients, decreased gastric volume caused by hepatomegaly, malabsorption due to edema and chronic hypoxia of the gut, pharmacologic agents, fluid restriction...

Increased in energy requirements can be due to increased respiratory rate accompanying congestive heart failure, cardiac hypertrophy, recurrent infections, increased activity of sympathetic nervous system, increased basal temperature...

The development of malnutrition depends on the type and severity of the cardiac lesion and associated disease condition. Infants with cyanotic heart lesions (tetralogy of Fallot) frequently have decreased weight and height compared with healthy infants. Chronic hypoxia is an important factor in anorexia and inefficient processing of nutrients at the cellular level. Atrioventricular septal defect and septal defect, the most common forms of CHD in DS, are acyanotic heart lesions but if there is a large left-to-right shunt, have reduced weight gain but growth may be maintained during infancy. However, in the presence of elevated pulmonary presure, severe growth failure frequently develops (Varan et al, 1999).

Associated genetic condition, Down syndrome, is another crucial factor and also influence energy intake, gastrointestinal absorption, expenditure, and growth expectations (Nydegger and Bines, 2006).

Most treatment strategies aim to facilitate "catch-up" growth, providing extra calories and protein that exceed the Recommended Dietary Allowance for age. However, there is no generally accepted set of guidelines that define appropriate caloric intake for catch-up growth. Early diagnosis of CHD in DS, brings out the nutrition challenge, the most effective nutrition strategies for children with CHD (Forchielly et al, 1994). Nutritional support via percutaneous endoscopic gastrostomy allows the safe delivery of the caloric intke needed in children with CHD and significant feeding-realed difficulties (Ciotti et al, 2002).

5.3 Prevention of infective endocarditis

It is recommended that parents and carers of all children with CHD should be given information about infective endocarditis preventive measures. Infective endocarditis is an

uncommon but life-threatening infection. Despite advances in diagnosis, antimicrobial therapy, surgical techniques, and management of complications, patients with infective endocarditis still have high morbidity and mortality rates related to this condition.
The development of infective endocarditis is the net result of the complex interaction between the bloodstream pathogen with matrix molecules and platelets at sites of endocardial cell damage.
The American Heart Association (AHA) guidelines for infective endocarditis prophylaxis were published in 1997. The 1997 document stratified cardiac conditions into high-, moderate- and low-risk (negligible risk) categories, with prophylaxis not recommended for the low-risk group. Nevertheless, since this document, many medical societies and physicians have questioned the efficacy of the prophylaxis. The quality of evidence was limited to a few case-control studies or was based on expert opinion, clinical experience, and descriptive studies that utilized surrogate measures of risk.
"The Committee" of AHA extensively reviewed data and published the updated recommendations in October 2007. This new document is intended to identify which, if any, patients and procedures may possibly benefit from infective endocarditis prophylaxis, and result in greater clarity for patients, healthcare providers, and consulting professionals (Wilson et al, 2007).

5.4 Prevention of Respiratory Syncytial Virus infection

Children with DS have an increased incidence of respiratory tract infections which might be associated with CHD, abnormal airway anatomy and physiology, hypotonia, and aspiration. However, children with DS and without CHD, also have a high incidence of respiratory morbidity and might be explained by an aberrant immune system as well (Bloemers et al, 2010).
Respiratory syncytial virus (RSV) is an enveloped, nonsegmented, negative-strand RNA virus of the family *Paramyxoviridae* that causes respiratory tract infections in children. In the North- ern Hemisphere, the peak infection season is November through April. By two years of age, most children will have had an RSV infection. Bronchiolitis, a lower respiratory tract infection, is often caused by RSV. An RSV infection is diagnosed based on patient history and physical examination. RSV is recognized as the leading cause of hospitalization among young children worldwide. Infants of young chronologic age and children with predisposing factors, such as premature birth, pulmonary disease, or hemodynamically significant congenital heart disease, are most susceptible to serious illness. Children with DS have an increased risk of being hospitalized for RSV-induced lower respiratory tract infection, indicating DS as a risk factor (Bloemers et al, 2010). Unlike other viruses, immunity to RSV infection is incomplete and short lived, and reinfection is common throughout life. RSV infection remains difficult to treat, and prevention is a worldwide goal. Initial infection with RSV affords limited protection to reinfection, yet repeated episodes decrease the risk for lower respiratory tract illness. The development of palivizumab, a monoclonal antibody that can bind to a specific antigenic site on the virus and prevent cell-to-cell spread of infection has since become the mainstay of RSV illness prevention in preterm infants and those with significant congenital heart disease. Palivizumab, the only monoclonal antibody approved for the prevention of RSV lower respiratory tract disease must be administered monthly throughout the RSV season and does not always prevent serious RSV illness. Palivizumab is administered intramuscularly at a dose of 15 mg/kg

once every 30 days, for a maximum of 5 doses. The American Academic of Pediatrics (AAP) published a policy statement on the use of palivizumab in November 1998, revised it in December 2003, and the last statement in the 2009 Red Book recommendations, safety and efficacy have been established for infants born at or before 35 weeks´ gestation with or without chronic lung disease of prematurity and for infants and children with hemodynamically significant heart disease (AAP, Committee on Infectious Diseases, 2009).

6. Conclusion

There is an increased incidence of congenital heart disease (CHD) and persistent pulmonary hypertension in Down syndrome (DS) neonates. A normal neonatal examination in children with DS does not therefore exclude a serious CHD. Clinical examination alone is insufficient to detect CHD in newborns. Failure to recognise these defects early in life can have serious consequences. The child´s future health, and indeed survival, may be severely compromised by late diagnosis. Neonatal echocardiography is the most effective single procedure and must be carried out by an appropiately trained person. A routine echocardiography should be performed in this population in the neonatal period.

7. References

Ainsworth, SB.; Wyllie, JP. & Wren, C. (1999). Prevalence and clinical significance of cardiac murmurs in neonates. *Arch Dis Child Fetal Neonatal Ed.* Vol.80, pp. F43-F45.

American Academy of Pediatrics Committe on Genetics. (2001). Helth supervision for children with Down syndrome. Pediatrics. Vol.107, Nº.2, (February 2001), pp.442-449, ISSN: 1098-4275.

Bloemers, BL.; van Furth, AM.; Weijerman, ME.; Gemke, RJ.; Broers CJ.; Kimpen, JL. & Bont, L. (2010). High incidence of recurrebt Wheeze in children with Down syndrome with and without previous Respiratory Syncitial Virus lower respiratory tract infection. *Pediatr Infect Dis J.* Vol.29, pp. 39-42, ISSN: 0891-3668/10/2901-0039.

Bloemers, BL.; Broers, CJ.; Bont, L.; Wiejerman, ME.; Gemke, RJ. & van Furth, AM. (2010). Increased risk of respiratory tract infections in children with Down syndrome: the consequence of an altered immune system. *Microbes and Infection.* Vol.12, pp. 799-808.

Ciotti, G. ; Holzer, R. ; Pozzi, M.& Dalzell,M. (2002). Nutritional support via percutaneous endoscopic gastrostomy in children with cardiac disease experiencing difficulties with feeding. *Cardiol Young.* Vol.12, Nº.6, (December 2002), pp.537-541.

Clark, EB. (2001). Etiology of congenital cardiovascular malformations : epidemiology and genetics, In : *Moss and Adams'heart disease in infants, children and adolescents, including the fetus and young adult,* Allen, HD. Gutgesell, HP. Clarck, EB. Driscoll, DJ. (Ed.), pp. 64-79, Lippincot Williams & Wilkins, ISBN 0-683-30742-8, Philadelphia, USA.

Committee on Infectious diseases, American Academy of Pediatrics. (2009). Modified recommendations for use of Palivizumab for prevention of respiratory syncitial virus infections. *Pediatrics.* Vol.124, Nº.6, (December 2009), pp.1694-1702.

Cua, CL. ; Blankenship, A. ; North, AL. ; Hayes, J. & Nelin, LD. (2007). Increased incidence of idiopathic persistent pulmonary hypertension in Down syndrome neonates. *Pediatric Cardiology.* Vol.28, (March 2007), pp. 250-254.

Dhannapuneni, RR.; Gladman, G.; Kerr, S.; Venugopal, P.; Alphonso, N. & Corno, AF. Complete atrioventricular septal defect: outcome of pulmonary artery banding improved by adjustable device. *The Journal of Thoracic and Cardiovascular Surgery*. Vol 141, (January 2011), pp. 179-182.

De Rubens, J. ; Del Pozzo, B. ; Bablos, JL, Calderon, C. & Castrejon, R. (2003). Heart malformations in children with Down syndrome. *Rev Esp Cardiol*. Vol.56, N°.9, pp.894-899.

Dennis , J. ; Archer, N. ; Ellis, J. & Marder, L. (2011). Recognising heart disease in children with Down syndrome. *Arch Dis Child Educ Pract*, Vol.95, pp. 98-104.

Du, ZD. ; Roguin, N. & Barak, M. (1997). Clinical and echocardiographic evaluation of neonates with heart murmurs. *Acta Paediatr*. Vol.86, pp. 752-756.

Evans, PR. (1950). Cardiac anomalies in mongolism. Br Heart J. Vol.12, pp. 258-262.

Fineman, JR. ; Heymann, MA. ; Morin, FC. (2001). Fetal and postnatal circulations : pulmonary and persistent pulmonary hypertension of the newborn, In : *Moss and Adams'heart disease in infants, children and adolescents, including the fetus and young adult*, Allen, HD. Gutgesell, HP. Clarck, EB. Driscoll, DJ. (Ed.), pp. 41-63, Lippincot Williams & Wilkins, ISBN 0-683-30742-8, Philadelphia, USA.

Forchielli, ML. ; McColl, R. ; Walker,WA. & Lo, C. Children with congenital heart disease : a nutrition challenge. *Nutr Rev*. Vol.52. pp. 348-53.

Freeman, SB. ; Bean, LH. ; Allen, E. ; Tinker, SW. ; Locke, AE. ; Druschel, C. ; Hobbs, CA. ; Romitti, PA. ; Royle, MH. ; Torfs, CP. ; Dooley, KJ. & Sherman, SL.(2008). Ethnicity, sex, and the incidence of congenital heart defects : a report from the National Down Syndrome Projet. *Genetics in Medicine*. Vol.10, N°.3, (March 2008), pp.173-180.

Fudge, JC. ; Li, S. ; Jaggers, J. ; O'Brien, SM. ; Peterson, ED. ; Jacobs, JP. ; Welke, KF. ; Jacobs, ML. ; Li, JS. & Pasqualli, SK. (2010). Congenital heart surgery in Down syndrome : analysis of a national clinical database. *Pediatrics*. Vol.126, No.2, (August 2010), pp. 315-322, ISSN 0031-4005.

Griebsch, I. ; Knowles, RL, Brown, J. ; Bull, C. ; Wren, C.& Dezateux, CA. (2007). Comparing the clinical and economic effects of clinical examination, pulse oximmetry, and echocardiography in newborn screening for congenital heart defects : a probabilistic cost-effectiveness model and value of information analysis. *Int J Technol Assess Health Care*. Vol.23, pp. 192-204.

Hawkins, A. ; Langton-Hewer, S. ; Henderson, J. & Tulloh, RM. Management of pulmonary hypertension in Down syndrome. *Eur J Pediatr*. Published online : 04 January 2011. DOI 10.1007/s00431-010-1378-1

Hoffman, J. (2009). Epidemiology of congenital heart disease : etiology, pathogenesis, and incidence, In : *Fetal cardiology. Embryology, genetics, physiology, echocardiographics evaluation, diagnosis and perinatal management of cardiac diseases*, Yaguel, S. Silverman, N. Gembruch, U, (Ed), pp. 101-110, Informa Healthcare, ISBN 978-0-415-43265-8, New York, USA.

Khairy, P. ; Ionescu-Ittu, R. ; Mackie, AS. ; Abrahamowicz, M. ; Pilote, L. & Marelli, AJ. (2010). Changing mortality in congenital heart disease. *Journal of the American College of Cardiology*. Vol.56, No.14, (September 2010), pp. 1149-1157, ISSN 0735-1097.

Hoohenkerk, GJ. ; Bruggemans, EF. ; Rijlaarsdam, M. ; Schoof, PH. ; Koolbergen, DR. & Hazekamp, MG. (2010). More than 30 years´experience with surgical correction of atrioventricular septal defects. *Ann Thorac Surg*. Vol.90, pp. 1554-1562.

Knowles, R. ; Griebsch, I. ; Dezateux, C. ; Brown, J. ; Bull, C. & Wren, C.(2005). Newborn screening for congenital heart defects: a systematic review and cost-effectiveness analysis. *Health Technol Assess*. 9(44), pp. 1-152, iii-iv.

Lange, R.; Guenther, T.; Busch, R, Hess J. & Schreiber, C. (2007). The presence of Down syndrome is not a risk factor in complete atrioventricular septal defect repair. *The Journal of Thoracic and Cardiovascular Surgery*. Vol 134, (August 2007), pp. 304-310.

Long, WA. (1990). Persitent pulmonary hypertension of the newborn syndrome (PPHNS), In : *Fetal & Neonatal Cardiology*, Long, WA (Ed), pp. 627-655, Sounders Company, ISBN 0-7216-1887-1, Philadelphia, USA.

Mackie, AS.; Jutras, LC.; Dancea, AB, Rohlicek, CV.; Platt, R. & Beland, MJ. (2009). Can cardiologists distinguish innocent murmurs from pathologic murmurs in neonates?. *The Journal of Pediatrics*. Vol.154, (January 2009), pp. 50-54.

Mahle, WT.; Newburger, JW.; Matherme, GP.; Smith, FC.; Hoke, TR.; Koppel, R.; Gidding, SS.; Beekman, RH.& Grosse, SD. (2009). Role of pulse oximetry in examining newborns for congenital heart disease: a scientific statement fron the American Heart Assiciation and American Academy Pediatrics. Circulation. Vol.120, pp. 447-458, ISSN 0009-7322.

Meberg, A.; Andreassen, A.; Brunvand, L.; Markestad, T.; Moster, D.; Nietsch, L.; Silberg, IE. & Skalevik, JE. (2009). Pulse oximetry screening as a complementary strategy to detect critical congenital heart defects. *Acta Paediatrica*. Vol.98, (April 2009), pp. 682-686.

Nydegger, A. & Bines, JE (2006). Energy metabolism in infants with congenital heart disease. *Nutrition*. Vol.22, pp. 697-704.

Paladini, D.; Tartaglione, A.; Agangi, A.; Teodoro, A.; Forleo, F.; Borghese, A. & Martinelli, P. (2000). The association between congenital heart disease and Down syndrome in prenatal life. *Ultrasound in Obstetrics and Gynecololy*. Vol.15, pp. 104-108.

Patton, C.; Hey, E. (2006). How effectively can clinical examination pick up congenital heart disease at birth?. *Arch Dis Child Fetal Neonatal Ed*. Vol.91, pp. F263-F267.

Reich, JD.; Connolly, B.; Bradley, G.; Littman, S.; Koeppel, W.; Lewycky, P. & Liske, M. (2008). Reliability of a single pulse oximetry reading as a screening test for congenital heart disease in otherwise asymptomatic newborn infants: the importance of human factors. *Pediatric Cardiology*. Vol.29, (March 2008), pp. 371-376.

Roguin, N.; Du, ZD, Barak, M.; Nasser, N.; Herschkowitz S & Milgram, E. (1995). High prevalence of muscular ventricular septal defect in neonates. *J Am Coll Cardiol*. Vol.26 (November 1995), pp. 1545-1548.

Sendelbach, DM.; Jackson, GL.; Lai, SS.; Fixler, DE.; Stehel, EK & Engle WD. (2008). Pulse oximetryscreening at 4 hoursof age to detect critical congenital heart defects. *Pediatrics*. Vol.122 (October 2008), pp. e815-820.

Suesaowalak, M.; Cleary, JP. & Chang, AC. (2010). Advances in diagnosis and treatment of pulmonary arterial hypertension in neonates and children with congenital heart disease. *World J Pediatr*. Vol.6, N°.1 , (February 2010), pp. 13-31.

Varan, B.; Tokel, K.& Yilmaz, G (1999). Malnutrition and growth failure in cyanotic ans acyanotic heart disease with and without pulmonary hypertension. *Arch Dis Child*. Vol.81, pp..49-52.

Vis, JC.; Duffels, MG.; Winter, MM.; Weijerman, M.; Cobben, JM.; Huisman, SA. & Mulder, BJ. (2009). Down syndrome: a cardiovascular perspective. Journal of Intellectual Disability Research. Vol.53, N°5, (May 2009), pp. 419-425.

Vohra, HA.; Chia, AX.; Yuen, HM.; Vettukattil, JJ.; Veldtman, G.; Gnanapragasam, J.; Roman, H.; Salmon, AP. & Haw, MP. Primary biventricular repair of atrioventricular septal defects: an analysis of reoperations. *Ann Thorac Surg*. Vol.90, pp. 830-838.

Weijerman, ME.; van Furth, AM.; Noordegraaf, AV.; van Wouwe, P, Broers, CJ.& Gemke, RJ. (2008). Prevalence, neonatal characteristics, and first-year mortality of Down syndrome: a national study. *The Journal of Pediatrics*. Vol.152, pp.15-19.

Weijerman, ME. ; van Furth, AM. ; van der Mooren, D. ; van Weissenbruch, MM. ; Rammeloo, L. ; Broers, CJ. & Gemke RJ. (2010). Prevalence of congenital heart defects and persistent pulmonary hypertension of the neonate with Down syndrome. Eur J Pediatr, Vol.169, pp. 1195-1199.

Wilson, W. ; Taubert, KA. ; Gewitz, M. ; Lockhart, PB. ; Baddour, LM. ; Levison, M. ; Bolger, A. ; Cabell, CH. ; Takahashi, M. ; Baltimore, RS. ; Newburger, JW. ; Strom, BL. ; Tani, LY. ; Gerber, M. ; Bonow, RO. ; Pallasch, T. ; Shulman, ST. ; Rowley, AH. ; Burns, JC. ; Ferrieri, P. ; Gardner, T. ; Goff, D. & Durack, DT. (2007). Prevention of infective endocarditis : Guidelines from the American Heart Association Rheumatic Fever, Endocarditis, and Kawasaki Disease Committee, Council on Cardiovascular Disease in the Young, and the Council on Clinical Cardiology, Council on Cardiovascular Surgery abd Anesthesia, and the Quality of Care and Outcomes Research Interdisciplinary Working Group. Circulation. Vol.116, N°9, (October 2007), pp. 1736-1754, ISSN : 0009-7322.

Wren, GL. ; Richmond, S. ; Donaldson, L. (1999). Presentation of congenital heart disease in infancy : implications for routine examination. *Arch Dis Child Fetal Neonatal Ed*, Vol.80, pp. F49-F53.

10

Down Syndrome in Nigeria Sub Saharan Africa

Olufemi Adebari Oloyede
Lagos State University Teaching Hospital, Ikeja, Lagos, Nigeria

1. Introduction

1.1 Burden

In his publication in 1866 titled 'Observation on an ethnic classification of idiots', John Langdon Down an English physician at the London Hospital, was the first to describe the external appearance of the genetic condition that was later to bear his name (Down, 1866). Following his description, scientists have conducted researches aimed at identifying the presence of the condition in various populations, race and ethnic groups as well as its incidence at birth and prevalence in the population. Most of the widely circulated reports on the incidence and prevalence of Down syndrome in Nigeria and other countries in sub Saharan Africa are estimates extrapolated from statistics obtained in developed countries such as the United Kingdom, United States of America, Canada or Australia. The studies did not consider the influence of factors such as socio cultural, genetic, racial and environmental characteristics on the prevalence of the condition, thus affecting the reliability of the data.

The earliest reported study on the incidence of Down syndrome by Adeyokunnu, in Ibadan, South Western Nigeria, reported an incidence of 1 in 865 live births (Adeyokunu, 1982). Prior to this time, it was believed that Down syndrome is rare or non - existent among Africans (Tompkins, 1964). This is collaborated by the reports of other clinicians that found no case of Down syndrome in their clinical practice over several years in Nigeria (Jelliffe, 1954a, Tooth, 1950). Rather, few cases reported were among Jamaicans and were postulated to be derived genetically from non African sources (Jelliffe, 1954b). While there may be other reports from Nigeria, the case report by Tompkins in 1964 was the first to draw attention to the occurrence of the condition among Nigerian children (Tompkins, 1964). After the report, it was now agreed that the condition is not as rare among Nigerians and Africans as was once believed. In spite of this however, there was still difficulty in achieving accurate data collection in Nigeria and other developing countries attributable to many factors. First, a large number of deliveries take place in non orthodox centres such as churches and traditional birth homes, most of which do not keep records. The government registered private maternity centres also have difficulty keeping accurate statistics (Oloyede, et.al, 2006). Secondly, within the community, cases of congenital malformations such as Down syndrome are not reported for record purpose because of the traditional belief that still associates them with witchcraft and witches. Consequently, true population based data are difficult to generate and most of the data reported are hospital based. In spite of this however, health planning are still based on these data with the assumption that they represent the actual situation.

Since the study by Adeyokunnu, there has been no other published report about the incidence in Nigeria till date. However, in South Africa, the Down Syndrome South Africa gave an incidence of about 1 in 500 live births in the country (DSSA). In same country, a study between January, 1974 and December, 1993, reported an overall prevalence rate of 1.49 per 1000, with a gradual decline to 1.3 per 1000 in the last 5 years of the study period, among the 3 study populations. The higher prevalence (1.88) among the white population compared with the prevalence in coloured (1.54) and blacks (1.29) could be attributed to the possibility that fewer blacks than whites undergo prenatal screened and diagnosis of the condition. This conclusion arose from the relative distribution of the number of terminations following prenatal diagnosis, being higher among whites (18.3%), intermediate in coloured (5.8%) and lowest in blacks (1.4%). The same study also confirms that the decline in the overall prevalence occur among the white population, while the blacks maintain their prevalence rate (Molteno, et, al., 1997). It should be noted that there is a fundamental difference in the statistical inferences from incidence and prevalence. Incidence is based on total birth in a year, while prevalence is based on actual population. While the difference is significant in developed countries because there is a better uptake of prenatal diagnosis services that influences the total birth incidence, same may not be true in Nigeria, where the uptake of such service is still poor. The incidence of Down syndrome could be higher in developing countries, with two factors as possible reasons. First the proportion of women that that conceive after 35 years is gradually rising in Nigeria compared to developed countries. Second, there is a higher mortality from complications of Down syndrome such as congenital heart defects in developing countries.

1.2 Down syndrome, maternal age and reproductive health

The commonest genetic mechanism for Down syndrome is maternal meiotic non disjunction and this has a very strong link with advance maternal age. Shuttleworth in 1909 was the first to observe the association between increased maternal age and Down syndrome after examining 350 cases. (Shuttleworth, 1909). Although no study from Nigeria has confirmed this trend, but a study on 'Down's syndrome in South Africa-incidence, maternal age and utilisation of prenatal diagnoses', reported that the prevalence of Down syndrome has been found to increase with advancing maternal age (Op't Hof J, et al., 1991). There are enough reasons to justify the expectation that the prevalence would continue to rise in future. The main factor that would explain this conclusion is the increasing maternal age at which more women in Nigeria now conceive. This follows the increasing strong desire to complete formal education before conception and the rising incidence of infertility (Oloyede and Osagie, 2003).

Although there are few studies on the epidemiology of Down syndrome in Nigeria and other sub Saharan African countries, its impact on reproductive health and quality of life is well documented. It is an important contributor to pregnancy wastage especially in early trimester. This is however difficult to ascertain because of the poor culture of follow-up diagnosis especially after spontaneous first trimester abortion in Nigeria. Various congenital malformations are associated with Down syndrome. Oloyede reported the occurrence of multiple congenital malformations in cases of Down syndrome in Sagamu, South Western Nigeria (Oloyede, et al., 2006). The pattern of congenital malformation seen in Ghana conforms to the well established pattern of malformations in Down syndrome. The main defect was atrioventricular defects and ventricular septal defects (Arthur, 1995). Other frequently reported anomalies are anorectal anomalies and speech disorders (Osei-Bagyina, 2000, Hesse, 2006). Majority present in early infancy, with features of congestive cardiac failure and cyanosis (Arthur, 1995).

Down syndrome has a lot of sociocultural colouration. Many local communities in Nigeria believed that all observable defects or early deaths which may occur in children with Down syndrome is traceable to parental misdeeds or links between the child and the evil world. In Ghana, it is believed that the Down child is given by the river gods and hence is called 'Nsuoba', meaning water children (Avoke, 1997). The pattern of response is similar in many other developing countries including Nigeria. Children that are affected by this syndrome are often times stigmatized by the society, treated with neglect and patronized. Lack of understanding and appreciation of the condition, makes the management of the individual with the condition difficult. The special educational and family support needed to optimize the well being of affected children are not usually available in many developing countries. The first coordinated effort at addressing the challenges of children with Down syndrome was provided through the National Down Syndrome Association of Nigeria and till date remains the only well coordinated group in West Africa. A similar organization is in South Africa called the Down Syndrome South Africa (DSSA). These bodies are non profit making. Like most other supportive organizations, the absence of community and governmental support is a strong limiting factor to their effectiveness. Overall, it is difficult for the child with Down syndrome child to realize the full potential in Nigeria and many other sub Saharan countries.

2. Strategies to reduce the incidence and impact of Down syndrome

The strategies to reduce the incidence and impact of Down syndrome should focus on 2 major areas

1. Implementation of acceptable and effective prevention programme in the prenatal period (Prevention)
2. Implementation of supportive health and non health initiatives for people affected by Down syndrome (Support)

2.1 Prevention programme

The seemingly rational way to prevent the birth of children with Down syndrome would be to prevent or reduce pregnancies in women above the cut off maternal age. There is however two issues involved in this policy. First, there is no clearly defined study from Nigeria that specifies the maternal age at which there is an exponential rise in the incidence of Down syndrome. Above this maternal age, the policy of no childbearing could be advocated based on the high incidence and also the risk of other complications of pregnancy above this age. Second, there are some considerations that influences the maternal age of conception such as the desire to complete educational pursuit, socioeconomic factors and increasing rate of infertility. These may altogether, increase the maternal age of conception in recent times. Having children is sometimes viewed from a completely different perspective in many rural communities in Nigeria, where it is a taboo for women to stop further childbearing till she either dies in the process or gets too old to continue, especially in communities where children are involved in economic activities such as farming. In the final analysis, this approach to preventing Down syndrome is not feasible in Nigeria and many other sub Saharan countries. A more acceptable compromise would be to advocate for the screening of women above the cut off maternal age.

Prevention strategy through screening and diagnosis is gradually becoming the hall mark of modern approach to the management and eradication of genetic condition in developed countries. It provides every woman an opportunity to determine the status of the fetus and takes decision on the future of affected pregnancies. This option of addressing the problem of Down syndrome is more relevant to developing countries where there is dearth of facilities to manage the physically challenged. In Nigeria, prenatal screening was considered the most feasible approach for the control of Sickle cell disorder (WHO, 1997). Genetic screening refers to the procedure to identify from within the population, individuals that are more likely to be produce offsprings with Down syndrome. Screening is not fool proof method as it merely suggests the propensity of occurrence of the condition. Its efficacy therefore improves as the number of tools used also increases.

The first and traditional screening method for the prevention of Down syndrome based on maternal age was introduced in the early 1970's, based on the observation by Shuttleworth (Shuttleworth, 1909). Although many physicians in Nigeria utilize maternal age in counselling women for the risk of Down syndrome, few utilize it for the purpose of screening. Op't Hof in South Africa shows that maternal age has influence on the risk of occurrence of Down syndrome in the country (Op't, 1991). The challenge is to arrive at an acceptable maternal age that can be used for screening in Nigeria, if it must differ from that used in Caucasians. This is because of the few reasons discussed earlier that contribute to increasing maternal age of conception. The decision about cut off maternal age also has economic and logistic implications. Because more women now achieve pregnancy at advance maternal age, it implies that the number that screens positive obtained using the traditional cut off maternal age of 35 years would also rise. This means additional logistics to cope with screening services. The logical step would be to further increase the cut off maternal age in other to maintain the recommended 5% screen positive rate. An important issue to contend with is the fact that the bulk of those that will end up having Down syndrome are in women below 35 years. Therefore maternal age would not suffice for effective screening in Nigeria.

A more common practice in Nigeria is the use of maternal serum hormones in the second trimester. Often times, it is not primarily intended for Down syndrome screening. The disadvantage of the present practice is that, screening is done at a gestational age when strong bonding has occurred between the mother and the fetus and the risk associated with extreme decisions such as termination of pregnancy is higher. Studies have indicated that, between 79.9 and 86% of women present either in the second trimester or third trimester for the first time in the antenatal period rather than in the first trimester, often times out of ignorance or misconceptions of the purpose and right time to commence antenatal care (Okunolola et al, 2008, Adekanle and Isawunmi, 2008, Ebeigbe and Igberase, 2005). The mean booking gestation in Nigerian is 20 weeks (Oladokun, et al., 2010). This observation is similar to reports from many sub-Saharan African countries but in sharp contrast to the practice in United Kingdom and United States of America, where women are advised to register within the first twelve weeks (National Institute for Health and clinical excellence, 2003, American Academy of Paediatrics, 2002). The late registration is believed from a study in Nigeria to the fact that most women do not perceive any advantage in early booking and viewed antenatal as curative rather than preventive (Ndidi, 2010). The physicians are therefore constrained by this reason. Standardized laboratory support that is peculiar for measuring hormones in pregnancy and calculating their deviations from median is also not available. There are no available statistics on the screen positive rate using these methods because there are no well defined criteria for their utilization.

Recently, another advance tool for screening of Down syndrome known as the nuchal translucency was introduced by Nicolaides and his team in the United Kingdom (Nicolaides, et al, 1992). The nuchal translucency refers to the fluid at the back of the neck of the fetus at 11 - 13 $^{+6}$ weeks of pregnancy. It is confirmed to have improved the detection rate for DS significantly for a much lower false positive rate (Nicolaides, et al, 1992). Generally, innovations in medicine are not rapidly incorporated into practice in Nigeria, especially public institutions, where the majority of women patronize (Oloyede, 2008). The Nuchal translucency scan screening was recently introduced into clinical practice in Nigeria in 2006. The benefits of the Nuchal translucency scan are in many folds. Its use was also reported in South Africa (Naidoo, et al., 2008)

1. It is a first trimester procedure
2. It does not rely on too many personnel or logistics to conduct and interpret unlike the MSB
3. Other congenital structural abnormalities can be ruled out at same time

More recent innovations in Down syndrome screening such as the nasal bone, and fronto maxillary facial (FMF) angle are yet to be incorporated into practice in Nigeria.

2.1.1 Factors affecting uptake and utilization of prenatal screening

Prenatal screening for Down syndrome has been shown to be an effective tool to reduce the prevalence of Down syndrome. In countries such as South Africa, where it is fairly available, studies have shown a reduction in the prevalence of Down syndrome especially among the white population that utilize the screening service (Molteno,1997). Prenatal screening for Down syndrome is not routine in many antenatal clinics in Nigeria. Therefore, most women do not benefit from this service (Oloyede, 2008). This in unlike the practice in many developed countries, where screening is widely incorporated into antenatal programs (Rosch,et al., 2000)

Several studies on the Nigerian population about the uptake of prenatal screening and attitude of women to prenatal screening were reviewed. The factors are broadly classified as

a. Health Service Factor
    - Skilled Manpower
    - Laboratory and Radiological Support
b. Non Health Service Factors
    - Awareness
    - Cost
    - Legal status of abortion
    - Religion
    - Sociocultural

Health Service Factor

Skilled Manpower

Several factors are known to affect the utilization of antenatal screening service in Nigeria. The first and perhaps the most important is that of physician appreciation of the condition at risk. Oloyede in 2008 showed that the bulk of obstetrician and antenatal care givers in Nigeria underwent training curriculum that places less emphasis on knowledge and skill to undertake screening and diagnosis of genetic conditions such as Down syndrome (Oloyede, 2008). The same study shows that most (66.1%) obstetricians in Nigeria consider training in prenatal screening and diagnosis for Down syndrome either below average or just average, majority (89.3%) do not conduct routine antenatal counseling and almost all (92.9%) do not have a standard screening protocol. It was also showed that maternal serum biochemistry in the second trimester was favoured against the nuchal translucency screening in the first trimester of pregnancy. It is known that the ability to know what to do after screening is an encouraging factor to undertake screening procedures. The skill to undertake nuchal translucency screening can be acquired within a reasonable time by most physicians and is therefore a method that should be encouraged in Nigeria.

Laboratory and Radiological Support

Laboratory analysis of maternal serum hormones for screening for Down syndrome has its peculiarities. A major influencing factor is the race. One of the challenges involved in the laboratory support is the absence of reference standards for blacks. Laboratory analyses are done without standard references that are acceptable and reproducible. There are automated machines that are designed to generate values, compare with multiples of median and report immediately. Maternal samples from Nigeria and many other countries are analysed in South Africa or Europe until very recently. This has to do with the huge cost of analysis machines that is beyond the capacity of many centres in Nigeria. The implication of analysing in a distant centre is that it takes longer days to transport samples and delay the time of decision making. This delay could be more tolerable if there are local regional centres in the country that could as well conduct first trimester analysis.
Another important factor that could affect the utilization is that of availability of ultrasound scan. In Nigeria, ultrasound scan is available in many obstetric units and mostly utilized by pregnant women (Lamina, et al., 2004).

Non Health Service Factors

Awareness

Awareness about prenatal screening and diagnosis in Nigeria among both the health practioners and public has been shown to be poor (Oloyede, et al., 2003, Oloyede, 2008). The role of health workers in the dissemination of appropriate information about prenatal diagnosis is very important (Oloyede,et al., 2003). This is what informs appropriate referral for utilization of screening service. Until after 2006, many health workers would refer women outside the country for prenatal diagnosis services or do nothing. Suggestions to improve awareness among the health workers include, incorporating education about prenatal screening and diagnosis into undergraduate education, wider dissemination of information in journals and scientific conferences and discussion in academic symposia (Oloyede, 2003).

Among pregnant women, there is a surprising good awareness of prenatal screening and diagnosis generally (Oloyede and Oyedele, 2008). Majority however, think only in terms of obvious structural defects that can be diagnosed through ultrasound scan. The traditional folk are also aware that advance maternal age is a risk factor to many fetal abnormalities and would therefore encourage early completion of procreation. Improvement in the awareness of Down syndrome screening could be achieved through information dissemination in local mass media in a manner that can be easily understood and appreciated. Information should address widely known preformed ideas and conceptions about the origin of conditions as well as the options of early diagnosis.

Cost

In Nigeria, cost is a major determinant of utilization of healthcare services. The majority of people live below poverty line and are struggling to cope with basic necessities of survival. Studies have demonstrated that the bulk (98.9%) of women that utilize prenatal diagnosis services are in the high socioeconomic group (Oloyede, 2005, Oloyede, 2008). Low utilization of prenatal screening was attributed to cost in 39.7% among other causes (Oloyede, 2008). Issues of subsidy from both governmental and non governmental agencies, bulk purchase of reagents for laboratory analysis are few suggestions to reduce cost (Oloyede, 2003). The introduction of scan screening would also reduce cost of screening in Nigeria.

Legal status of abortion

One of the controversial and ethical issues in Down syndrome screening is that of abortion. Most women that utilize prenatal screening have the issue of termination to contend with. In a study in Lagos, 70% of respondents would terminate a fetus that is affected (Oloyede, 2006). In taking a decision, few other factors may be important. Women with previously affected person in the family are much more likely to terminate than otherwise. Screening in the first trimester offers a better opportunity for safer termination than second trimester screening. Various associations such as the Down syndrome association of Nigeria and the Down syndrome South Africa are also cautious in the campaigning for or against abortion. This is because, it is viewed that the final decision is entirely a personal issue. Abortion law is restrictive in Nigeria and many other countries in sub Saharan Africa. Counseling following prenatal screening and diagnosis is largely non directional and leaves the option of termination in the hands of the couple.

Abortion following the screening and diagnosis of Down syndrome has been shown to reduce the prevalence of the condition in South Africa (Molteno, 1997). Considering the handicap in the care of the Down syndrome in the society in Nigeria and many other sub Saharan African countries, abortion may be a rational decision for affected cases.

Religion

Religion is sometimes a barrier to the wider utilization of prenatal screening services in Nigeria. It is responsible for poor utilization in about 28% of women in a Nigerian study (Oloyede and Oyedele, 2008). It is believed that the predominant religions in Nigeria are not well disposed to investigating the status of an unborn child, nor the decision to abort any fetus with genetic disorder (Oloyede, 2002).

The observation from Nigeria is that the influence of religion is modified by the occurrence of any previous congenital defect. Interestingly, another study in Nigeria showed that many couples underwent prenatal diagnosis for Sickle cell disorder solely to be informed and prepare for the birth and care of an affected child (Olatubosun, 2000).

2.2 Supportive measures

Supports should be offered to all people living Down syndrome to optimize their chances of survival and quality of life. There are three levels at which these supports could be offered in an integrated approach to achieve the best effect

1. Family level
2. Community/Society level
3. Governmental level

Family level

The family system in Nigeria is more of extended rather than nuclear based. The benefit from such system is that family burdens can be shared. Unfortunately, it has the opposite effect in respect of children with Down syndrome. Consequently, many families would not share such information with other families. Indeed, it is as ridiculous in some situation as to necessitate hiding Down child from neighbours and visitors. The level of support from the family is perhaps the most important determinants of outcome in children with Down syndrome. The family should realize that love, affection and tolerance are the very key to successful outcome and perhaps this would help to discourage the usual habit of child abandonment. The children need special learning skills which have to be started very early from the home. This is because of the generally lower IQ compared with normal children. The coming together of families with Down syndrome children should be encouraged for exchange of knowledge and skill in the management of the condition.

Community/Society level

The society is to complement the roles of both the family and the government. This is better achieved through nongovernmental organizations such as the Down Syndrome Associations. In Nigeria, the Down syndrome Association of Nigeria serves as the main rallying point for all activities about Down syndrome. In particular, the body initiates and encourages the implementation of all measures that improves the survival of the Down syndrome child. Outside the body, few other organizations have come up as homes for the less privilege that try to address the challenges associated with Down syndrome.

A problem that is common to all these initiative is lack of societal support as well as governmental assistance to function optimally. In addition to this, many communities in Nigeria, patronize and discriminate against children with Down syndrome. Recently, there has been noticeable positive change in the societal attitude to Down syndrome. More public programmes are now organized to increase awareness about the condition and solicit for support in the care of those affected.

Governmental level

In Nigeria, major health policies and implementation are government driven. In particular, health problems that are considered rare in occurrence and impact are given little attention. The peculiar educational need of the Down syndrome child requires that special school curriculum is designed to optimize their potential.

The area of support would be:

Incorporation of health programmes that relates to prenatal screening and diagnosis of Down syndrome as well as screening and management of health complications into the national health system

Provision of subsidy to Down syndrome associations and other related bodies for better execution of programmes

Establishment of schools with special curriculum for those physically challenged by Down syndrome. This is considered more advantageous than educating them in regular schools in Nigeria

Organization of special events to draw attention to the plight of those with Down syndrome and to encourage community assistance. This could be in form of activities such as yearly marathon race

Design of social infrastructures that makes daily living easy for people with Down syndrome such as walk ways and bus lifts.

3. Conclusion

The up to date statistics about Down syndrome in Nigeria and many other sub Saharan countries is difficult to determine. However, empirical evidences from the few scientific publications available suggest that the condition is equally important and may even be more prevalent in the country than previously insinuated. The challenges faced in Nigeria include

1. Determine the exact magnitude of the problem
2. Early detection of cases through prenatal screening and diagnosis
3. Effective care for those affected in the population.

There are evidences to suggest that statistics can be updated in the next few years.

The last challenge is the most worrisome. This is because of the apparent lack of enthusiasm and slow response to initiatives to effectively care for the effected. In addition, there are inadequate facilities to adequately manage and optimize the survival and quality of lives of those affected.

Early detection appears the most feasible short term option in Nigeria. It gives the benefit of choice to the women. This approach involves both prenatal screening and diagnosis. Though not widely available, it has been shown to be favoured by many women. It will take a long time before a wide array of screening options become available in Nigeria. The cost, manpower and other logistics are prohibiting factors. In the meantime, the nuchal translucency scan holds the best promise for a wide scale screening. it is relatively cheaper to undertake and with less logistic required. Moreover a strong desire has been expressed by women for first trimester screening, with preference for the ultrasound scan (Oloyede and Oyedele, 2008). Efforts to improve on its availability and utilization would among other initiative involve review of training local curriculum to better emphasize prenatal medicine and collaboration between local and foreign postgraduate medical colleges for exchange and update of knowledge and skills.

4. References

Down L. J. (1866). Observation on an ethnic classification of idiots. *Clinical Lectures and Reports*, London Hospital. Vol. 3, pp. 259-62

Adeyokunnu A.A. (1982). The incidence of Down's syndrome in Nigeria. *Journal of Medical Genetics*. Vol. 19, pp.277-279.

Tompkins, A.B (1964). Down's Syndrome in Nigerian Children. *Journal of Medical Genetics*. Vol. 1, pp.115- 117.

Jelliffe, D. B. (I954a). Aetiology of mongolism. *Lancet*, Vol. 2, p. 871.

Tooth, G. (I950). Studies in mental illness in the Gold Coast. *Colonial Res. Pub. Ser.*, No. 6. H.M.S.O., London.

Jelliffe, D. B. (I954b). Mongolism in Jamaican children. *W. Indian Med. J.*, Vol. 3, p. I64. Down Syndrome South Africa.
http://www.downsyndrome.org.za/main.aspx?artid=53 accessed 14th March, 2011.

Molteno C, Smart R, Viljoen D, Sayed R, Roux A. (1997). Twenty-year birth prevalence of Down syndrome in Cape Town, South Africa. *Paediatr Perinat Epidemiol*, Vol. 4, pp.428-35.

Shuttleworth G.E.(1909). Mongolian Imbecility. *British Medical Journal*, Vol. 2, 661-665

Op't Hof J, Venter PA, Louw M. (1991). Down's syndrome in South Africa-incidence, maternal age and utilisation of prenatal diagnosis. *South African Medical Journal*, Feb 1991, Vol. 79, pp.213-6.

Oloyede, O.A.O, Giwa- Osagie, O.F. (2003). The New Techniques of Assisted Reproduction. *Tropical Journal of Obstetrics and Gynaecology*. 20 (1), April 2003, pp. 67-73

Oloyede O.A.O, Fetuga M.B, Iyaniwura C.A, Jagun E.O. (2006). Profile of Congenital Malformations in Sagamu, Nigeria. *The Nigerian Medical Practitioner*, Vol. 49, pp. 65-67.

Arthur, J.T. (1995). Cardiac lesions in 'Trisomy 21' Ghanian Children. *Ghana Medical Journal*. Vol. 29, pp. 617-620.

Osei-Bagyina, A. (2000). Causes of child language disorders in patients at KATH, Kumasi, Ghana. *Journal of Science and Technology*, Vol. 20, Nos. (1, 2 and 3), pp.132-138

Hesse,A.A., Appeadu-Mensah, W. (2006). Anorectal Anomalies in Ghana - A Review Of 54 Cases. *African Journal of Paediatric Surgery*, Vol. 3, No. 1, pp.4-8.

Avoke, M. (1997). Introduction to Special Education for Universities and Colleges. Accra: City Publishers

W.H.O (1997). Proposal for a feasibility study on the control of Sickle cell disease in Africa. Report of a WHO informal consultation. WHO document. WHO/HDP/SCD/87.3 Geneva.

Okunlola M.A, Owonikoko K.M, Fawole A.O et al. (2008). Gestational age at antenatal booking and delivery outcome. *African Journal Medical Medical Science*, Vol. 37, No. 2, pp.165 -169.

Adekanle D A, Isawumi A I. (2008). Late antenatal care booking and its predictors among pregnant women in South Western Nigeria. *Online Journal of Health and Allied Sciences*, Vol. 7, No. 1, pp.4-7

Ebeigbe P N, Igberase GO. (2005). Antenatal Care: A comparison of demographic and Obstetric Characteristics of early and late attendees in the Niger delta, Nigeria. *Medical Science Monitor,* Vol. 11, No. 11, pp. 529-32.

Oladokun A, Oladokun RE, Morhason-Bello I, Bello AF, Adedokun B. (2010). Proximate predictors of early antenatal registration among Nigerian pregnant women. *Annals of African Medicine* [serial online],[cited Mar 11, 2011], Vol. 9, pp.222-5

National Institute for Health and Clinical Excellence: Antenatal care: Routine care for healthy pregnant women. 2003.

American Academy of Pediatrics, American College of Obstetricians and Gynaecologists. Guidelines for perinatal care. 5th ed. Elk Grove Village, (IL): American Academy of Paediatrics, American College of Obstetricians and Gynaecologists; 2002.

Ndidi, E. P and Oseremen, I.G. (2010). Reasons Given by pregnant women for late initiation of antenatal care in Niger Delta, Nigeria. *Ghana Medical Journal.* Vol. 44, No. 2, pp. 47-51

Nicolaides, K.H, Azar, G, Byme, D, Mansur,C, Marks, K (1992). Fetal nuchal translucency ultrasound screening for chromosomal defects in first trimestrer of pregnancy. *British Medical Journal.* 304, pp. 867-869.

Oloyede O.A.O (2008). Down syndrome screening in Nigeria. *International Journal of Gynaecology and Obstetrics,* Vol.100, No. 1, pp. 88-89.

Naidoo P, Erasmus I, Jeedbodh J, Nicolaou E, van Gelderen CJ. (2008). Nuchal translucency as a method of first-trimester screening for aneuploidy. *South African Medical Journal,* 2008, Vol. 98: pp.295-299.

Rosch C, Steinbicker V, Kropf S. (2000). Down's syndrome: the effects of prenatal diagnosis and demographic factors in a region of the eastern part of Germany. *European Journal of Epidemiology,* Vol. 16, pp. 627-32.

Lamina, M.A, Oloyede O.A.O, Adefuye P.O. (2004). Should Ultrasonography be done Routinely for all Pregnant Women?. *Tropical Journal of Obstetrics and Gynaecology,* Vol.21, No. 1, pp. 11- 14

Oloyede, O.A.O, Akinde, J.A, Emuveyan, E., Odusoga, O.L, Lamina, M.A, Ibidapo, M.O. (2003). Prenatal Diagnosis: Appraisal of Awareness and Utilization among Health Workers in Southwestern, Nigeria. *Nigerian Journal of Clinical Practice.* June, 2003; Vol. 5, No. 1, pp. 41-47

Oloyede, O.A.O, Oyedele, R.A. (2008). Women's attitude to prenatal screening services for congenital abnormalities in Nigeria. *Journal of Obstetrics and Gynaecology.* 2008; Vol. 28, No. 4, pp. 406-407.

Oloyede, O.A. O (2005). Influence of Socio - Demographic Characteristics on the Utilization of Chorionic Villus Sampling Service in Nigeria *Tropical Journal of Obstetrics and Gynaecology.* Vol.22, No. 2, pp. 116-119.

Oloyede O.A.O. (2006). Psychological Impact of Prenatal Diagnosis and Post Procedure Options. *Nigerian Journal of Health and Biomedical Sciences.* Vol 5, No. 2, pp.: 83-86

Oloyede O.A.O, Akinde J.A, Emuveyan E.E, Ibidapo M.O, Adewole T.A. (2002). Review of Chorionic Villus Sampling in Prenatal Diagnosis. *Nigerian Journal of Clinical Practice.* Vol. 5, No. 1, pp. 45-51.

Olatubosun A.O (2000). Contemporary Approach to Prenatal diagnosis. *Achives of Ibadan Medicine*. Vol.1. No. 3, pp.12-15.

11

Non Invasive Prenatal Diagnosis of Down Syndrome

Dimitra Kappou[1], Eleftheria Papadopoulou[2] and Stavros Sifakis[1]
[1]*Department of Obstetrics & Gynecology, University Hospital of Heraklion, Crete*
[2]*Department of Pediatrics, University Hospital of Heraklion, Crete*
Greece

1. Introduction

Down syndrome (trisomy 21), which has an incidence of 1 in 800 live births, is considered to be the most frequent etiology of mental retardation and it is the predominant reason for women seeking prenatal diagnosis [Driscoll & Gross, 2009]. Trisomy 21 is used as a benchmark because it is the most common aneuploidy compatible with life and is associated with mental retardation and serious congenital anomalies. Currently used screening tests for aneuploidy are based on the assessment of fetal sonographic markers and/or the evaluation of biochemical markers in the maternal circulation during the first and second trimester. Screening test based on the combination of nuchal translucency assessment and biochemical markers at 11^{+0}-13^{+6} weeks of gestation may detect 90-94% of pregnancies affected by Down syndrome at a false positive rate of 5% [Kagan et al., 2008]. The current gold standard for diagnosis of trisomy 21 is provided by invasive sampling of fetal genetic material through chorionic villus sampling (CVS) or amniocentesis followed by conventional cytogenetic or DNA analysis; however, both procedures are associated with an increased risk of fetal loss of about 1% and therefore they are recommended for pregnancies considered to be at high risk of fetal trisomy 21 [Alfirevic et al., 2003].
Since 1997, when cell free fetal DNA in maternal circulation was discovered, the research interest has focused on the development of reliable techniques for non-invasive prenatal diagnosis (NIPD) that would allow the direct analysis of fetal genetic material based on the discovery of cell-free fetal (cff) DNA and RNA in the maternal circulation. Current investigation fields of NIPD include fetal Rhesus D genotype determination in RhD negative women, fetal sex determination for sex-linked disorders and the role of cffDNA in pregnancy disorders such as preeclampsia but the holy grail of NIPD remains the detection of fetal aneuploidies [Honda et al., 2002; Bianchi et al., 2005]. The direct analysis of circulating fetal DNA for the NIPD of chromosomal aneuploidies is mainly complicated by the presence of the coexisting background maternal DNA. NIPD will hopefully overcome the limitations of the currently used methods for diagnosing Down syndrome antenatally and make prenatal testing safer for pregnant women and their fetuses. However, irrespective of which strategy is selected for isolating or distinguishing fetal genetic material in maternal plasma, the small quantity of cffDNA and cff mRNA poses severe technical challenges; all these issues should be addressed before the clinical application of these methods as screening test with high sensitivity, specificity and reproducibility.

In this chapter, we focus on recent advances in the NIPD of Down syndrome via the use of fetal cells or cell-free nucleic acids, and provide an overview of the future perspectives in terms of improvement of enrichment technologies and assaying methods and possibilities for clinical applications as well.

2. Intact fetal cells and cell-free fetal DNA in the maternal circulation

It has been established for over a century that fetal cells circulate in the maternal blood throughout gestation although the rarity of these cells limits eventually the practicability of a diagnostic process based on their enumeration in maternal plasma. A considerable challenge for the researchers in this field is to enrich or isolate these rare fetal cells, either for cytogenetic analysis by fluorescence in situ hybridization (FISH) or for analysis of fetal cell DNA by other molecular techniques [Bianchi and Hanson, 2006; Mavrou et al., 2007]. Several studies have reported that the number of fetal cells in maternal blood is markedly increased up to six times in women bearing aneuploid fetuses [Falcidia et al., 2004]. A large-scale study for this cell-based approach, conducted by the National Institute of Child Health and Human Development in the USA, demonstrated that detection of trisomy in these fetal nucleated erythrocyte cells is difficult possibly due to the fact that the chromosomes in these cells disintegrate some time before the nucleus is eliminated from the cell, making FISH analysis of samples from maternal circulation unreliable [Bianchi et al., 2002; Babochkina et al., 2005]. The use of fetal cells other than fetal nucleated red blood cells also found in maternal circulation has been studied, however these cells are able to persist for years, or even decades, following previous pregnancies and this persistence limits their potential value for NIPD [Guetta et al., 2003]. Possible explanations include a simple presence of these fetal cells or the fact that the maternal hematopoietic system becomes engrafted with fetal stem cells during pregnancy [Puszyk et al., 2008].

The first experimental demonstration of cffDNA in the maternal plasma and serum of women carrying male fetuses by Lo et al., (1997), opened up new possibilities in NIPD. Lo et al. were inspired by previous reports that documented the presence of tumour-derived DNA in the plasma of women suffering from a variety of cancer types. Potential sources of cffDNA include the fetal nucleated red blood cells which undergo apoptosis in the maternal circulation but the most likely source of origin is the placenta [Alberry et al., 2007]. Paternally derived DNA sequences in cffDNA can be reliably identified in maternal plasma, from as early as 5 weeks after conception and there is a positive correlation with gestational age. In particular, the median values of the quantity of cffDNA are 15.9, 21.5 and 52.0 genome equivalents/ml of blood in the first, second and third trimester respectively; the accumulation of cffDNA as pregnancy progresses lends further support to the placental origin of cffDNA [Lo et al., 1998; Sekizawa et al., 2001; Birch et al., 2005]. In particular, cytotrophoblasts (CTBs) are a likely candidate as a source of cffDNA; however, the increased rate of hyperploidy in these cells and the yet unknown relationship between the ploidy status of these cells and the ploidy of cffDNA in maternal circulation could make a diagnostic test problematical [Weier et al., 2005]. Moreover, there is a link between hypoxia and an increasing release of cffDNA that led to the suggestion that it may be a useful biomarker to assess well-being of the placenta during pregnancy [Tjoa et al., 2006]. It is known that cffDNA represents a mean of 3-6% of the DNA that is present in maternal plasma while the bulk of the DNA is derived from the mother herself and a rapid clearance occurs post partum with a half-life in the order of 16 minutes despite the narrow conflicting results [Invernizzi et al., 2002; Rijnders et al., 2004]. First applications of cffDNA included prenatal determination of fetal sexing based on paternally derived DNA sequences such as SRY, determination of Rhesus-D status of the fetus and detection of paternally inherited genetic abnormalities [Lo, 2006; Van der Schoot et al., 2006].

3. Detection of trisomy 21 from nucleic acids in the maternal plasma

There are two approaches for the detection of trisomy 21 based on the use of cffDNA in maternal circulation. The first is defined as the relative chromosome dosage (RCD) method and compares the quantity of a chromosome 21-derived DNA sequence in cffDNA with the amount of a reference DNA sequence in cffDNA derived from a chromosome other than chromosome 21 [Lo et al., 2007a]. In a normal pregnancy the RCD of chromosome 21 is 2:2, whereas in trisomy 21 the RCD is expected to be 3:2. The second method is defined as the allele ratio (AR) method and involves the allelic ratio of single nucleotide polymorphisms (SNPs) present in a fetal-specific nucleic acid marker [Tong et al., 2006]. In a normal pregnancy where the fetus is heterozygous for a particular gene sequence, the AR in cffDNA is expected to be 1:1 whereas in a case of trisomy 21 the AR of chromosome 21 would be 2:1. The main disadvantage of this approach is that it is applicable only to heterozygous fetuses for the analyzed SNP.

3.1 Fetal DNA enrichment methods

The detection of fetal chromosomal aneuploidies with the aid of cffDNA presents considerable technical challenge: first, to select a subset of nucleic acid in maternal plasma that is completely fetal specific and second, to determine the chromosomal dosage in this subset. The major technical challenge that makes NIPD a demanding task is that cffDNA makes up a low proportion in maternal plasma in a high background of maternal DNA. Currently, several assay procedures are developed in order to enrich and enhance the fractional concentration of fetal DNA or just to distinguish the cffDNA in maternal blood samples. One point of differentiation between cffDNA and cell-free maternal DNA (cfmDNA) is that the first has a shorter size distribution (the majority being 145 bp in length or shorter whereas cfmDNA is significantly longer) [Li et al., 2004]. Based on this observation, researchers try to apply methods of size fractionation with the aid of various kits and columns that rely on the inability of large molecular weight DNA to pass through or by retention of low molecular weight DNA in a gel or column [Legler et al., 2007]. Main disadvantages of this approach are: a) the currently used electrophoretic method is labor-intensive and probably prone to contaminations and b) it is unknown if the provided DNA enrichment is enough satisfactory for the prenatal diagnosis of chromosomal aneuploidies [Lo, 2008]. In 2004, Dhallan's group proposed a specific blood processing protocol in which the addition of formaldehyde in maternal blood samples before centrifugation dramatically increased the percentage of fetal DNA recovered with the concurrent suppression of the maternal DNA background [Dhallan et al., 2004]. There are two speculations about the role of formaldehyde in increased yield of fetal DNA: a) prevention of maternal cell lysis and subsequent reduction of the amount of cfmDNA, and b) prevention of the degradation of cffDNA via its nuclease inhibitory effect [Dhallan et al., 2004]. The same research group supported that the application of this technique resulted in a significant increase in the proportion of cffDNA present from a maximum of about 6% to mean values of 20.2-25% in samples collected during various stages of gestation [Dhallan et al., 2004]. In an attempt to reproduce these results, other investigators confirmed the previous results and reported a similar or a less pronounced increase of cffDNA (1-3%) whereas other studies yielded inconsistent results [Costa et al., 2004; Chinnapapagari et al., 2005]. A possible reason for this discrepancy is that the sample processing time differs between the studies and it is known that the amount of time spent in the tube affects the concentration of total cell-free DNA [Zhang et al., 2008]. Zhang et al. (2008) proposed that the formaldehyde addition will offer a beneficial effect if there is a delay > 6 hours in sample processing as they demonstrated no maternal blood lysis or released extra maternal free DNA into plasma within the first six hours. Future studies should be conducted to clarify the contribution of elapsed time between blood-taking and processing on the recovery of cell-free DNA from maternal plasma and determine other confounding factors in the effect of formaldehyde. The quantification of cffDNA in maternal circulation from women carrying Down syndrome fetuses could also serve as a prognostic marker for trisomy 21 as quantitative aberrations in biochemical markers of placental origin that contribute to the aneuploidies screening tests. Previous studies present conflicting results as both a two-fold increase and no significant difference in maternal concentration of cffDNA have been reported [Lee et al., 2002; Spencer et al., 2003]. Possible explanations of the observed discrepancy between the reported results include the small number of samples examined, the variable degree of placental apoptosis, the broad ranges of cffDNA concentration at each stage of pregnancy and other sampling or methodological variables that might affect the level of circulating cffDNA. In a recent study, DNA from pre-CVS maternal samples was extracted from 72 trisomy 21 and 264 control pregnancies and authors concluded that there is no difference in first trimester cffDNA levels and the quantification of cffDNA (studied only in pregnancies with male fetuses) has no prognostic value at least in the early stages of pregnancy [Gerovassili et al., 2007]. However, quantification of cffDNA in maternal plasma might be a valuable second-trimester serum marker of Down syndrome pregnancy. Farina et al., found that the maternal serum fetal DNA concentrations were elevated in 15 Down syndrome cases during the second trimester and that fetal DNA could give a 21% detection rate at a 5% false positive rate; in addition, fetal DNA increased the estimated detection rate of quadruple test from 81% to 86% at a 5% false positive rate [Farina et al., 2003]. Main limitation of this approach is that its screening performance has been evaluated only in pregnancies with male fetuses with the aid of unique DNA sequences on the Y chromosome and when a reliable gender-independent fetal DNA marker will be assayed, its clinical utility should be reassessed.

3.2 The role of epigenetic markers in rapid detection of Down syndrome

The term epigenetics refers to the molecular processes that affect gene expression with the concurrent avoidance of any change in DNA sequence or content. The most studied epigenetic process is the DNA methylation, which involves the addition of a methyl group to the cytosine residues of a DNA sequence and when it occurs in the promoters of genes has an inhibitory effect on the gene expression. Epigenetic markers for cffDNA have been discovered for other aneuploidies; these are *SERPINB5* (serpin peptidase inhibitor, clade B, member 5; also known as maspin) on chromosome 18 and *RASSF1A* (Ras association [RalGDS/AF-6) domain family 1] on chromosome 3 [Lun et al., 2007]. In addition, the allelic ratio for placental-derived hypomethylated *SERPINB5* molecules in maternal plasma was further shown to be valuable in the non-invasive detection of trisomy 18 [Tong et al., 2006]. Nowadays, there is intense interest to identify differentially methylated DNA patterns on chromosome 21 between the placenta and maternal blood cells in order to

develop a similar method for the NIPD of Down syndrome. Such epigenetic markers could be useful either via the analysis of the epigenetic allelic ratios or directly compared with a placenta-derived DNA methylation marker on a reference chromosome [Tong et al., 2006].
A potential issue for any epigenetic approach to NIPD is the interindividual epigenetic variation as it has been documented in monozygotic twins; moreover, this process is regulated in a dynamic manner as epigenetic differences seem to increase over time in a process described as "epigenetic drift". However, epigenetic biomarkers sequences whose methylation has a functional significance may be subject to less individual variation than others with no functional constraint. The discovery of a number of DNA sequences that are differentially methylated between maternal and fetal DNA could provide novel markers for cffDNA via the quantification of fetal-specific DNA sequences derived from chromosome 21. One previous study described the methylation status for chromosome 21 in placenta and blood samples after the selection of sequences in promoter and non-promoter regions but it relied on an assay that used a methylation-sensitive restriction enzyme, HpaII that enables the analysis of a small proportion of all the CpG sites in the human genome [Old et al., 2007]. Differentially methylated sequences located at 21q22.3 (AIRE, SIM2 and ERG genes), 1q32.1 (CD48 gene and FAIM3 gene), 2p14 (ARHGAP25 gene) and 12q24 (SELPLG gene) were identified. Moreover, it was demonstrated that the methylation status for the sequences tested was not altered between early and term pregnancy [Old et al., 2007]. Recently, Chim et al. have performed a systematic search of 114 studied genomic regions (CpG islands) on chromosome 21 in a search for loci that were differentially methylated in placental tissue and blood cells and identified 22 (19%) that showed epigenetic differences between the maternal and fetal tissues [Chim et al, 2008]. The next step was to propose two new fetal-DNA epigenetic markers, *U-PDE9A* and *U-CGI137* found in the maternal circulation only during pregnancy and rapidly cleared upon delivery of the fetus [Chim et al, 2008]. This research group used a high resolution approach via bisulphite sequencing that increased the number of applicable CpG sites by 5-fold compared with the above-mentioned HpaII-based approach. These promising results suggest that fetal-specific epigenetic markers on chromosome 21 may provide a rich source of markers for NIPD. A novel method of trisomy 21 detection measures the ratio of a fetal-specific epigenetic marker on chromosome 21 (the putative promoter of the holocarboxylase synthetase (HLCS) gene) that is hypermethylated in the placenta and a genetic marker (ZFY, zinc finger protein, Y-linked) to determine the chromosome-dosage comparison in 5 maternal plasma samples from women carrying a fetus with Down syndrome [Tong et al., 2010]. Instead of ZFY, any other Y-chromosomal markers or any fetal-specific genetic targets that will be applied in female fetuses could also be used. Also, the placenta-specific epigenetic signature could be combined with the RNA transcripts of placental origin. This epigenetic-genetic chromosome dosage approach appears to be more precise compared to an approach based purely on epigenetic markers that will be extensively affected by the variability in the level of DNA methylation of individual molecules. Another group of investigators presented an alternative approach using methylation-dependent immunoprecipitation (MeDiP) that captures methylated sites combined with real-time quantitive PCR and identified 14 trisomy 21 cases and 26 euploid controls from pregnancies of 11-14 weeks old [Papageorgiou et al., 2011]. The accurate diagnosis of fetuses with Down syndrome was based on the ratio of a subset of fetal-specific methylated regions located on chromosome 21 compared with normal cases and regarding the clinical performance of the method both the sensitivity and

specificity were 100% [Papageorgiou et al., 2011]. The main methods performed for the study of DNA methylation are methylation-dependent immunoprecipitation (MeDiP), bisulphite conversion of DNA, and methylation sensitive restriction endonuclease assay to digest away the maternal sequneces. Main limitations of the most commonly used methods for DNA methylation analysis are that the use of bisulphite-based reagents results in DNA degradation (up to 96%) and thus in reduction of target DNA available for subsequent analysis and the methylation sensitive restriction endonuclease assay is limited to the differentially methylated regions that contain a restriction site [Grunau et al., 2001].

4. Chromosome 21-encoded mRNA of placental origin in maternal circulation

In 2000, Poon et al. showed that mRNA transcribed from the Y chromosome could be detected in the plasma of women carrying male fetuses [Poon et al., 2000]. Since then, a series of reports confirmed that cell-free fetal m RNA (cffRNA) circulates in the maternal plasma in a relatively protected form and is predominately placental in origin; therefore, it could be valuable in NIPD for Down syndrome [Tsui et al., 2002]. The underlying mechanisms by which mRNA appears in the maternal plasma remain unknown, although programmed cell death (apoptosis) seems to be involved. The transfer of cffRNA is unidirectional from the placenta to the maternal circulation and microarray-based studies of the placenta are conducted to investigate the global m RNA expression profiles in placenta, a tissue type that is only present in the fetus [Maron et al., 2007]. The m RNA transcripts of two genes expressed in the placenta, human placental lactogen (h PL) and human chorionic gonadotrophin (β HCG) have already been detected and quantified throughout gestation in maternal circulation [Chiu et al., 2006].

The potential utilization of cffRNA in detecting fetal trisomy is based on the assumption that the allelic ratio in mRNA matches the chromosomal AR; therefore, the research interest is focused on the discovery of single nucleotide polymorphisms (SNPs) as biomarkers that will exhibit the 2:1 ratio of alleles in trisomy 21 to ascertain the aneuploidy status [RNA-SNP allelic ratio approach]. Candidate m RNA markers should be encoded from genes located on chromosome 21 and be detectable in maternal plasma during early pregnancy. The first valuable cffRNA marker shown to be highly accurate in assessing trisomy 21 is PLAC4 (placenta-specific 4) m RNA transcribed from the PLAC4 gene on chromosome 21 and originating exclusively from fetal cells in the placenta and cleared following delivery of the fetus [Lo et al., 2007 b]. If the fetus is euploid, that is containing two copies of chromosome 21 and thus two copies of the PLAC4 gene, the ratio of the two candidate SNP alleles would be 1:1. Similarly, the ratio of placental mRNA in maternal plasma that is transcribed from each of these two alleles would also be 1:1. However, if the fetus has trisomy 21, then the RNA-SNP allelic ration would become 1:2 or 2:1 [Lo, 2009]. Compared with the epigenetic approach, the evaluation of RNA-SNP allelic ratio has two advantages; first, the transcription of a gene in the placenta will produce multiple copies of m RNA and second, application of reverse transcriptase PCR to detect m RNA markers is less complicated technique than bisulfite conversion methods used for the identification of epigenetic markers. The main drawback of this RNA-SNP allelic ratio approach is that it relies upon the fetus inheriting two different SNP alleles in a region which is transcribed into m RNA and therefore only fetuses heterozygous for the analysed SNP can be successfully diagnosed. Another candidate gene for this purpose is LOC90625 within the Down syndrome critical region that is over expressed in trisomy 21 placentas even from the first

trimester [Oudejans et al., 2003]. RNA from this chromosome was found to be present in 60-100% of maternal samples depending on the volume of plasma sample analysed leading to the conclusion that the detection of encoded m RNA could be used in NIPD.
This approach seems to be quite promising as in a recent study Lo et al. recruited a sample of 119 pregnancies and trough the use of a mass spectrometry-based method for measuring the RNA-SNP allelic ratio precisely, demonstrated that this strategy could achieve a high diagnostic sensitivity and specificity for trisomy 21 (90% and 96.5% respectively) [Lo et al., 2007b]. The application of novel molecular techniques as digital PCR in which individual target molecules are amplified will possibly improve the protocols for plasma RNA processing and extraction and further increase the diagnostic yield. This method could also be useful in the detection of other fetal-derived m RNA species in maternal plasma. Hopefully, the reproducibility of these success rates maybe with the addition of other markers of similar value to that of PLAC4 in large-scale clinical trials will open up new avenues in NIPD.

5. Novel techniques for the prenatal detection of Down syndrome

The urgent need for the widespread application of NIPD in the detection of trisomy 21 has created strong interest in rapid and accurate single-molecule counting methods [digital PCR, multiplexed maternal plasma sequencing] which could be used in routine clinical diagnosis in the form of automated platforms. These methods will be gender-and polymorphism-independent and will detect trisomy 21 cases based on the presence of an elevated amount of chromosome 21 sequences in maternal blood. The main disadvantage of these approaches is that they require the counting of an extremely large number of molecules for markers that are not fetal-specific (random sequences from chromosome 21) and their use demands expensive equipment and reagents and complex bioinformatics methods. We present an overview of the currently proposed techniques that have been associated with encouraging results in the detection of fetuses with Down syndrome and will hopefully be moved into the practical application.

5.1 Digital polymerase chain reaction (PCR) technology

The above-mentioned approaches (the fetal enrichment techniques, the epigenetic markers, the RNA-SNP allelic ratio method) try to resolve the issue of the low fractional concentration of fetal DNA in maternal circulation and the technical challenges that it poses in the direct detection of chromosomal aneuploidies with conventional methods, for example by real-time PCR [Lo et al., 1998]. Recent reports have indicated that digital PCR, a method that was initially applied in the determination of the allelic frequencies of oncogenic alterations in samples from patients with cancer, could be a valuable new tool in NIPD of trisomy 21 [Zimmermann et al., 2008]. In 2007, Lo et al., used digital PCR to discriminate trisomy 21 placental DNA samples from euploid ones after having applied this method in the measurement of the RNA-SNP allelic ratio for non-invasive detection of fetal aneuploidy in microwell plates [Lo et al., 2007]. In particular, they were able to distinguish four aneuploid fetuses from nine normal ones based on the PLAC4 m RNA SNP approach. In their second trial, the same research group applied a dosage approach and compared the dosage of a locus on chromosome 21 to a locus on the reference chromosome 1 and tried to detect fetal aneuploidy in artificial mixtures of euploid and aneuploidy DNA with as low as 25% trisomic material (a concentration that could be obtained in clinical samples using enrichment strategies for cffDNA sequences). The innovation of digital PCR is that multiple PCRs are performed in parallel and each PCR will contain either a single or no target molecule. Subsequently, the counting of the number of the positive reactions at the end of amplification will lead to the estimation of the number of input target molecules. The same research group has also defined the number of molecules needed for trisomy detection in different fetal DNA concentrations. Digital PCR does not depend on allelic distribution or gender and is able to detect signals in the presence of mosaics or contaminating maternal DNA; the widespread application of this method is still limited by that the fact that a large number of digital PCRs are needed for each analysis [Fan and Quake, 2007]. Fan and Quake used for their assay material obtained from a cell line with trisomy 21 and genetic material from cells with a normal genomic complement on a microfluidic chip [Fan and Quake, 2007]. The next step was to compare the dosage of an amyloid gene sequence on chromosome 21 to that of the GAPDH [glyceraldehydes 3-phosphate dehydrogenase) on chromosome 21 which was used as reference sequence. Their preliminary results suggest that digital PCR should be indicated for the discrimination between aneuploid and normal samples. It is noteworthy that the discrimination was possible even when the aneuploidy material represented a low proportion (10%) of the total material being examined, indicating the clear advantage of this method over conventional techniques such as real-time PCR or fluorescent quantitive PCR (QF-PCR). A significant barrier for using digital PCR is the small fraction of cffDNA in maternal plasma but an approach like size-fractionation that enriches cffDNA could overcome it. So far the reported encouraging results come from few preliminary studies and the question whether this method could be introduced as a screening tool has not yet been answered. In the near future, it seems likely that the efficacy of novel applications as microfluidic digital PCR and emulsion PCR that allow the simultaneous performance of few thousands of reactions in a single PCR step will be assessed [Zimmermann et al., 2008].

5.2 Shotgun sequencing DNA

Shotgun sequencing DNA technology is based on the massively parallel sequencing of DNA that produces tens of millions of short sequence tags in a single run followed by mapping to the chromosome of origin and measurement of the over- and underrepresentation of chromosomes from an aneuploidy fetus [Mardis 2008]. Fan et al., used this method and successfully identified all nine cases of trisomy 21 in their study population at gestational ages as early as the 14th weeks [Fan et al., 2008]. Further studies are required to specify technical features as the sample-volume limitations and the variations in the counts of sequenced fragments from sample to sample; in addition, this technology will contribute to current knowledge about cell-free nucleic acids revealing unknown features about plasma mRNA distributions and epigenetic features of plasma DNA.

5.3 Multiplexed maternal plasma DNA sequencing

Multiplexed maternal plasma sequencing can overcome the difficulty that poses the small proportion of fetal DNA in maternal circulation as it can identify and quantify millions of DNA fragments in biological samples in a span of days [Schuster 2008]. The feasibility and the diagnostic performance of this alternative approach has already been explored in three cohort studies that recruited few Down syndrome cases with promising results [Chiu et al., 2008; Fan et al., 2008; Chiu et al., 2010]. A recent large-scale validity study used multiplexed maternal plasma DNA sequencing analysis in 753 pregnant women at high risk for fetal trisomy 21 according to the results of conventional screening who underwent invasive procedures for full karyotyping [Chiu et al., 2011]. Two different protocols (2-plex protocol and 8-plex protocol) were used with different levels of sample throughput followed by the measurement of the proportion of DNA molecules that originated from chromosome 21. The 2-plex protocol achieved 100% sensitivity and 97.9% specificity to rule out trisomy 21 with a positive predictive value of 96.6% and negative predictive value of 100% while the 8-plex protocol with which less plasma DNA molecules were analyzed, exhibited a relatively moderate diagnostic performance. The researchers also concluded that if the referrals for amniocentesis or CVS were based on the sequencing tests results, invasive diagnostic procedures could be avoided in about 98% of the cases in a high-risk population [Chiu et al., 2011]. Further studies will confirm the suitability of this method as first trimester screening test in the general population and its cost-effectiveness as it is currently expensive and not easily accessible to diagnostic laboratories.

6. Prenatal detection of Down syndrome through detection of trophoblasts in cervical smears

Fetal cells are also present in the uterine cavity from 5 to 15 weeks of pregnancy and are most probably exfoliated extravillous trophoblasts (shed from the placenta) [Holzgreve and Hahn, 2000]. Trophoblast cells can be retrieved from the cervical canal using aspiration, cryobrush or cotton wool swabs, endocervical lavage, and intrauterine lavage. Initial approaches using endocervical samples obtained by mucus aspiration or by cryobrush resulted in higher success rates of fetal sex prediction [Griffith-Jones et al, 1992; Falcinelli et al, 1998]. However, direct PCR amplifications from unpurified transcervical cells are likely to result in maternal cell contamination. A more recent study using PCR and FISH analyses on transcervical cells resulted in poor detection of fetal cells [Cioni et al, 2003]. To distinguish trophoblast cells from the predominant maternal cell population in transcervical cell samples, antibodies directed against placental antigens were employed [Koumantaki et al, 2001; Bulmer et al, 2003]. These analyses resulted in an overall detection rate of trophoblasts of 25 to 93%.

Another suggestion is that fetal cell search can be improved through better and faster recognition of fetal cells with the aid of automated scanning (automated microscope systems). Theoretically, the automated microscope could work faster and continuously and thus process more cells or more samples than the fatigued human. Analysis of interphase nuclei by FISH, can be used to detect numerical chromosome aberrations (Evans et al., 1992; Ward et al., 1993). The attraction of FISH as a relatively simple approach is based on experience with peripheral blood, amniocentesis samples, and transcervical samples, which have large numbers of cells to examine so that occasional poor signals are only a nuisance. With the few fetal cells available in fetal cell work, FISH quickly shows limitations. It seems necessary to further develop automated microscope systems, which would robotically identify and analyse putative target fetal cells. A recent study tested the hypothesis that fetal cells retrieved from the distal endocervical canal during the first trimester (as early as 5 weeks) may be a source of fetal genetic material for NIPD of trisomy 21 [Sifakis et al., 2011]. The hybridization of fetal cells with chromosome 21 specific probes followed by analysis with an automated fluorescence microscope led to the successful detection in 5 out of 5 trisomy 21 pregnancies [Sifakis et al., 2011]. Examples of the trisomy 21 cells detected, one from a male and the other from a female trisomy 21 pregnancy are shown in the Figure 1.

Additional studies with larger sample size are required to verify the potential of the utilization of fetal cells obtained via cervical samples for NIPD.

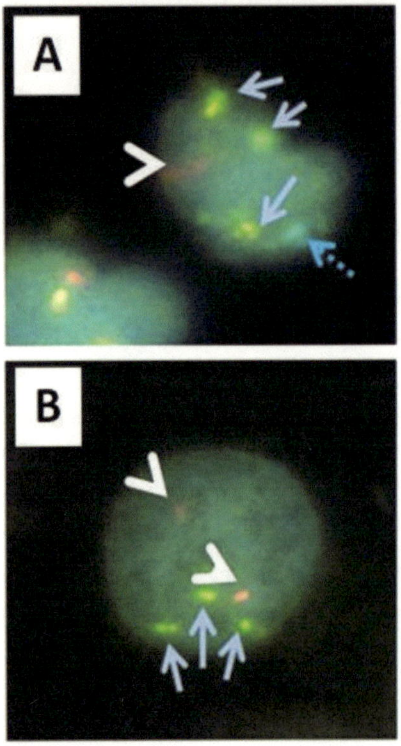

Fig. 1. Identification of trisomy 21 cells in cervical samples from trisomy 21 pregnancies. Panel A: Male trisomy 21 nucleus exhibiting X signal (white arrowhead), Y signal (broken blue arrow) and chromosome 21 signals (arrows). Panel B: Female trisomy 21 nucleus exhibiting two X signals (white arrow heads) and three chromosome 21 signals (arrows).

7. Conclusion

The development of a non-invasive genetic test for Down syndrome that would provide true genetic information without carrying risk for the progress of the pregnancy will continue to be an actively researched area in prenatal diagnosis. The trials performed so far highlight the medical and commercial potential of NIPD but the proposed techniques are not yet applicable in clinical practice. A major obstacle in the widespread application of NIPD in clinical diagnostics is that fetal DNA constitutes a small percentage of total DNA in maternal blood and intact fetal cells are even rarer. In the previous years the researchers were trying to discover Y chromosomes sequences or paternally inherited polymorphisms as targeted fetal DNA markers in maternal plasma but still there is no such a single marker that can be applied in all fetal-maternal pairs. One promising alternative approach appears to be the development of gender- and polymorphism- independent fetal DNA markers with a unique methylation pattern that will characterize the placental-derived free DNA in the maternal circulation. In parallel, the refinement of novel sequencing methods will create a universal test for fetal aneuploidy by using maternal plasma DNA that will not depend on the presence of specific genetic polymorphisms at specific loci but on the enrichment and quantification of cffDNA in maternal peripheral blood. Also, an important goal of the ongoing research is to develop laboratory protocols with the aid of bioinformatics algorithms that will allow their application in large sample numbers. Nevertheless, large-scale studies will need to be performed to confirm the diagnostic efficacy of these methods and subsequently lead to introduction of the experimentally validated strategies into the clinical practice of fetal medicine.

8. References

Alberry M, Maddocks D, Jones M, Abdel Hadi M, Abdel-Fattah S, Avent N, et al. Free fetal DNA in maternal plasma in anembryonic pregnancies: confirmation that the origin is the trophoblast. Prenat Diagn 2007;27:415–8.

Alfirevic Z, Sundberg K, Brigham S. Amniocentesis and chorionic villus sampling for prenatal diagnosis. Cochrane Database Syst Rev 2003;(3):CD003252.

Babochkina T, Mergenthaler S, Dinges TM, Holzgreve W, Hahn S. Direct detection of fetal cells in maternal blood: a reappraisal using a combination of two different Y chromosome-specific FISH probes and a single X chromosome-specific probe. Arch Gynecol Obstet 2005;273:166–9.

Bianchi DW, Hanson J. Sharpening the tools: a summary of a National Institutes of Health workshop on new technologies for detection of fetal cells in maternal blood for early prenatal diagnosis. J Matern Fetal Neonatal Med 2006;19:199–207.

Bianchi DW, Simpson JL, Jackson LG, Elias S, Holzgreve W, Evans MI, et al. Fetal gender and aneuploidy detection using fetal cells in maternal blood: analysis of NIFTY I data. National Institute of Child Health and Development Fetal Cell Isolation Study. Prenat Diagn 2002;22: 609–15.

Bianchi DW, Avent ND, Costa JM, van der Schoot CE. Noninvasive prenatal diagnosis of fetal Rhesus D: ready for Prime(r) Time. Obstet Gynecol 2005;106:841-4.

Birch L, English CA, O'Donoghue K, Barigye O, Fisk NM, Keer JT. Accurate and robust quantification of circulating fetal and total DNA in maternal plasma from 5 to 41 weeks of gestation. Clin Chem 2005;51:312–20.

Bulmer JN, Cioni R, Bussani C, Cirigliano V, Sole F, Costa C, et al. HLA-G positive trophoblastic cells in transcervical samples and their isolation and analysis by laser microdissection and QF-PCR. Prenat Diagn 2003;23:34-9.

Chim SSC, Jin S, Lee TYH, Lun FMF, Lee WS, Chan LYS, et al. Systematic search for placental epigenetic markers on chromosome 21:towards noninvasive prenatal diagnosis of fetal trisomy 21. Clin Chem 2008;54:500-11.

Chinnapapagari SK, Holzgreve W, Lapaire O, Zimmermann B, Hahn S. Treatment of maternal blood samples with formaldehyde does not alter the proportion of circulatory fetal nucleic acids (DNA and mRNA) in maternal plasma. Clin Chem 2005;51:652–5.

Chiu RWK, Lui W, Cheung M, Kumta N, Farina A, Banzola I, et al. Time profile of appearance and disappearance of circulating placenta-derived mRNA in maternal plasma. Clin Chem 2006;52:313–6.

Chiu RKW, Chan KCA, Gao Y, Lau VYM, Zheng W, Leung TY, et al. Noninvasive prenatal diagnosis of fetal chromosomal aneuploidy by massively parallel genomic sequencing of DNA in maternal plasma. Proc Natl Acad Sci USA 2008;105:20458-63.

Chiu RWK, Sun H, Akolekar R, Clouser C, Lee C, McKerman K, et al. Maternal plasma DNA analysis with massively parallel sequencing by ligation for noninvasive prenatal diagnosis of trisomy 21. Clin Chem 2010;54:459-63.

Chiu RW, Akolekar R, Zheng YW, Leung TY, Sun H, Chan KC, et al. Non-invasive prenatal assessment of trisomy 21 by multiplexed maternal plasma DNA sequencing: large scale validity study. BMJ 2011;342:c7401.

Cioni R, Bussani C, Scarselli B, Bucciantini S, Barciulli F, Scarselli G. Fetal cells in cervical mucus in the first trimester of pregnancy. Prenat Diagn 2003; 23:168-71

Costa JM, Gautier E, Benachi A. Genetic analysis of the fetus using maternal blood. Gynecol Obstet Fertil 2004;32:646–50.

Dhallan R, Au WC, Mattagajasingh S, Emche S, Bayliss P, Damewood M, et al. Methods to increase the percentage of free fetal DNA recovered from the maternal circulation. JAMA 2004;291:1114–9.

Driscoll DA, Gross S. Clinical practice. Prenatal screening for aneuploidy. N Engl J Med 2009;360:2556-62.

Evans MI, Klinger KW, Isada NB, Shook D, Holzgreve W, McGuire N, et al. Rapid prenatal diagnosis by fluorescent in situ hybridization of chorionic villi: an adjunct to long term culture and karyotype. Am J Obstet Gynecol 1992;167:1522–5.

Falcidia E, Parano E, Grillo A, Pavone P, Takabayashi H, Trifiletti RR, et al. Fetal cells in maternal blood: a six-fold increase in women who have undergone amniocentesis and carry a fetus with Down syndrome: a multicenter study. Neuropediatrics. 2004 ;35:321-4.

Falcinelli C, Battafarano S, Neri C, Mazza V, Ranzi A, Forabosco A. Analysis of fetal sex in TCC sample DNA: a contribution to the validation of this approach. Prenat Diagn 1998;18:1109-16

Fan HC, Quake SR. Detection of aneuploidy with digital polymerase chain raction. Anal Chem 2007;79:7576-9.

Fan HC, Blumenfeld YJ, Chitkara U, Hudgins L, Quake SR. Noninvasive diagnosis of fetal aneuploidy by shotgun sequencing DNA from maternal blood. Proc Natl Acad Sci USA 2008;105:16266-71.

Farina A, LeShane ES, Lambert-Messerlian GM, Canick JA, Lee T, Neveux LM, et al. Evaluation of cell-free fetal DNA as a second-trimester maternal serum marker of Down syndrome pregnancy. Clin Chem 2003;49:239-42.

Gerovassili A, Garner C, Nicolaides KH, Thein SL, Rees DC. Free fetal DNA in maternal circulation: a potential prognostic marker for chromosomal abnormalities? Prenat Diagn 2007;27:104-10.

Griffith-Jones MD, Miller D, Lilford RJ, Scott J, Bulmer J. Detection of fetal DNA in trans-cervical swabs from first trimester pregnancies by gene amplification: a new route to prenatal diagnosis? Br J Obstet Gynaecol 1992; 99:508-11.

Grunau C, Clark SJ, Rosenthal A. Bisulfite genomic sequencing: systematic investigation of critical experimental parameters. Nucleic Acids Res 2001;29:E65-5.

Guetta E, Gordon D, Simchen MJ, Goldman B, Barkai G. Hematopoietic progenitor cells as targets for non-invasive prenatal diagnosis: detection of fetal CD34+ cells and assessment of postdelivery persistence in the maternal circulation. Blood Cells Mol Dis 2003;30:13–21.

Holzgreve W, Hahn S. Fetal cells in cervical mucus and maternal blood. Baillieres Best Pract Res Clin Obstet Gynaecol 2000;14:709-22.

Honda H, Miharu N, Ohashi Y, Samura O, Kinutani M, Hara T, et al. Fetal gender determination in early pregnancy through qualitative and quantitative analysis of fetal DNA in maternal serum. Hum Genet 2002;110:75-9

Invernizzi P, Biondi ML, Battezzati PM, Perego F, Selmi C, Cecchini F, et al. Presence of fetal DNA in maternal plasma decades after pregnancy. Hum Genet 2002;110:587–91.

Kagan KO, Wright D, Baker A, Sahota D, Nicolaides KH. Screening for trisomy 21 by maternal age, fetal nuchal translucency thickness, free beta-human chorionic gonadotropin and pregnancy-associated plasma protein-A. Ultrasound Obstet Gynecol 2008;31:618-24.

Koumantaki Y, Sifakis S, Dragatis G, Matalliotakis I, Froudarakis G, Papadopoulou E, et al. Microsatellite analysis provides efficient confirmation of fetal trophoblast isolation from maternal circulation. Prenat Diagn 2001;21: 566-70

Lee T, LeShane ES, Messerlian GM, Canick JA, Farina A, Heber WW, et al. Down syndrome and cell-free fetal DNA in archived maternal serum. Am J Obstet Gynecol 2002;187:1217-21.

Legler TJ, Liu Z, Mavrou A, Finning K, Hromadnikova I, Galbiati S, et al. Workshop report on the extraction of foetal DNA from maternal plasma. Prenat Diagn 2007;27:824–9.

Li Y, Holzgreve W, Page-Christiaens GC, Gille JJ, Hahn S. Improved prenatal detection of a fetal point mutation for achondroplasia by the use of size-fractionated circulatory DNA in maternal plasma–case report. Prenat Diagn 2004;24:896–98.

Lo YM, Corbetta N, Chamberlain PF, Rai V, Sargent IL, Redman CW, et al. Presence of fetal DNA in maternal plasma and serum. Lancet 1997;350:485–7.

Lo YM, Tein MS, Lau TK, Haines CJ, Leung TN, Poon PM, et al. Quantitative analysis of fetal DNA in maternal plasma and serum: implications for noninvasive prenatal diagnosis. Am J Hum Genet 1998;62:768–75.

Lo YM. Recent developments in fetal nucleic acids in maternal plasma: implications to noninvasive prenatal fetal blood group genotyping. Transfus Clin Biol 2006;13:50–2.

Lo YMD, Lun FMF, Chan KCA, Tsui NB, Chong KC, Lau TK, et al. Digital PCR for the molecular detection of fetal chromosomal aneuploidy. Proc Natl Acad Sci USA 2007a;104:13116–21.

Lo YM, Tsui NB, Chiu RW, Lau TK, Leung TN, Heung MM, et al. Plasma placental RNA allelic ratio permits noninvasive prenatal chromosomal aneuploidy detection. Nat Med 2007b;13:218–23.

Lo YM. Fetal nucleic acids in maternal plasma. Toward the development of noninvasive prenatal diagnosis of fetal chromosomal aneuploidies. Ann NY Acad Sci 2008;1137:140-3.

Lo Y. Noninvasive prenatal detection of fetal chromosomal aneuploidies by maternal plasma nucleic acid analysis: a review of the current state of the art. BJOG 2009;116:152-7.

Lun FM, Chiu RW, Leung TY, Leung TN, Lau TK, Lo YM. Epigenetic analysis of RASSF1A gene in cell-free DNA in amniotic fluid. Clin Chem 2007;53:796–8.

Maron JL, Johnson KL, Slonim D, Lai CQ, Ramoni M, Alterovitz G, et al. Gene expression analysis in pregnant women and their infants identifies unique fetal biomarkers that circulate in maternal blood. J Clin Invest 2007;117:3007–19.

Mavrou A, Kouvidi E, Antsaklis A, Souka A, Kitsiou Tzeli S, Kolialexi A. Identification of nucleated red blood cells in maternal circulation: a second step in screening for fetal aneuploidies and pregnancy complications. Prenat Diagn 2007;27:150–3.

Mardis ER. Next-generation DNA sequencing methods. Annu Rev Genomics Hum Genet 2008;9:387-402.

Old RW, Crea F, Puszyk W, Hultén MA. Candidate epigenetic biomarkers for non-invasive prenatal diagnosis of Down syndrome. Reprod Biomed Online 2007;15:227-35.

Oudejans CB, Go AT, Visser A, Mulders MA, Westerman BA, Blankenstein MA, et al. Detection of chromosome 21-encoded mRNA of placental origin in maternal plasma. Clin Chem 2003;49:1445-9.

Papageorgiou EA, Karagrigoriou A, Tsaliki E, Velissariou V, Carter NP, Patsalis PC. Fetal-specific DNA methylation ratio permits noninvasive prenatal diagnosis of trisomy 21. Nat Med 2011;17:510-3.

Poon LL, Leung TN, Lau TK, Lo YM. Presence of fetal RNA in maternal plasma. Clin Chem 2000;46:1832-4.

Puszyk WM, Crea F, Old RW. Noninvasive prenatal diagnosis of aneuploidy using cell-free nucleic acids in maternal blood: promises and unanswered questions. Prenat Diagn 2008;28:1-6.

Rijnders RJ, Christiaens GC, Soussan AA, van der Schoot CE. Cell-free fetal DNA is not present in plasma of nonpregnant mothers. Clin Chem 2004;50: 679–81.

Schuster SC. Next-generation sequencing transforms today's biology. Nat Methods 2008;5:16-8.

Sekizawa A, Kondo T, Iwasaki M, Watanabe A, Jimbo M, Saito H, et al. Accuracy of fetal gender determination by analysis of DNA in maternal plasma. Clin Chem 2001;47:1856–8.

Sifakis S, Ghatpande S, Seppo A, Kilpatrick MW, Tafas T, Tsipouras P, et al. Prenatal diagnosis of trisomy 21 through detection of trophoblasts in cervical smears. Early Hum Dev 2010;86:311-3.

Spencer K, de Kok JB, Swinkels DW. Increased total cell-free DNA in the serum of pregnant women carrying a fetus affected by trisomy 21. Prenat Diagn 2003;23:580-3.

Tjoa ML, Cindrova-Dvaies T, Spasic-Boskovic O, Bianchi DW, Burton GJ. Trophoblastic oxidative stress and the release of cell-free feto-placental DNA. Am J Pathol 2006;169:400-4.

Tong YK, Ding C, Chiu RWK, Gerovassili A, Chim SS, Leung TY, et al. Noninvasive prenatal detection of fetal trisomy 18 by epigenetic allelic ratio analysis in maternal plasma: theoretical and empirical considerations. Clin Chem 2006;52:2194–202.

Tong YK, Jin S, Chiu RW, Ding C, Chan KC, Leung TY, et al. Noninvasive prenatal detection of trisomy 21 by an epigenetic-genetic chromosome-dosage approach. Clin Chem 2010;56:90-8

Tsui NB, Ng EK, Lo YM. Stability of endogenous and added RNA in blood specimens, serum, and plasma. Clin Chem 2002;48:1647–53.

Van der Schoot CE, Soussan AA, Koelewijn J, Bonsel G, Paget- Christiaens LG, de Haas M. Non-invasive antenatal RHD typing. Transfus Clin Biol 2006;13:53–7.

Ward BE, Gersen SL, Carelli MP, McGuire NM, Dackowski WR, Weinstein M, et al. Rapid prenatal diagnosis of chromosomal aneuplodies by fluorescence in situ hybridization: clinical experience with 4,500 specimens. Am J Hum Genet 1993;52:854–65

Weier JF, Weier HU, Jung CJ, Gormley M, Zhou Y, Chu LW, et al. Human cytotrophoblasts acquire aneuploidies as they differentiate to an invasive phenotype. Dev Biol 2005;279:420–32.

Zhang Y, Li Q, Hui N, Fei M, Hu Z, Sun S. Effect of formaldehyde treatment on the recovery of cell-free fetal DNA from maternal plasma at different processing times. Clin Chim Acta 2008;397:60-4.

Zimmermann BG, Grill S, Holzgreve W, Zhong XY, Jackson LG, Hahn S. Digital PCR: a powerful new tool for noninvasive prenatal diagnosis? Prenat Diagn 2008;28:1087-93.

12

Prenatal Examinations for Down Syndrome and Possible Effects on Maternal-Fetal Attachment

Susanne Georgsson Öhman
Sophiahemmet University College, Stockholm, Sweden and Karolinska Institutet, Department of women's and children's health, Stockholm Sweden

1. Introduction

The pregnancy and the adaptation to motherhood is one of the most signifcant events during a woman's life time. The pregnancy is associated with major psychological and physical changes. The woman expects to attach to the fetus and prepare for the life as a mother. Interventions during pregnancy must be implemented with respect for the sensitive period as a pregnancy is.

The aim with this chapter is to describe and discuss possible effects of prenatal examinations for Down syndrome during pregnancy on maternal-fetal attachment. Additional aims are to illuminate experiences and reactions during the waiting-time for test results, the experience of false positive results from screening examinations and the perception of complex information from prenatal examinations. There is of great importance to explore and highlight these questions to minimize the risk for negative affection on the maternal-fetal attachment by prenatal screening or diagnosis for Down syndrome.

2. Maternal-fetal attachment

One of the basic prerequisite for the survival of a new-born baby is that there is a relation of attachment to the parents. This means a lasting emotional relation to a person who will secure the baby's trust and safety. The theory about attachment was developed by John Bowlby in England in the 50s. Maternal-fetal attachment (MFA) is a concept used to describe the relationship between a pregnant woman and the fetus. It describes the process in which the pregnant woman experience feelings and emotions for the fetus. At the same time her maternal identity is developed. This concept is rather new and is still not well studied or fully defined. MFA is based on representations of the fetus according to qualitative descriptions of maternal attitudes and adaption to pregnancy (Salisbury et al., 2003). The attachment between the pregnant woman and the fetus during the pregnancy had been described as the first important relation to the baby and has strongly been associated with the following mother-child relation after the birth. The attachment to the fetus and later to the baby is developing successively. It starts in early pregnancy and increases during the pregnancy to be most intensive during the last trimester (Alhausen, 2008, Yercheski, 2008). The concept maternal-fetal attachment was defined by professor

Mecca S. Cranley and are described as "the extent to which women engage in behaviors that represent affiliation and interaction with their unborn child" (Cranley, 1981, s 282).

There is not consensus about the concept attachment/bonding during pregnancy. The definitions are in generally split in definitions which describe attachment as emotions and those who describes attachment as behaviours during pregnancy which indicates the pregnant woman's attachment to the fetus. Three scales based on each definition of the concept have been developed to quantify MFA. The original maternal-fetal attachment scale (MFAS), developed by Cranley (1981) contains 24 items and intends to measure maternal-fetal attachment. The scale measures to what extent the mother-to-be is engaged in behaviour which is expressing a sense of belonging and an interaction with the unborn baby. The attachment is defined as how the mother-to-be cope with the development as the pregnancy means. It was developed from the attachment theory of Bowlby (Bowlby, 1969). The 24 items were divided into five subscales; differentiation of self from fetus, interaction with the fetus, attributing characteristics to the fetus, giving of self, and role taking. The response format is Likert-like with scores of 1 (definitely no), 2 (no), 3 (uncertain), 4 (yes) and 5 (definitely yes). Regarding the reliability of the scale, in previous studies. In previous studies the Cronbach's alpha for the total scale ranged from .82 to .91 and for the subscales .52 to .73 (Bloom, 1995; Lindgren, 2001; Shieh, 2006).

In 1990 another, the second, instrument intending to measure prenatal attachment was developed by Müller. This instrument - prenatal attachment inventory (PAI) was designed to measure the relationship that develops between the mother-to-be and the fetus. Müller defined prenatal attachment as the unique, affectionate relationship that develops between the pregnant woman and the fetus (Müller, 1993).

According to Condon & Corkindale, 1997, the concept prenatal attachment include the following five factors; wishing for knowledge about the unborn baby, happiness for the interplay with the baby, wishing for protecting the baby and satisfying its needs, worrying about losing the baby or that something will be wrong with the baby, and that the baby's needs have priority over the own needs. They developed the instrument MAAS (maternal antenatal attachment scale). Condon's definition was closer to the attachment theory of Bowlby. Condon described attachment as love, his definition of attachment was "the core experience of attachment is love" and proposed five subjective experiences of love.

The disposition to:

1. Know
2. Be with and to interact
3. To avoid separation or loss
4. To protect and
5. To identify and to gratify the needs of the object (Condon, 1993; Condon & Corkindale, 1997).

There are some difficulties to measure maternal-fetal attachment with the self assessment instruments which are available today. One difficulty is the limitation of the scales in their sensitivity to cultural differences and experiences. An adaption of the existing scales may be possible. Cranley's maternal-fetal attachment scale has been modified to a Japanese version with 20 items. The results of that study of 275 women confirmed previous studies. MFA increased significantly from gestational week 5 to gestational week 40. Feeling fetal movements had a particularly positive effect. Women with ambivalent feelings responded lower in the scale (Narita & Maehara, 1993).

Another close concept to maternal-fetal attachment is maternal/fetal interaction. A questionnaire to measure maternal/fetal interaction was developed in 1997 by Nelson. By this instrument the mothers spontaneous talk to herself or to the fetus assessed and emotional words such as "happy", "sad", "bored", "excited", "calm" or "anxious". Higher scores on the scale indicate higher level of maternal/fetal interaction (Ji & Han, 2010).

3. Factors which may affect maternal-fetal attachment

The development of the technologies which are used in the context of pregnancy and child birth may have psychological consequences for the expecting mother. There are normal psychological changes during pregnancy. It is a period of psychological and physiological adaptation and causes strong emotional reactions and sometimes even ambivalent feelings. It is a complex process. It is also related to the partner, the own mother and friends (Bibring et al., 1961; Shereshefsky & Yarrow, 1975). The first part of a pregnancy is characterized as a vulnerable period when the woman has to accept the fetus as a part of herself (Raphael-Leff, 1992). All interventions during pregnancy must be done with the normal psychological changes in mind.

Some factors are known as such which may facilitate the attachment; the experience of fetal movements, support from family, friends and the partner. Higher age of the expectant mother, depression, worry and abuse may affect the attachment in a negative way. Higher levels of maternal-fetal attachment are reported when the woman has a positive relationship with the expectant father. Women with high- risk pregnancies do not seemed to attach to their fetus in a lower extent than women with normal pregnancies. Failure to attach to the fetus during pregnancy seems to be more common in women from poor social and economic conditions (Alhausen, 2008). Patient education courses seem to positively influence the prenatal attachment (Bellieni et al., 2007).

In a study of 252 pregnant women MFA had a positive relationship with positive health practices, such as diet exercise, drug and alcohol use (Lindgren, 2001).The author discuss the practical problems about interventions intended to increase maternal-fetal attachment. There is not yet evidence which effects different interventions have on MFA. However, some reasons for delayed or low levels of maternal-fetal attachment are well-known, for example self-protection for emotional trauma suffering during a previous loss. In the antenatal care the care givers can try to identify women with poor maternal-fetal attachment and help them improve their health practices trying to improve woman's health and pregnancy outcome.

Effects of an intervention based on mind and body interconnectedness, called Qi, on maternal-fetal interaction were studied. Totally 70 women were included in the study. Qi exercise was carried out in the second half of the pregnancy. The exercise lasted for 90 minutes, twice a week. This study showed effect of Qi on maternal/fetal interaction as well as on maternal depressive symptoms and physical comfort. In this study the maternal/fetal interaction was measured by the Interpersonal Communication Questionnaire (Talking to the baby) (Ji & Han, 2010).

Hyperemesis gravidarum is a rather rare complication of pregnancy, which means a severe form of nausea and vomiting. This may lead to problems to intake food and fluid. Among women with hyperemesis gravidarum there were an association with less developed maternal-fetal attachment in gestational weeks 7-16, but this negative effect was very small compared to pregnant women without hyperemesis gravidarum. At follow-up after 26th

weeks of gestation this negative effect could not be proved anymore (McCormack et al., 2011).
Maternal-fetal attachment is not studied in developing countries. It is reasonable to assume that the MFA is affected of the high mortality rate for both women and infants (Salisbury et al., 2003).
When using assistance with IVF – in vitro fertilization to get pregnant there may be stressful for the woman compared to getting pregnant the "normal" way. However, it does not seem to affect the attachment to the baby during pregnancy (McMahon et al., 1997, Stanton & Golombok, 1993). Prenatal attachment was in a study by Hjelmstedt and colleagues (2006) compared between 56 women who had underwent IVF and 41 controls. A self-rating scale was completed in gestational weeks 26 and 36. As the pregnancy progressed the prenatal attachment was increased in the same way in both groups. A conclusion of this study was that marital satisfaction, age, ambivalence and detachment was significant contributors to prenatal attachment. As proved in other studies the same results are presented regarding women who get pregnant with assistance. When women are less positive about pregnancy, childbirth and childcare they show weaker attachment to their unborn child (Stanton & Golombok, 1993).
When having an increased risk for having a child with a genetic condition one possibility is PGD (prenatal genetic diagnosis). In vitro fertilization is used to produce embryos which are genetic tested and selected on the absence of particular genetic conditions. There is often a need for repeated cycles of ovarian stimulations, IVF and transfers of an embryo. This is trying and results in fluctuations in the woman's anxiety (Karatas et al., 2011), which may affect the attachment.

4. Prenatal examinations in general and its possible effects on maternal-fetal attachment

An ultrasound examination in the second trimester is offered to all pregnant women in Sweden. This examination is accepted of the vast majority (SBU 1998). To many expecting parents the ultrasound examination has such a strong confirming effect that they wait until after the examination before they tell family and friends about the pregnancy (Ekelin, 2004). The possibility to see the fetus on the ultrasound screen has shift the focus from the time point when the pregnant woman felt the movements of the baby by herself to the time point when you can see the fetus on the screen.
If, and in what extent, prenatal examinations affects the attachment are fairly insufficient explored. Ultrasound examination usually takes place before the woman recognizes the first movements of the baby and may be a facilitator for maternal-fetal attachment. However, studies of ultrasound examination and its effects on the maternal-fetal attachment show contradictory findings. The relationship between the expectant mother, and even the expectant father may start earlier in pregnancy (Stormer, 2003, Zeichmeister, 2001). The time point when the woman reported movements from her baby, so called quickening, used to be a very important moment, but have in those days been replaced by seeing the fetus on the ultrasound screen. Studies of attachment between the expecting mother and the fetus in relation to ultrasound examination have showed contradictory results (Lumley, 1990). Some studies do not present any differences between the attachment to the fetus (Heidrich & Cranley, 1989), whereas other studies present a positive effect (Caccia, 1991), especially the first ultrasound examination during pregnancy (Sandbrook & Adamson-Macedo, 2004) and ultrasound examination early in pregnancy (Stormer, 2003). According to a meta-analysis of

the effects of ultrasound examination on maternal-fetal attachment, the attachment increased to some extent (Yercheski et al., 2008). Several studies of the effects of 3 D- or 4 D ultrasound have not proved any improved attachment compared to 2 D ultrasound (Righetti et al., 2005; Rustico et al., 2005, Sedgmen et al., 2005), but may cause a positive change in the parents-to-be's feelings for the fetus (Pretorius et al., 2006). The attachment seems to increase and the worry about the health of the fetus decrease when the ultrasound examination is combined with a discussion with a health care professional. The discussion contained an explanation of the woman's and the fetuses anatomy and a demonstration of fetal movements. Except the discussion in relation to the examination the strategy also contained a follow-up discussion (Boukydis et al., 2006). When assessing the ultrasound examination's effects on the maternal-fetal attachment there are, except the general difficulties to measure maternal-fetal attachment, some methodological factors to take into consideration. The length of the examination, the information related to the examination and the communication between the health care giver and the parents-to-be affects the experience of the examination and may even the maternal-fetal attachment (Alhausen, 2008). Comparing studies are difficult to perform due to the fact that almost all women undergo ultrasound examination during pregnancy (Lumley, 1990).
The aim of an ultrasound examination in the second trimester is not primarily screening for Down syndrome but it is possible to detect malformations soft markers or anomalies which are associated with Down syndrome.

5. Prenatal examinations for Down syndrome and its possible effects on maternal-fetal attachment

Today, many of the prenatal examinations and screening such as nuchal translucency measurement in early pregnancy, maternal serum screening, combined ultrasound examination and biochemical screening and invasive diagnostics are aimed to find risk pregnancies for Down syndrome or Down syndrome. The invasive test being used are amniocentesis or chorion villous biospy. To be offered early screening, either early ultrasound examination including measurement of nuchal translucency or maternal serum screening has in one study showed an increase of the maternal-fetal attachment. However, this increase seemed to be small and temporary (Kleinveld et al., 2007). A conceivable reason that the attachment will increase may be that the women receive information about the examination which lead to improved awareness about the unborn baby. The awareness will, of course, be improved if the woman undergoes the examination. Even following invasive test may the attachment to the fetus increase. Among women who underwent chorion villus biopsy the attachment increased five week earlier than for those who underwent amniocentesis. When the women received normal test results the attachment increased. However, there are even results from studies which show the opposite. Women who had underwent serum screening on the indication advanced maternal age showed less attachment than those who underwent amniocentesis for the same indication or those who refused the test. The reason for that may, due to the discussion by the authors, that screening do not result in a diagnosis but a probability for Down syndrome which may lead to an additional feeling of insecurity (Lawson & Turiff-Jonasson, 2006).
There is insufficient research in the field of how risk or perceived risk for the baby during pregnancy influences the MFA. One study which had the underlying assumption that women in high risk groups would have less MFA than women in low-risk groups failed to

proved that (Cannella, 2005). In a qualitative study by Hedrick (2005) of women who expected a child with a nonlethal abnormality, the participants did not express less maternal fetal attachment, rather a feeling of a wish to protect the baby who was not perfect. However, information about an increased risk for carrying a baby with Down's syndrome from an early ultrasound examination including nuchal translucency measurement strongly implies the worry about the baby (Georgsson Öhman et al., 2006).

In a sub study of large randomized controlled trial aiming at evaluating the effects of screening for Down syndrome by means of an ultrasound scan including measurement of nuchal translucency in early pregnancy (gestational weeks 12 to 14), the aim was to investigate how the early scan compared to a ultrasound examination in second trimester, may have affected maternal-fetal attachment in mid-pregnancy. There were 2026 women included in the study. Women were randomly allocated either o the intervention or to a control group where the routine care with an ultrasound scan in gestational week 17 to 20 was offered. Data were collected by questionnaires before randomization and in gestational week 24. MFA was measured by a modified version of the Cranley maternal-fetal attachment scale. One item (I grasp my baby's foot through my tummy to move it around) was excluded in the present study because it seemed irrelevant to use in gestational week 24. Another item (I enjoy watching my tummy jiggle as the baby kicks inside) was replaced with "I like to read about the development of the baby, how it grows, how it looks like". Mean scores were used for comparisons and were calculated for the total scale and individual subscales. The results of the study showed that the mean score of MFA was 3.50 in the intervention group compared to 3.44 in the control group (p=0.04). The mean scores on all subscales were slightly higher in the intervention group, but only statistically significant regarding "Differentiation of self from fetus" $p = 0.01$. The conclusion of this study was that ultrasound screening for Down syndrome in the first trimester may have a modest positive effect on MFA in mid-pregnancy, compared with a ultrasound scan in the second trimester (Georgsson Öhman & Waldenström (2010).

In a study by Berryman and Windridge (1996) a lower attachment to the fetus among older women was shown. The authors interpreted this result as they restrain the attachment because they were aware about the risk of Down syndrome associated to high maternal age and as a consequence a possible loss of the pregnancy.

6. Reactions and experiences during waiting-time for test results

To wait for results from invasive testing, such as amniocentesis and chorion villous biopsy, seems to be worrying and a period full of concerns. This seems to be a difficult time period irrespective of nothing is expected to deviate, and irrespective of the invasive test has preceeded of information about increased risk for chromosomal abnormalities or not (Cederholm et al., 2001). Women who have undergone an amniocentesis described that they had an emotional distance to the pregnancy until the health of the fetus had been confirmed by the result of the test (Rothman, 193). The waiting time are often experienced as hard irrespective of normal test result or not (Cederholm et al., 2001, Green & Statham, 1996).

Many women who had received information about risk for the fetus having Down syndrome in relation to an early ultrasound examination including nuchal translucency measurement, describes the waiting time for having an amniocentesis and further to wait for the test result as a time when they repressed the pregnancy. They avoided to think about the baby, and denied their pregnancy in different ways. This can be interpreted as a strong feeling but still the question if this period of repression of the pregnancy affects the attachment is unanswered. Information about increased risk for something being wrong with the baby may lead to great consequences for the pregnant women, such as denying the pregnancy - taking a "time-out", until the test shows normal results. The women did not feel happiness about the pregnancy, they didn't tell anyone about it, didn't look for baby equipment or thought about names for the baby. This "time-out" lasted until a normal result from the invasive test was received in about one month. Considering one month of denying the pregnancy it is still reasonable to assume that prenatal examinations may affect the attachment (Baillie, 2000; Georgsson Öhman et al., 2006).

7. False positive results

To receive false positive results that there is an increased risk for the baby having a chromosomal abnormality lead to unnecessary worry about the health of the baby. Women have describes the time from receiving an increased risk that the baby have Down syndrome until they receive a normal result from the invasive test as a "time-out" a repression of the pregnancy as mentioned above (Baillie et al., 2000; Georgsson Öhman et al., 2006). There are reasons to assume that this time with decreased interaction with the fetus may affect the attachment and the feelings for the unborn child in some way. This is an important question for further research. Including waiting-time for the invasive test and the test result this period when the women repressed pregnancy could last for about a month.

In general, to reduce the number of false positive results is an important ethical issues about screening. Even after a reassuring diagnostic test can some worry remain (Green et al., 2004). In a study by Baillie et al. (2000), 24 women who received a false positive result from an ultrasound examination including measurement of nuchal translucency and a calculation of the probability for having a baby with Down syndrome were interviewed. Two thirds of the women in the study still experienced anxiety up to four weeks following the normal diagnostic test. In a study by Weinans and colleagues in 2004 anxiety in association with false positive results from nuchal translucency screening and from serum screening was compared. There were 20 women in each group in both groups the risk was presented as a numerical value. In this study the women in the group who underwent nuchal translucency screening stated they were more worried about the health of the baby than those who underwent maternal serum screening. A possible explanation to this finding is that the fetus was visualized in the "NT-group". In a study including 33 women who received false positive results from serum screening, 20% remained worried two months after a normal diagnostic test (Santalahti et al., 1996). Feelings of worry could easily be recalled as long as ten years after maternal serum screening (Smedler & Bremme, 1992). In a study of 102 families who had received false positive results from screening for congenital hypothyreoidism, 78 families experienced strong emotional reactions. As many as 18 of these families stated that they still felt insecure about the baby's health after a period of 6 to 12 months (Bodegård, Fyrö & Larsson, 1983). This link of studies presented above, all show that false positive results make a deep mark on those who are affected. There are still no studies which explore the effect of those strong feelings on the maternal fetal attachment.

8. Importance of information

Information about prenatal screenings and diagnostic is very complicated and complex. To give equal information in early pregnancy to all women who want to have the information is a great challenge. The ambition is to give equal information to all women irrespective of social and cultural background, education and age. The information will be standardize, evidence based, comprehensible and not generate worry (SFOG, 2008).

The content of the information will be;

- that most of the newborn children are healthy,
- the purpose with the screening or the examination,
- the pros and cons,
- that the participation is voluntary
- about the methods - the procedure, possibilities, limitations
- that a assessment of probability is not a diagnosis
- the meaning of the test results
- the probability for false positive and false negative results
- possible consequences and possible alternatives after the test results
- that the parents-to-be will be faced difficult decisions and dilemmas in cases were a abnormality is detected
- how common the abnormalities are and possible consequences for the child
- alternatives after diagnosis
- references to were additional information can be reached. (Halsey Lee et al., 2005)

The aim with the information about prenatal diagnosis is to enable the woman to make an informed choice (Dormandy et al., 2002). One common definition of informed choice adapted from O'Connor et al. (2009) is that "the informed choice is based on relevant knowledge, consistent with the decision makers' values and behaviourally implemented". When talking about prenatal screening or diagnosis this means that an informed choice to undergo prenatal examinations is when the woman has relevant knowledge about the test, a positive attitude towards it and actually undergoes it (Marteau et al., 2001, Michie et al., 2002, Potter et al., 2008). Sufficient knowledge is not enough to be able to make an informed choice. The choice should also reflect one's values and attitudes towards undergoing the test.

There are several difficulties with information regarding prenatal examination. Many pregnant women do not know that prenatal screening is an option; they do not know the meaning of false positive and false negative results and what it means to live with DS but they have more knowledge of practical aspects of prenatal screening (Dahl et al., 2008). Pregnant women can receive information about prenatal screening from different sources such as health care, pamphlets, books, the internet, friends and family (Park & Matthews, 2009). Film as a source of information has shown to increase the knowledge (Björklund et al., 2011, Hewison et al., 2001).

Regarding information about prenatal screening, a study was performed with the aim to compare the growth of maternal-fetal emotional attachment in groups of women whose decisions about participation in screening were informed or not informed. The result of the study showed that the group who made an informed choice had significantly lower attachment scores than the group who had not made an informed choice. The authors pointed out that the findings of this study have uncertain consequences. Delayed emotional attachment can be interpreted as a psychological defense, a way to keep distance from the fetus in case if the pregnancy will be terminated due to diagnosis of fetal abnormality

(Rowe, 2009). Delayed attachment may prevent positive behaviour which protects well-being of both the woman and the fetus such as good diet; non smoking and alcohol use (Rowe et al., 2009). On the other hand is it an important purpose in the antenatal care to strive for so many women as possible to been able to make an informed choice (Halsey Lee et al., 2005).

9. Conclusion

The human being is malleable and most difficulties and crisis we are able to cope with. Despite traumatic experiences, such as information about something may be wrong with the baby, with following crisis and repressing of the pregnany most of the women seem to recover and develop a stromg attachment to the fetus and bonding to the new born baby. However, some women may show stronger reactions such as depression or considerable worry. There is also a risc for remaining distrustfulness for the health of the child during the childhood. So far, there is a lack of concordant methods to measure maternal-fetal attachment, with some contraditiry results from research. Further development, validation and assessment of the available scales for self assessment of matrnal feta attachment are in a great demand. Further research is required to verify possible effects of prenatal examinations on the maternal fetal attachment in general. Additionally, there is a need for scrutinizing the field of information, and the possibility for the expectant mothers to make an informed choice regarding prenatal examinations. There is a lack of knowledge about conceivable adverse effects of prenatal examinations for detecting Down syndrome during pregnancy.

10. References

Alhausen, J.L. (2008). A literature update on maternal-fetal attachment. JOGNN, 37,315-328.

Baillie, C., Smith, J., Hewison, J. & Mason, G. (2000). Ultrasound screening for chromosomal abnormality: women's reactions to false positive results. British Journal of Health Psychology, 5, 377-94.

Bellieni, C.V., Ceccarelli, D., Rossi, F., Buonocore, G., Maffei, M., Perrone, S. and Petriaglia, F. (2007). Is prentatal bonding enhanced by prenatal education courses? Minerva Ginecol., 59(2):125-9.

Berryman J. & WIndridge, K. (1996). Pregnancy after 35 and attachment to the fetus. J Reprod Infant Psychol, 14:133-143.

Bibring, G., Dwyer, T., Huntington, D.S. & Valenstein, A.F. (1961). A study of the psychological processes in pregnancy and of the earliest mother-child relationship: some propositions and comments. Psychoanalytic Study of the child, 16, 9-27.

Björklund, U., Marsk, A., Levin, C. & Georgsson Öhman, S. (2011). Audiovisual information affects informed choice and expereince of information in antenatal Down syndrome screening - A randomized controlled trial. Patient Educ Couns. Doi:10.1016/j.pec.2011.07.004

Bloom, K.C. (1995). The development of attachment behaviors in pregnant adolescents. Nurs Res, 44 (5):284-9.

Bodegård, G. Fyrö, K. & Larsson, A. (1983). Psychological reactions in 102 families with a newborn who has a falsely positive screening test for congenital hypothyreoidism, Acta Pediatrica, 304. 1-21.

Boukydis, C.F., Treadwell, M.C., Delaney Black, V., Boyes, K., King, M., Robionson, T. et al. (2006). Women's responses to ultrasound examinations during routine screens in obstetric clinic. J Ultrasound Med, 25,721-728.

Bowlby, J. (1969). Attachment and loss: Volume 1. Attachment, New York: Basic Books.

Bricker, L., Garcia, J., Henderson, J., Mugford, M., Neilson, J., Roberts, T. & Martin, M.A. (2000). Ultrasound screening in pregnancy: a systematic review of the clinical effectiveness cost-effectiveness and women's views, Health Technology Assessment, 4(16), 1-093.

Caccia, N., Johnsson J.M., Robinsoon, G.E. & Barna, T. (1991). Impact of prenatal testing on maternal-fetal bonding: chorionic villus sampling versus amniocentesis. An J Obstet Gynecol, 165:1122-25.

Cannella, B. (2005). Maternal-fetal attachment: an integrative review. J Adv Nurs 50 (1):60-68.

Cederholm, M., Sjödén, P-O. & Axelsson, O. (2001). Psychological distress before and after prenatal invasive karyotyping. Acta Obstet Gynecol Scand, 80(6):539-545.

Condon, J.T. (1993). The assessment of antenatal emotional attachment: development of a questionnaire instrument. Br J Med Psychol, 66:167-183.

Condon, J.T. & Corkindale, C. (1997). The correlates of antenatal attachment in pregnant women. Br J Med Psychol 70 (4):359-172.

Cranley, M.S. (1981). Development of a tool for the measurement of maternal attachment during pregnancy, Nursing Research, 30: 281-284.

Dahl, K., Kesmodel, U., Hvidman, L.& Olesen F. (2006). Informed consent: attitudes, knowledge and information concerning prenatal examinations. Acta Obstet Gynecol Scand. 85:1414-19.

Dormandy, E., Hooper, R., Michie, S., Marteau, TM. (2002). Informed choice to undergo prenatal screening: a comparison of two hospitals conducting testing either as a part of a routine visite or requiring a separate visit. J Med Screen, 9:109-14.

Ekelin, M., Crang-Svalenius, E. & Dykes, A-K. (2004). A qualitative study of mothers' and fathers' experiences of routine ultrasound examination in Sweden. Midwifery, 20:335-344.

Georgsson Öhman, S. & Waldenström, U. (2010). Effect of first-trimester ultrasound screening for Down syndrome on maternal-fetal attachment - A randomized controlled trial. Sexual & reproductive Healthcare. 1:85-90.

Georgsson Öhman, S., Saltvedt, S., Waldenström, U., Grunewald, C.& Olin-Lauritzen, S. (2006). Pregnant women's responses to information about an increased risk of carrying a baby with Down syndrome. Birth, 33:1,664-73.

Green, J.M. & Statham, H. (1996). Psychological aspects of prenatal screening and diagnosis. T. Marteau & M. Richards (red.). The troubled helix: Social and psychological implications of the new human genetics. Cambridge: University Press.

Green, J.M., Hewison, J., Bekker, H.L., Bryant, L.D. & Cuckle, H.S. (2004). Psychological aspects of genetic screening of pregnant women and newborns: a systematic review. Health Technology Assessment, 8(33),1-109.

Halsey Lee, D, Williams, J. & Donahue, P. (2005). Ethical issues in genetic testing. Journal of midwifery & Women's health, 50:234-240.

Hedrick, J. (2005). The lived experience of pregnancy while carrying a child with a known, nonlethal congenital abnormality. J Obstet Gynecol Neonatal Nurs. Nov-Dec; 34(6):732-40.

Hewison, J., Cuckle, H., Baillie, C., Sehmi, L., Jackson, F. & Batty J. Use of videotapes for viewing at home to inform choice in Down syndrome screening: a randomised controlled trial. Prenat Diagn. 2001;21:146-49.

Hjelmstedt, A., Widström, A.M. & Collins, A. (2006). Psychological correlates of prenatal attachment in women who conceived after in vitro fertilization and women who conceived naturally. Birth, 33(4):303-10.

Ji, E.S. & Han, H-R. (2010). The effects of Qi exercise on Maternal/Fetal interaction and maternal well-being during pregnancy. JOGNN, 39, 310-318.

Kleinveld, J.H., van den Berg, M., van Eijk, J.T.H., van Vugt, J.M.G van der Val, G. & Timmermans, D.R.M. (2008). Does offering prenatal screening influence pregnant women's attitudes regarding prenatal testing? Community Genet. 11:368-374.

Lawson, K.L. & Turriff-Jonasson, S.I. (2006). Maternal serum screening and psychosocial attachment to pregnancy. Journal of Psychosomatic Research, 60:371-378.

Lindgren, K. (2001). Relationships among maternal-fetal attachment, prenatal depression, and health practices in pregnancy. Research in Nursing & Health, 24:203-217.

Lumley, J. (1990). Through a glass darkly: ultrasound and prenatal bonding. Birth, 17(4):214-17.

McCormack, D., Scott-Heyes, G. & McCusker, C. (2011). The impact of hyperemesis gravidarum on maternal mental health and maternal-fetal attachment. Journal of Psychosomatic Obstetrics & Gynecology, Early Online, 1-9.

McMahon, CA., Ungerer, J.A., Beaupaire, J., Tenant, C. & Saunders, D. (1997). Anxiety during pregnancy and fetal attachment after in-vitro fertilization conception. Hum Reprod., 12(1):176-82.

Marteau, T.M., Dormandy, E. & Michie, S. (2001) A measure of informed choice. Health Expect. 4:99- 108.

Michie, S., Dormandy, E., Marteau, T.M.(2002) The multi-dimensional measure of informed choice: a validation study.

Patient Educ Couns. 48:87-91.

Müller, M.E. (1993). Development of the prenatal attachment inventory. West J Nurs Res 15: 199-211.

Narita, S. & Maehara, S. (1993). The development of maternal-fetal attachment during pregnancy. Nihon Kango Kagakkaishi, 131:1-9.

O'Connor A.M, Bennett, C.L, Stacey, D., Barry, M, Col, N.F., Eden, K. B et al. (2009) Decision aids for people facing health treatment or screening decisions (Review). The Cochrane Collaboration.

Park, A., & Mathews, M. (2009). Women's decisions about maternal serum screening testing: A qualitative study exploring what they learn and the role prenatal care providers play. Women and Birth, 22:73-8.

Potter, B.K., O'Reilly, N., Etchegary, H., Howley, H., Graham, I.D., Walker, M. et al. (2008). Exploring informed choice in the context of prenatal testing: findings from a qualitative study. Health Expect. 11:355-65.

Pretorius, D.H., Gattu, S., Ji, E., Hollenbach, K., Newton, R., Hull, A. et al. (2006). Preexamination and postexamination assessment of parental-fetal bonding in patients undergoing 3-/4-dimensioanl obstetric ultrasonography. J Ultrasound Med, 25, 1411-1421.

Raphael-Leff, J. (1992). Psychological processes of childbearing. London: Chapman & Hall.

Rothman, B.K. (1993). The tentative pregnancy: how amniocentesis changes the experience of motherhood. New York: W.W. Norton & Company.

Rowe, H., Fisher, J. & Quinlivan, J. (2009). Women who are well informed about prenatal genetic screening delay emotional attachment to their fetus. J Psychosom Obst & Gyn. 30(1):34-41.

Salisbury, A., Law, K., LaGasse, L. & Lester, B. (2003). Maternal-Fetal Attachment. JAMA, 289, 13, 1701.

Sandbrook, S.P. & Adamson-Macedo, E.N. (2004). Maternal-fetal attachment: searching for a new definition. Neuro Endocrinol Lett. 25, 169-82.

Santalahti, P., Latikka, A-M., Ryynänen, M. & Hemminki, E. (1996). On what grounds do women participate in prenatal screening? Birth, 23(2), 101-7.

SBU. Swedish Council on Technology Assessment in Health Care. (1998). Rutinmässig ultraljudsundersökning under graviditet (Routine ultrasound screening during pregnancy) (SBU-rapport nr 139). In Swedish. Stockholm: SB Offset AB.

SFOG. (2008). Swedish association for obstetrics and gynecology. Maternal care, sexual and reproductive health. Report no 59.

Shereshefsky, P. & Yarrow, L. (1975). Psychological aspects of a first pregnancy and early postnatal adaptation. New York: Raven Press.

Shieh, C. & Kravitz, M. (2006). Severity of drug use, initiation of prenatal care and maternal-fetal attachment in pregnant marijuana and cocaine/heroin users. J Obstet Gynecol Neonatal Nurs 35(4):499-508.

Smedler, A. & Bremme, K. (1992). Screeningundersökta gravid måste få hjälp att bearbeta oroande besked (Pregnant women participating in screening must be helped with anxiety generated by alarming information). In Swedish. Läkartidningen 59, 652-3.

Stanton, F. & Golombok, S. (1993). Maternal-fetal attachment during pregnancy following in vitro fertilization. J Psychosom Obstet Gynecol., 14(2):153-8.

Stormer, N. (2003). Seeing the fetus: The role of technology and image uin the maternal-fetal relationship. Journal of the American Medical Association, 289,1700.

Righetti, P.L., Dell'Avanzo, M.D., Grigio, M. & Nicolini, U. (2005). Maternal/paternal antenatal attachment and fourth-dimensional ultrasound technique: a preliminary report. British Journal of Psychology, 96:129-137.

Rustico, M.A., Mastromatteo, C., Grigio, M., Maggionin, C., Gregori D. & Nicolini, U. (2005). Two-dimensional vs. two-plus four dimensional ultrasound in pregnancy and the effect on maternal emotional status. A randomized study. Ultrasound Obstet Gynecol, 25, 468- 472.

Watson, M.S., Hall, S., Langford, K. & Marteau, T.M. (2002). Psychological impact of the detection of soft markers on routine ultrasound scanning: a pilot study investigating the modifying role of information. Prenatal Diagnosis, 22(7), 569-75.

Zeichmeister, I. (2001). Foetal images: The power of visual technology in antenatal care and the implications for women's reproductive freedom. Health Care Analysis, 93:387-400.

Yercheski, A., Mahon, N.E., Yercheski, T.J., Hank, M.M. & Cannella, B.L. (2008). A meta-analytic study of predictors of maternal-fetal attachment. Int Journal of Nursing Studies, doi:10.1016/j.ijnurstu.2008.10.013.

13

Gender Affects Clinical Suspicion of Down Syndrome

Natalia V. Kovaleva
St. Petersburg State Pediatric Medical Academy under the Federal Agency of Health Care and Social Development Russian Federation

1. Introduction

It is known that the Down syndrome phenotype can result from a triplication of a small portion of chromosome 21. In the majority of cases diagnosed as Down syndrome (90%), free trisomy for chromosome 21 is found; in some 6% of the cases translocations are observed, and about 3% are mosaics with normal cell line; other aberrations involving chromosome 21 are rare and found in less than 1% [Mikkelsen, 1988]. In a huge literature on the epidemiology of Down syndrome, there are two features undoubtedly established, a strong association of free trisomy 21 frequency with advanced maternal age, and male prevalence among patients with Down syndrome due to regular trisomy 21.
Generally, the clinical diagnosis is straightforward and well-known to all medical workers [Mikkelsen, 1988]. However, misdiagnosis (false positive diagnosis) of Down syndrome was reported in numerous publications [Ahmed et al., 2005; Baccichetti et al., 1990; Ballesta et al., 1977; Engel et al., 1970; Fried et al., 1980; Hamerton et al., 1965; Melve et al., 2008; Szollar et al., 1983], being particularly high in neonates [Devlin & Morrison, 2004; Hindley & Medakkar, 2002]. Factors which alter suspicion of trisomy 21 are known to be early delivery and prematurity [Mikkelsen, 1988].
Previous studies reported a significant female prevalence among Down syndrome patients with clinical diagnosis only which suggested that gender also may alter a suspicion of Down syndrome in infants [Kovaleva et al., 1999; Kovaleva, 2002]. Therefore, the main objectives of this study were to evaluate a rate of false positive diagnosis of Down syndrome in a large well-defined geographically population and to determine male-to-female ratio (sex ratio, SR) among patients with false-positive diagnosis.

2. Materials and methods

St. Petersburg is a large city with a population of about 5 million, and an average of 50 000 births a year. Almost all births take place in a hospital. There is one major clinical genetic unit in the city which provides the service to the target population, the St. Petersburg Centre for Medical Genetics. The overwhelming majority of live born babies suspected to have genetic disease have been examined by clinical geneticists from the Centre within the first several days after birth and prior to discharge from a hospital. Medical personnel at children hospitals and special institutions for handicapped children may also call for a clinical geneticist for suspected genetic condition. It is mandated that few cases born in private hospitals and tested cytogenetically elsewhere, must be reported to the Centre. Older patients or their parents can arrange an appointment to the Centre themselves after being referred to by medical specialists. Only certified clinical geneticists at St. Petersburg Centre for Medical Genetics can request karyotyping to confirm or refute a suspected chromosomal abnormality.

In St. Petersburg, due to global social transition, the birth rate fell dramatically from about 73 thousand in 1987 to 29 thousand in 1999 which caused a decline in the number of live born patients with Down syndrome over time. Since 2000, the birth rate begun to increase steadily, reaching more than 50 thousand in 2009. However, at the same time, since 2000, the impact of prenatal diagnosis on the prevalence of Down syndrome prevalence has been expanding rapidly, affecting the number of live born babies with Down syndrome.

The completeness of cytogenetic confirmation of trisomy 21 varied significantly, increasing from 21% in 1970 to almost 100% currently. Therefore, for the sake of sufficient sample size, the author has chosen for the analysis the period of 1986-2009, when data completeness had begun improving from 82% in 1986 to about 100% in 1999 and upward.

All cases of Down syndrome delivered during the period January 1, 1986 to December 31, 2009 were abstracted from a population-based registry, the St. Petersburg Down Syndrome Register, founded and run by the author. The Register has been collecting data on all Down syndrome patients residing in St. Petersburg, whether diagnosed antenatally or live born since 1970. The method for data collection has been described elsewhere [Kovaleva et al., 2001].

Data on patients suspected to have Down syndrome but with a normal karyotype were retrieved from logbooks of the cytogenetic laboratory at the St. Petersburg Centre for Medical Genetics and from logbooks of the cytogenetic laboratory at the Leningrad Oblast Children Hospital which provides service to the regions surrounding St. Petersburg. The degree of certainty of the Down syndrome diagnosis was determined by presence of question mark(s) in the records of indication for karyotyping in the logbooks. When the diagnosis at clinical examination seemed obvious, the question mark was absent. In doubtful cases, sometimes up to three question marks presented in the record. In some cases, suspected mosaicism was an indication. The data obtained were analyzed using standard statistics including binomial test and Chi-square test with Yates correction.

3. Results

Over a period of twenty-four years (from 1.01.1986 to 31.12.2009), 1257 children had been referred to cytogenetic investigation for either confirmation or exclusion of trisomy 21. The Down syndrome diagnosis was confirmed in 1129 (89.8%) of them and 120 (9.5%) children had a normal karyotype. The remaining eight children with another chromosomal abnormality were excluded from the analysis (Table 1). 1119 cases of trisomy 21 were diagnosed in the St. Petersburg Centre for Medical Genetics and ten cases were diagnosed elsewhere. The sex ratio among children with confirmed DS diagnosis was skewed, with a surplus of males (612 males/517 females, SR=1.18). In contrast, among children with a normal karyotype, there was a strong female prevalence (25 males/95 females, SR=0.26), the difference is highly significant, $p \ll 0.0001$.

Neonates constituted 94% of patients with confirmed Down syndrome while a proportion of neonates among those with false positive diagnosis was appreciably smaller (65%).

Therefore a proportion of false positive cases among neonates was 6.8% compared to 35% in patients aged one month and older (Table 1). The annual rate of false positives among neonates varied from 0% in 1990, 1995, and in 2000 to 21% in 2008 (Figure 1). There was an apparent trend with an increase in false positives in relation to a reduction in the number of cases tested. This variation did not depend on the clinical experience of the referring doctors. For example, 8 of 9 false positive cases in 2008 were referred to cytogenetic testing by clinical geneticists whose experience had exceeded 15 years, and the remaining one case was suspected to have Down syndrome by a clinical geneticist with 7 years of experience.

Age of patients	True Down syndrome (trisomy 21)	False positive diagnosis		Total
		Normal karyotype	Other chromosomal abnormality	
Neonates	1063	77	6 [a]	1146
Patients under 1 yo	59	20	2[b]	81
Patients aged 1 yo and older	7	23		30
Total	1129	120	8	1257

[a] 46,XY,18p-; 46,XX,t(11;22); 46,X,t(X;16)(p11;q13); 46,XX,r(18); 46,XX, r(18); 47,XXX
[b] 46,XY,add(10)(q26); 46,XX,inv(22)(p13;q12)

Table 1. Proportion of false positive diagnosis according to the patients' age at cytogenetic examination

Among false positive neonates, there was a very strong female prevalence, with 11 males/ 66 females, SR=0.17. Notable female predominance was also found in both patients aged under 1 year old (7 males/13 females, SR=0.54) and in older patients (7 males/16 females, SR=0.44).

Further analysis was performed regardless of the date and place of birth of the patients. Overall, a normal karyotype was diagnosed in 103 neonates (17 males/86 females, SR = 0.20, different from population value of 1.06, $p < 0.0001$), in 68 children of the age group up to 1 year old (24M/44 females, SR = 0.55, $p = 0.0052$), and in 64 children aged 1 year and older (29M/35 females, SR = 0.83, $p > 0.05$).

Data on the level of certainty in false positives cases is presented in Table 2. The diagnosis at clinical examination seemed obvious in 22% of neonates and in only 6% of children 1 year and older. In two cases, since features of Down syndrome were obvious, chromosome testing was requested twice. The proportion of suggested mosaicism was increased with the patients' age, from 3% in neonates to about 10% in the oldest group of patients. Request for excluding Down syndrome was noted in two cases only. Unquestionable Down syndrome diagnosis was stated in 20% and mosaicism was suspected in about 9% of males, while in females these figures were 14% and 4% correspondingly (Table 3).

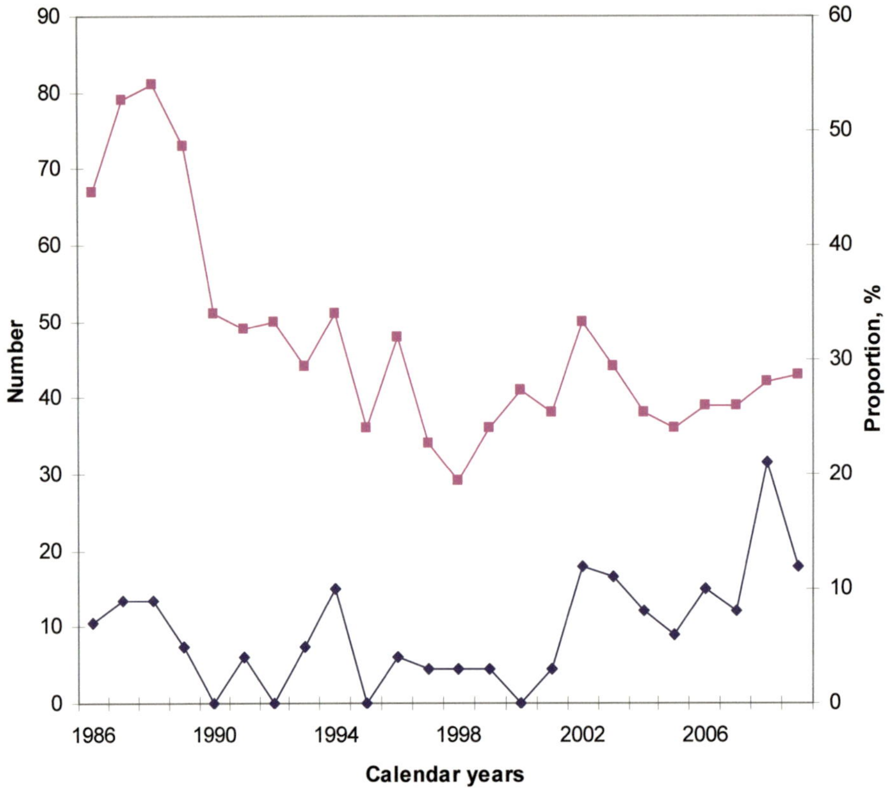

Fig. 1. Total number of cytogenetically tested cases (red line) and proportion of cases with false positive diagnosis (blue line).

Expression of certainty	Patients with false positive diagnosis of Down syndrome			
	Neonates	Under 1 yo	1 yo and older	Total
Down syndrome	22 (22%)	11 (16%)	4 (6%)	37
Mosaicism?	3 (3%)	3 (4.5%)	6 (9.5%)	12
Down syndrome?	60 (58%)	51 (75%)	53 (83%)	164
Down syndrome??	14 (14%)	2 (3%)	1 (1.5%)	17
Down syndrome???	2 (2%)	1 (1.5%)		3
Request for excluding Down syndrome	2 (2%)			2
Total	103	68	64	235

Table 2. Degree of certainty in requesting for cytogenetic testing according to the age of the patients

Expression of certainty	Patients with false positive diagnosis of Down syndrome		
	Males	Females	Total
Down syndrome	14 (20%)	23 (14%)	37
Mosaicism?	6 (8.5%)	6 (4%)	12
Down syndrome?	47 (67%)	117 (71%)	164
Down syndrome??	2 (3%)	15 (4%)	17
Down syndrome???	1 (1.5%)	2 (1%)	3
Request for excluding Down syndrome	0	2 (1%)	2
Total	70	165	235

Table 3. Degree of certainty in requesting for cytogenetic testing according to the gender of patients with false positive diagnosis

Data on distribution of both true Down syndrome patients and false positives by maternal age is presented in Table 4. The analysis of maternal age distribution in false positive patients was complicated since maternal ages were available in only a small proportion of the sample. There is some increase (13%) in the proportion of mothers aged 35 years old and older compared to general population (6% to 9%), due to a higher proportion (23.5%) of mothers of advantaged ages in the group of patients 1 year old and older. The overall figure of 13% in false positives is significantly lower compared to about 33% in true Down syndrome (p = 0.0003).

Maternal age	Down syndrome		Patients with false positive diagnosis of Down syndrome							
			Neonates		Under 1 yo		1 yo and older		Total	
< 20	87		6		3		1		10	
20-24	378		6		7		5		18	
25-29	367		15		3		5		23	
30-34	324		10		4		2		16	
35-39	352	33%	2	7.5%	2	15%	3	23.5%	7	13%
40+	213		1		1		1		3	
Total	1721		40		20		17		77	

Table 4. Maternal ages in Down syndrome and in false positive diagnosis, 1970-2009

4. Discussion

4.1 Proportion of false positive cases

Over the study period, 1129 postnatal cases of Down syndrome were identified. Regular trisomy 21 was observed in 90.9%, translocation trisomy in 5.4%, and mosaicism in 3.7% of the cases. These figures are in accordance with previous data worldwide. One hundred-twenty cases, referred for cytogenetic examination for suspicion of Down syndrome, displayed a normal karyotype, while eight children were diagnosed with another chromosome abnormality. Therefore, the proportion of misdiagnosed cases was 10.2% (128/1129). Analysis of the literature (Table 5) showed these data to be in agreement with majority of previous studies. Data from Spain [Ballesta et al., 1997] is of particular interest regarding the object of the present publication. The authors performed rigorous clinical screening of patients with suspected Down syndrome followed by cytogenetic testing. Eleven of 71 (15.5%) patients with psychomotor delay and features of Down syndrome were found to have a normal karyotype. On subsequent fluorescent in situ hybridization (FISH) testing, only one of them had triplication of the Down syndrome region on FISH testing.

When neonates were analyzed separately, the false positive rate has improved up to 7.2%. Among publications where data on accuracy of Down syndrome diagnosis can be found there are some reporting on the prevalence of false positive diagnosis in neonates [Devlin & Morrison, 2004; Fried, 1980; Hall, 1964; Hindley & Medakkar, 2002; Melve et al., 2008; Sivakumar & Larkins, 2004]. The rate of false positives in our sample appeared to be the lowest, being closer to figure of 9.6% in Norway [Melve et al., 2008]. Annual rate of false positive diagnosis varied significantly, from 0% in 1990, 1995, and in 2000 to 21% (9 of 42) in 2001 (Figure 1). Obviously this variation did not depend on the clinical experience of the referring doctors. Similar figures were reported by Melve et al. [2008], the highest annual number of false positives in neonates was 18 (18.9%) and the lowest was 4 (4.8%).

False positive diagnosis implies a great undue mental stress for parents, therefore maximizing clinical diagnostic accuracy is of importance [Hindley & Medakkar, 2002]. Significance of expert clinical assessment of a patient before cytogenetic testing was explored by Sivakumar & Larkins [2004]. They reported a more favorable accuracy rate from Birmingham Women's Hospital (25 of 29 suspected cases had trisomy 21) compared to the West Midland region (false positive rate 14% and 36%, correspondingly). "This can be explained by the fact that the tertiary hospital may have more experienced neonatologists compared to the broad cohort of junior and senior pediatricians… We believe that an assessment by a senior pediatrician before testing may minimize the risk of negative results."[Sivakumar & Larkins, 2004]. The data from the present study, that is a low false positive rate as the result of expert clinical assessment by clinical geneticists, support this suggestion.

4.2 Degree of certainty about the diagnosis of Down syndrome

4.2.1 Degree of certainty about the diagnosis of Down syndrome in false positive cases

Despite the widely held belief that the clinical diagnosis of Down syndrome is very obvious, some publications report on difficulties of clinical judgment arising in the neonatal period [Druce et al., 1995; Fried, 1980; Hall, 1966; Hindley & Medakkar, 2002; Lee et al., 1961]. Factors which alter suspicion of Down syndrome are known to be early delivery and prematurity [Mikkelsen, 1988]. No data on sex difference in suspicion of Down syndrome or in degree of certainty of DS diagnosis were reported before.

Source	Country	Study period	Age of patients	Number of tested patients	Proportion of false positive diagnosis
Hamerton et al, 1965	UK	1960-1964	not specified	173	16 (9%)
Engel et al., 1970	Germany	1963-1968	various ages	365	6 (15%)
Johnson et al., 1985	Ohio, USA	1970-1981	various ages	769 [a]	48 (6%)
	New York, USA	1980-1983	various ages	126 [b]	10 (8%) [c]
Szollar et al., 1983	Hungary	1970-1979	under 1 yo	214	16 (7.5%)
			1 yo and older	85	3 (3.5%)
Czeizel, 1988	Hungary	1973-1982	various ages	81	4 (5%)
Baccichetti et al., 1990	Italy	1988	teenagers and adults predominantly	116	14 (12%)
Ballesta et al., 1997	Spain	not specified	not neonates	71	11 (15.5%) [d]
Ahmed et al., 2005	Pakistan	1998-2001	various ages	325	30 (9%) [e]

[a,b] cytogenetic confirmation in about 77% of the patients; [c] including one case with trisomy 18; [d] FISH study of 11 cases detected a partial trisomy 21 in one case; [e] including 12 cases with other chromosomal anomalies

Table 5. Accuracy of the clinical diagnosis of Down syndrome in patients of various ages

Data presented in Table 2 suggests that the level of certainty in false positives cases was comparably low, decreasing with the patients' age. The diagnosis at clinical examination seemed obvious in 22% of neonates and in only 6% of children 1 year and older. However a proportion of clinical diagnosis suggestive of mosaicism increased with the patients' age, from 3% in neonates to about 10% in the oldest group of patients. Surprisingly, despite a strong prevalence of females among false positive children, a higher level of certainty of Down syndrome diagnosis was given to male patients (Table 3). In males, unquestionable Down syndrome or suspected mosaicism were indications for cytogenetic testing in 20% and in 8.5 %of the cases, while in females these figures were 14% and 4% respectively.

4.2.2 Degree of certainty about the diagnosis of Down syndrome in confirmed cases

The data reported above prompted the author to taking a quick look at degree of certainty of the clinical diagnosis in the cases of true Down syndrome. It was found that 17 of 106 (16%) neonates with Down syndrome born during 2007-2009 had a questionable clinical diagnosis (including one diagnose accompanied with three question marks), among them there were 8 males and 9 females. Thus, at least in neonates with Down syndrome, there was no association of clinical suspicion of the diagnosis with the gender of the patient.

Source	Geographic area	Study period	Number of tested patients	Proportion of false positive diagnosis
Hall, 1964	Sweden	1961-1962	43	5 (11.6%)
Fried, 1980	Israel	1973-1977	30	4 (13.3%)
Hidley, & Medakkar, 2002	UK	1999-2000	962	307 (32%) [a]
Devlin & Morrison, 2004	Northern Ireland	1969-2001	268 [d]	82 (31%) [b]
Sivakumar & Larkins, 2004	UK	2000-2002	233	85 (36%)
Melve et al., 2008	Norway	2001-2005	376	36 (9.6%)
Present study	Russia	1986-2009	1146	83 (7.2%) [c]

[a] including one case with 49,XXXXY; [b] including 5 females with another chromosomal abnormality; [c] including 2 males and 6 females with another chromosomal abnormality; [a] neonates constitute 90% of the patients

Table 6. Accuracy of the clinical diagnosis of Down syndrome in neonates

4.3 Sex ratio in Down syndrome

4.3.1 Sex ratio in cases considered or proved to be true Down syndrome

Sex ratio in true Down syndrome is well known to be skewed towards males [Mikkelsen, 1988; Mutton et al., 1996]. Meta-analysis of publications reporting cytogenetic profile of Down syndrome worldwide [Kovaleva, 2002] showed typical male prevalence (SR ~1.3) among both patients with regular trisomy 21 and carriers of translocation trisomy 21, either sporadic or inherited. The only exception is mosaic variant of trisomy, where some prevalence of females was documented (SR~0.96).

Several hypotheses have been put forward to explain the skewed sex ratio in Down syndrome. Meiotic disturbance (non-homologous co-orientation in male meiosis) [Kovaleva, 1992; Petersen et al. 1993], fertilization event (greater accessibility of Y-bearing sperm to ova disomic for chromosome 21 or promotion of non-disjunction in the ova by Y-bearing sperm) [Ferguson-Smith & Yates, 1984; Kovaleva & Mutton, 2005], and post-fertilization events (intrauterine selection against females) [Huether et al., 1996; Hook et al., 1999] have been discussed. Data from recent studies supports suggestion that male excess among live born with non mosaic trisomy 21 might be due to selection against female fetuses [Oliver et al., 2009; Kovaleva, 2010]. Female prevalence among carriers of mosaic trisomy was suggested to be a result of sex-specific chromosome loss in early embryogenesis [Kovaleva, 2005].

The trigger of the present study was an observation of an intriguing dynamics of sex ratio in Down syndrome in St. Petersburg (former Leningrad) within period of 1970-1996 [Kovaleva et al., 1999] subsequently confirmed by the meta analysis of the literature [Kovaleva, 2002]. It was a steady increase in sex ratio from a population figure of 1.05 or even less in the earliest studies in 1940's to 1.3 - 1.6 in the studies conducted during late 1980's (Figure 2). Analysis showed that this increase was accounted for by the growing use of karyotyping to confirm the diagnosis. Among individuals with a clinical diagnosis only, sex ratio was 0.97 (1160 males/1198 females) [Collman & Stoller, 1962; Davidenkova et al., 1965; Huether, 1990; Kovaleva et al., 2001; Staples et al., 1991] while among individuals with confirmed trisomy 21 this figure was 1.31 (1918 males/1466 females) [Huether, 1990; Kovaleva et al., 2001; Mikkelsen et al., 1976; Mikkelsen et al., 1990; Sharav, 1991; Staples et al., 1991; Stoll et al., 1990; Wahrman & Fried, 1970]. Correspondingly, in samples where proportion of clinical diagnosis only was 30% and more, intermediate figure of 1.12 (1950 males/1742 females) [Baird & Sadovnik, 1987; Christoderescu et al., 1977; Johnson et al., 1996; Kallen et al., 1996; Kovaleva et al., 2001; Staples et al., 1991] was observed. These observations raised a suggestion that low sex ratio in Down syndrome patients with clinical diagnosis only might be accounted by a large proportion of false positive diagnosis in females [Kovaleva, 2002].

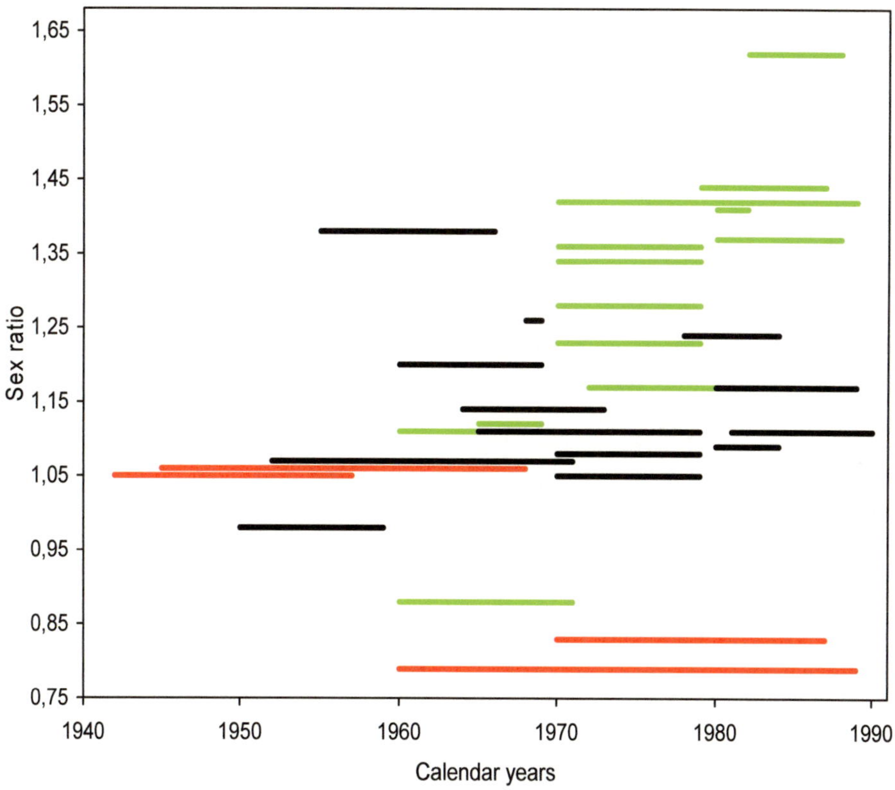

Fig. 2. Sex ratio in Down syndrome, data from epidemiological studies worldwide (adapted from Kovaleva [2002]). Red line: clinical diagnosis only; black line: clinical diagnosis or trisomy 21, green line: trisomy 21

4.3.2 Sex ratio in false positive diagnosis

Though theoretically, misdiagnosis should occur uniformly in both sexes, data from the present study demonstrates a significant female prevalence among false positive patients. In neonates, a five-fold prevalence of females over males was detected (17 males/86 females, SR = 0.20, different from population value of 1.06, $p < 0.0001$). Female excess diminished with older children; two-fold prevalence was found among children of the age up to 1 year old (24 males/44 females, SR = 0.55, p = 0.0052), and notable but statistically insignificant prevalence among patients aged 1 year and older (29 males/35 females, SR = 0.83, p > 0.05). Therefore, data from the present study supports the suggestion of low sex ratio in Down syndrome patients with clinical diagnosis only as the result of a large proportion of false positive diagnosis in females. However the reason of female predominance among the clinically suspected Down syndrome remains unclear.

Patients with clinical features of Down syndrome but without trisomy 21 were reported occasionally before the advent of molecular technologies allowing definite detection of Down syndrome critical region located at chromosome 21 [Hall, 1961; Hamerton & Polani, 1962; Bowen et al., 1974]. As an explanation for absence of trisomy 21 in different tissues of patients with apparent manifestations of the syndrome, several suggestions were proposed: (1) low-level mosaicism, (2) the presence of the trisomic cell line in tissues other than those investigated, (3) elimination of the aberrant cell line *in vivo* or selective regress *in vitro* [Engel et al., 1970], and (4) gene mutation that might cause a "phenocopy" [Hall, 1962].

Subsequent studies showed the presence of a cryptic duplication of the Down syndrome critical region in individuals with clinical diagnosis of Down syndrome and an apparently normal karyotype [see for reference Forster-Gibson et al., 2001]. However several patients with mental retardation and Down syndrome phenotype, but without molecularly detectable duplication of the critical region, have been reported [McCormick et al., 1989; Ahlbom et al., 1996]. The majority of them were females. For example, a woman with clinically typical Down syndrome but apparently normal chromosomes, was extensively examined for the presence of any partial trisomy for any segment of chromosome 21. Since the proposita's parents were half-sibs, and her sister suffered from the same disorder as the proposita, the authors suggested an autosomal recessive disorder which is phenotypically indistinguishable from Down syndrome [Ahlbom et al., 1996]. As it was mentioned above, FISH testing of 11 patients with developmental delay and clinically obvious Down syndrome revealed only one of them who had triplication of the critical Down syndrome region. Unfortunately the gender of the patients was not reported [Ballesta et al., 1997].

The data obtained in the present study suggest that gender in particularly significantly affects clinical suspicion of Down syndrome in neonates. Since characteristic features allowing suspicion of Down syndrome include facial dysmorphisms, one may hypothesize sex differences in the normal process of facial cranium ontogenesis during perinatal period.

In patients aged one year and older, sex ratio (0.83) appeared to be close to sex ratio typical to carriers of mosaic trisomy 21 (0.96). In this group, proportion of mothers of advanced age seemed to be increased which might support a suggestion of undetected mosaicism in some of these patients. An abnormal condition(s) specific to females might also be implicated in a proportion of the misdiagnosed cases.

4.4 Implications of false positive-female-prevalence-phenomenon to Down syndrome epidemiology

The observation of female prevalence in false positive clinically diagnosed cases allows an insight into the ground for reported sex ratio variability in Down syndrome. For example, the ECLAM (Estudio Colaborativo Latinoamericano de Malformaciones Congenitas) group reported as "an unusual finding" a markedly low sex ratio (0.98) found in 3,157 newborn Down syndrome patients in South America populations [Carothers et al., 2001]. Only 13% of the patients were reported to have confirmed diagnosis, therefore, in the light of the data presented in this paper, a low sex ratio among patients mostly clinically diagnosed as Down syndrome, is a well expected finding.

Moreover, based on data on sex ratio in both all clinically diagnosed cases and true Down syndrome cases in a population where sufficient completeness of cytogenetic confirmation is not readily achievable, it is realizable to calculate a crude rate of false positives [Kovaleva, 2002]. For example, assuming all males among clinically diagnosed cases in ECLAM's sample to be true Down syndrome (which can not be absolutely correct since some false positive cases might be found among males) and typical for Down syndrome sex ratio to be 1.3, for 1563 males, 1203 females (not 1594) are expected, with odd number of 391 females. Resulted proportion of misdiagnosed cases is 391/3,157=12%.

The results from the present study might have some further implications. (1) Overestimation of maternal age-specific rates due to false positive cases, in young women predominantly, might take place in the early years of monitoring of Down syndrome, as well as in populations with a high proportion of unconfirmed cases (those covered by Chernobyl fallout in the Former Soviet Republics). (2) It was generally accepted that maternal age specific risks were stable over time, and variations in population rates were explained by changing in maternal age composition [Huether et al., 1998; Carothers et al., 2001]. However if age-specific rates stay stable over long time, irrespective of increase in proportion of confirmed cases, it might indicate an increase in real rates. (3) The results from this study would suggest that the use of epidemiological data collected on Down syndrome prior to routine cytogenetic analysis, should be reconsidered in meta-analyses of Down syndrome population data.

5. Conclusion

The present study is the largest study to address the accuracy of clinical diagnosis of Down syndrome and the first one demonstrating that gender may affect a clinical suspicion of a chromosomal disease. The advantages of this study are well-defined geographical population, clinical screening of the cases suspected to have a chromosomal disease by experienced clinical geneticists prior to requesting for cytogenetic testing, a high completeness of cytogenetic confirmation of the Down syndrome diagnosis, and perfect recording of the cases on logbooks of the cytogenetic laboratory at the St. Petersburg Centre for Medical Genetics. Apparent limitations of this study are a lack of detailed clinical description of the cases and absence of follow-up. Additional studies, both clinical and genetic, would be reasonable for uncovering mechanism(s) responsible for the remarkable sex bias in clinical suspicion of Down syndrome.

6. Acknowledgment

The author's greatest thanks belong to Prof. Virginia C. Thurston (Indiana University School of Medicine) for helpful comments and amending the English in this paper.

7. References

Ahmed, I.; Ghafoor, T.; Samore, N.A. & Chattha M.N. (2005). Down syndrome: clinical and cytogenetic analysis. *Journal of the College of Physicians and Surgeons – Pakistan,* Vol. 15, No.7 (July 2005), pp. 426-429, ISSN 1022-386X

Baccichetti, C.; Lenzini, E. & Pegoraro, R. (1990). Down syndrome in the Belluno district (Veneto Region, northeast Italy): age distribution and morbidity. *American Journal of Medical Genetics. Supplement,* No. 7, (n.d.), pp. 84-86, ISSN 1040-3787

Baird, P.A. & Sadovnick, A.D. (1987). Life expectancy in Down syndrome. *The Journal of Pediatrics,* Vol. 110, No.6, (June 1987), pp. 849-854, ISSN 0022-3476

Ballesta, F.; Antich, J.; Aledo, R.; Milà, M.; Sanchez, A. & Moreno, J. (1997). Down syndrome: genotype-phenotype correlation in 71 patients. *Cytogenetics and Cell Genetics,* Vol.77, Suppl. 1, (June 1997), p. 6, ISSN 0011-4537

Bowen, P.; Chernick, B.C.; Campbell, D.J. & Rouget, A. (1974). Mild characteristic of Down syndrome with normal karyotype in cultured lymphocytes and skin fibroblasts. *Birth Defects Original Articles Series,* Vol.10, No.10, pp. 43-48, ISSN 0547-6844

Carothers, A.D.; Castilla, E.E.; Dutra, M.G. & Hook, E.B. (2001). Search for ethnic, geographic, and other factors in the epidemiology of Down syndrome in South America: Analysis of data from the ECLAMC Project, 1967-1997. *American Journal of Medical Genetics,* Vol.103, No.2, (October 2001), pp. 149-156, ISSN 1040-3787

Christoderescu, D.; Berbescu, C.; Retereanu, A.; Constantinescu, E.; Ciupitu, A.; Urse M. & Radu M. (1977). The incidence of Down's syndrome in Bucharest. A retrospective survey. *Revue roumaine de medicine. Neurologie et psychiatrie.* Vol.15, No.2, (April-June 1977), pp.147-154, ISSN 0377-502X

Collman, R.D. & Stoller, A. (1962). A survey of mongoloid births in Victoria, Australia, 1942-1957. *American Journal of Public Health and the Nation's Health,* Vol.52, May 1962, pp. 813-829, ISSN 0002-9572

Czeizel, E. (1988). Some epidemiological characteristics of Down's syndrome in Hungary. *Acta morphologica Hungarica,* Vol.36, No.1-2, pp. 63-77, ISSN 0236-5391

Davidenkova, E.F.; Shtilbans, I.I. & Verlinskaia, D.K. (1965). Some data on 181 newborn infants with Down's disease. *Pediatriia,* Vol.44, February 1965, pp. 67-72, ISSN 0031-403X

Devlin, L. & Morrison, P.J. (2004). Accuracy of the clinical diagnosis of Down syndrome. *The Ulster Medical Journal,* Vol. 73, No.1, (May 2004), pp. 4-12, ISSN 041-6193

Druce, M.; Cohen, I.J.; Naor, N. & Shohat, M. (1995). Late diagnosis of Down syndrome due to incorrect cytogenetic diagnosis and extreme prematurity. *Clinical Genetics,* Vol.48, No. 4, (October 1995), pp. 192-194, ISSN 0009-9163

Engel, W.; Reinwein, H.; Müller, I. & Kunze, G. (1970). Chromosomenbefunde bei 365 patienten mit Down-syndrome oder Verdacht auf Down-syndrome. *Humangenetik,* Vol.8, No.4, (March 1970), pp. 307-311, ISSN 0018-7348

Ferguson-Smith, M.A. & Yates, J.R.W. (1984). Maternal age-specific rates for chromosome aberrations and factors influencing them: report of a collaborative European study on 52 965 amniocenteses. *Prenatal Diagnosis,* Vol.4, Special No, (Spring 1984), pp. 5-45, ISSN 0197-3851

Forster-Gibson, C.J.; Davies, J.; MacKenzie, J.J. & Harrison, K. (2001). Cryptic duplication of 21q in an individual with a clinical diagnosis of Down syndrome. *Clinical Genetics,* Vol.59, No.6, (June 2001), pp. 438-443, ISSN 0009-9163

Hall, B. (1962). Down's syndrome (mongolism) with normal chromosomes. *Lancet,* Vol. 2, November 17, pp. 1026-1027, ISSN 0140-6736

Hall, B. (1964). Mongolism in newborns. A clinical and cytogenetic study. *Acta Paediatrica Scandinavica. Supplementum,* No.154, (n.d.), pp. 1-95

Hamerton, J.L. & Polani, P.E. (1962). Down's syndrome (mongolism) with normal chromosomes. *Lancet,* Vol.2, December 8, p. 1229, ISSN 0140-6736

Hamerton, J.L.; Gianelli, F. & Polani, P.E. (1965). Cytogenetics of Down's syndrome (Mongolosm) I. Data on consecutive series of patients referred for genetic counseling and diagnosis. *Cytogenetics,* Vol.4, No.3, (n.d.), pp. 171-185, ISSN 0011-4537

Hindley, D. & Medakkar, S. (2002). Diagnosis of Down's syndrome in neonates. *Archives of Disease in Childhood. Fetal and Neonatal Edition,* Vol.87, No. 3, (November 2002), pp. F220-F221, ISSN 1359-2998

Hook, E.B.; Cross, P.K. & Mutton, D.E. (1999). Female predominance (low sex ratio) in 47,+21 mosaics. *American Journal of Medical Genetics,* Vol.84, No.4, (June 1999), pp. 316-319, ISSN 1040-3787

Huether, C.A. (1990). Epidemiological aspects of Down syndrome: sex ratio, incidence, and recent impact of prenatal diagnosis. *Issues and Reviews in Teratology.* Vol.5, (n.d.), pp. 283-316, ISSN 0740-8242

Huether, C.A.; Martin, R.L.M.; Stoppelman, S.M.; D'Souza, S.; Bishop, J.K.; Torfs, C.P.; Lorey, F.; May, K.M.; Hanna, J.S.; Baird, P.A. & Kelley, J.C. (1996). Sex ratio in fetuses and live born infants with autosomal aneuploidy. *American Journal of Medical Genetics,* Vol.63, No.3, (June 1996), pp. 492-500, ISSN 1040-3787

Huether, C.A.; Ivanovich, J.; Goodwin, B.S.; Krivchenia, E.L.; Hertzberg, V.; Edmonds, L.D.; May, D.S. & Priest, J.H. (1998). Maternal age specific risk rate estimates for Down syndrome among live births in whites and other races from Ohio and Metropolitan Atlanta, 1970-1989. *Journal of Medical Genetics,* Vol.35, No.6, (June 1998), pp. 482-490, ISSN 0022-2593

Johnson, K.M.; Huether, C.A.; Hook, E.B., Crowe, C.A.; Reeder, B.A.; Sommer, A.; McCorquodale, M.M. & Cross, P.K. (1985). False positive reporting of Down syndrome on Ohio and New York birth certificates. *Genetic Epidemiology,* Vol.2, No.2, (n.d.), pp. 123-131, ISSN 0741-0395

Johnson, Z.; Lillis, D.; Delany, V.; Hayes, C. & Dack, P. (1996) The epidemiology of Down syndrome in four counties in Ireland 1981-90. *Journal of Public Health Medicine,* Vol.18, No.1, (March 1996), pp.78-86, ISSN 0957-4832

Kallen, B.; Mastroiacovo, P. & Robert, E. (1996). Major congenital malformations in Down syndrome *American Journal of Medical Genetics,* Vol.65, No.2, (October 1996), pp. 160-166, ISSN 1040-3787.

Kovaleva, N.V. (1992). Distributive pairing and aneuploidy in man. *Genetika,* Vol.28, No.10, (n.d.), pp. 5-15, ISSN 0016-1993

Kovaleva, N.V. (2002). Sex ratio in Down syndrome. A review. *Tsitol Genet,* Vol.36, No.6, (November-December 2002), pp. 54-69, ISSN 0563-3783

Kovaleva, N.V. (2005). Sex-specific instability in early human development. *American Journal of Medical Genetics,* Vol.136A, No.1, (April 2005), pp. 401-413, ISSN 1040-3787

Kovaleva, N.V. (2010, March 18). Germ-line transmission of trisomy 21: data from 80 families suggest an implication of grandmaternal age and a high frequency of female-specific rescue. *Molecular Cytogenetics, BioMed Central,* Retrieved from http://www.molecularcytogenetics.org/content/3/1/7

Kovaleva, N.V.; Butomo, I.V.; Verlinskaya, D.K.; Ilyashenko, N.Y.; Pantova, I.G.; Prozorova, M.V.; Khitrikova, L.E. & Shandlorenko, S.K. (1999). Karyological characterization of Down syndrome: clinical and theoretical aspects. *Tsitologiia,* Vol.41, No.12, (n.d.), pp. 1015-1021, ISSN 0041-3771

Kovaleva, N.V.; Butomo, I.V. & Körblein, A. (2001). Sex ratio in Down syndrome. Studies on patients with confirmed trisomy 21. *Tsitologiia i Genetica,* Vol.36, No.6, (November-December 2001), pp. 43-49, ISSN 0564-3783

Kovaleva, N.V. & Mutton, D.E. (2005). Epidemiology of double aneuploidies involving chromosome 21 and sex chromosomes. *American Journal of Medical Jenetics*, Vol.134A, No.4, (August 2005), pp. 24-32, ISSN 1040-3787

Lee, C.H.; Schmid, W. & Smith, P.M. (1961). Definitive diagnosis of mongolism in newborn infants by chromosome studies. *JAMA*, Vol.178, December 9, (December 1961), pp. 1030-1032, ISSN 0098-7484

Melve, K.K.; Lie, R.T.; Skjaerven, R.; Van Der Hagen, C.B.; Gradek, G.A.; Jonsrud, C.; Braathen, G.J. & Irgens, L.M. (2008). Registration of Down syndrome in the Medical Birth Registry of Norway: validity and time trends. *Acta Obstetrica et Gynecologica Scandinavica*, Vol.87, No.8, (n.d.), pp. 824-830, ISSN 0001-6349

McCormick, M.K.; Schinzel, A.; Petersen, M.B.; Stetten, G.; Driscoll, D.J.; Cantu, E.S.; Tranebjaerg, L.; Mikkelsen, M.; Watkins, P.C. & Antonarakis, S.E. (1989). Molecular genetic approach to the characterization of the "Down syndrome region" of chromosome 21. *Genomics*, Vol.5, No. 2, (August 1989), pp. 325-331, ISSN 0888-7543

Mikkelsen, M.; Fischer, G.; Stene, J.; Stene, E. & Petersen, E. (1976). Incidence study of Down's syndrome in Copenhagen, 1960-1971: with chromosome investigation. *Annals of Human Genetics*, Vol.40, No.2, (November 1976), pp.177-182, ISSN 0003-4800

Mikkelsen, M. (1988). The incidence of Down's syndrome and progress towards its reduction. *Philosophical Transactions of the Royal Society. Biological Sciences*, Vol.319, No.1194, (June 1988), pp. 315-324, ISSN 0962-8436

Mikkelsen, M.; Poulsen, H. & Nielsen, K.G. (1990). Incidence, survival, and mortality in Down syndrome in Denmark. *American Journal of Medical Genetics. Supplement*, No. 7, (n.d.), pp. 75-78, ISSN 1040-3787

Mutton, D.; Alberman, E. & Hook, E.B. (1996). Cytogenetic and epidemiological findings in Down syndrome, England and Wales 1989 to 1993. *Journal of Medical Genetics*, Vol.33, No.3, (May 1996), pp. 387-394, ISSN 0022-2593

Oliver, T.R.; Bhise, A.; Feingold, E.; Tinker, S.; Masse, N. & Sherman, S.L. (2009). Investigation of factors associated with paternal non disjunction of chromosome 21. *American Journal of Medical Genetics*, Vol.149A, No.8, (August 2009), pp. 1685-1690, ISSN 1040-3787

Petersen, M.B.; Antonarakis, S.E.; Hassold, T.J.; Freeman, S.B.; Sherman, S.L.; Avramopoulos, D. & Mikkelsen, M. (1993). Paternal non disjunction in trisomy 21: excess of male patients. *Human Molecular Genetics*, Vol.2, No.10, (October 1993), pp. 1691-1695, ISSN 0964-6906

Sharav, T. (1991). Aging gametes in relation to incidence, gender, and twinning in Down syndrome. *American Journal of Medical Genetics*, Vol.39, No.1, (April 1991), pp.116-118, ISSN 1040-3787

Sivakumar, S. & Larkins, S. (2004). Accuracy of clinical diagnosis in Down's syndrome. *Archives of Diseases in Childhood.* Vol.89, No.7, (July 2004), p. 691, ISSN 0003-9888

Staples, A.J.; Sutherland, G.R.; Haan, E.A. & Clisby, S. (1991). Epidemiology of Down syndrome in South Australia (1960-89). *American Journal of Human Genetics*, Vol.49, No.5, (November 1991), pp.1014-1024, ISSN 0002-9297

Stoll, C.; Alembik, Y.; Dott, B. & Roth, M.P. (1990). Epidemiology of Down syndrome in 118, 265 consecutive births. *American Journal of Medical Genetics. Supplement*, No. 7, (n.d.), pp. 79-83, ISSN 1040-3787

Szollar, J.; Osztovics, M.; Pazonyi, I. & Balogh, L. (1983). The frequency of Down syndrome in a Budapest study during 1970-1979. *Clinical Genetics*, Vol. 23, No.3, p. A249, ISSN 0009-9163

Wahrman, J. & Fried, K. (1970) The Jerusalem prospective newborn survey of mongolism. *Annals of New York Academy of Sciences*, Vol.171, No.2, (October 1970), pp. 341-360, ISSN 0077-8923

14

Down Syndrome Screening in Pregnancies Conceived after Assisted Reproductive Technologies

Maarit Sahraravand and Markku Ryynanen
Department of Obstetrics and Gynecology, Oulu University Hospital
Finland

1. Introduction

Over the last three decades, prenatal screening for Down syndrome and other chromosomal abnormalities has become routine during antenatal care. Down syndrome screening has changed from the second to the first trimester of pregnancy because of the higher detection rate and earlier diagnosis. Second-trimester screening, based on the combination of maternal serum human chorionic gonadotropin (hCG), alpha-fetoprotein (AFP), and unconjugated estradiol (uE3) as a function of maternal age, yields a detection rate of 60% with a false-positive rate (FPR) of 5% (Wald et al., 1988). In standard practice, first-trimester screening, which combines maternal age, nuchal translucency thickness (NT), and maternal serum free beta-human chorionic gonadotropin (fβ-hCG), and pregnancy-associated plasma-protein-A (PAPP-A), can achieve a detection rate 90% with a FPR of 5% (Snijders et al., 1998; Nicolaides, 2004; Wojdemann et al., 2005; Spencer, 2007).

Down syndrome screening among women pregnant after assisted reproductive technologies (ART) is complicated by several factors. Pregnancies conceived after ART represent a group of high-risk pregnancies, which carry a higher psychological and financial burden compared to spontaneous pregnancies (Oddens et al., 1999). The proportion of women aged 35 years or more is higher in ART pregnancies, therefore, they a more likely to be carrying a child affected by Down syndrome (Geipel et al., 1999; Pinborg et al., 2004; Weisz and Rodeck, 2006, Gjerris et al., 2008). Studies have also shown that foetuses conceived after intracytoplasmic sperm injection (ICSI) are known to have an increased risk of chromosomal aberrations (Aboulghar et al., 2001; Bonduelle et al., 2002; Jozwiak et al., 2004; Gjerris et al., 2008). Pregnancies conceived after ART are also associated with a higher rate of multiple pregnancies (Weisz and Rodeck, 2006, Gjerris et al., 2008). Maternal and fetal complications, such as foetal growth restriction, preeclampsia, preterm birth, congenital abnormalities, and low birth weight occur more often in assisted reproduction pregnancies (Helmerhorst et al., 2004; Amor et al., 2009; Williams and Sutcliffe, 2009; Henningsen et al., 2011). Women who have conceived after assisted reproductive techniques usually prefer to avoid invasive diagnostic procedures, such as amniocentesis and villus biopsy, due to the risk of miscarriage. Rather, they choose non-invasive screening before making a decision about invasive testing (Meschede et al., 1998; Schover et al., 1998; Geipel et al., 1999; Geipel et al., 2004).

Pregnancies conceived by assisted reproduction techniques have also been reported to be associated with changes in the biochemical parameters of screening for Down syndrome, leading to an increased false-positive rate in the second trimester (Barkai et al., 1996; Ribbert et al., 1996; Frishman et al., 1997; Wald, 1999; Raty et al., 2002: Lambert-Messerlian et al., 2005). The effect of ART on first-trimester Down syndrome screening has been examined, but the results are inconclusive. The majority of the studies have reported that nuchal translucency screening is not affected by the mode of conception (Liao et al., 2001; Nieminen et al., 2001; Wojdemann et al., 2001; Orlandi et al., 2002; Ghisoni et al., 2003; Lambert-Messerlian et al., 2006; Matilainen et al., 2011). Yet, some studies suggested that NT measurements are altered in pregnancies conceived with ART (Maymon et al., 2002; Hui et al., 2005; Amor et al., 2009; Gjerris et al., 2009). Several studies have found that serum marker levels, especially PAPP-A levels, seem to be altered in ART pregnancies, leading to the higher false-positive rate, whereas other studies have been unable to confirm this.

In this chapter, we present the recent findings of first-trimester Down syndrome screening in singleton and twin pregnancies conceived after assisted reproductive technologies.

2. The effect of ART on nuchal translucency thickness and other ultrasound markers

Measurement of nuchal translucency thickness as a single marker may be the most effective screening test, and is thought to be least affected by the mode of conception. Down syndrome screening, which combines maternal age and fetal nuchal translucency thickness measurement, can achieve a detection rate of 75 - 80% with a false-positive rate of 3 - 5% (Kagan et al., 2010). There are several studies which have been examined, whether the nuchal translucency measurements are altered in pregnancies conceived by ART.

In the study by Gjerris et al., (2009) the median NT in entire ART group (n = 992) was smaller when compared with spontaneous pregnancies (n = 2532). They also found that the mode of the conception had an effect on NT: the nuchal translucency thickness was thinner in *in-vitro* fertilization (IVF) cases when compared with intracytoplasmic sperm injection (ICSI) cases. They also found that a smaller nuchal translucency thickness was noted in pregnancies treated with a long protocol hormone treatment compared with those with the short hormone treatment protocol. There was not any obvious biological explanation for these findings; any significant differences might be due to chance as several statistical analyses were performed. Opposite findings were reported by Amor et al., (2009); they found that in ART pregnancies (n = 833) the nuchal translucency thickness was increased compared with the controls. There was no difference between IVF and ICSI group.

In our own study (Matilainen et al., 2011), we investigated 282 pregnancies conceived after assisted reproductive technologies, and in which only one fetus was noted in early ultrasound examination, and who participated in first trimester combined screening. There were 24.783 spontaneous singleton pregnancies in our control group. Patients were divided into four groups according to the type of conception, as follows: controls, hormonally stimulated *in-vitro* fertilization or intracytoplasmic sperm injection group, spontaneous non-stimulated frozen embryo transfer (FET) group, and hormonally stimulated FET group (HRT-FET). In our study population, NT or NT MoMs (multiples of the medians) were not significantly different between the different type of ART pregnancies and spontaneous pregnancies.

The majority of the studies found no difference in the size of NT in ART pregnancies compared with spontaneous pregnancies (Liao et al., 2001; Nieminen et al., 2001; Wojdemann et al., 2001; Orlandi et al., 2002; Ghisoni et al., 2003; Lambert-Messerlian et al.,

2006 and Matilainen et al. 2011), and no influence on the screening performance and the false-positive rate by compining maternal age and NT for Down syndrome risk assessment (Liao et al., 2001; Ghisoni et al., 2003; Bellver et al., 2005; Lambert-Messerlian et al., 2006; Tul and Novac-Antolic, 2006; Ancaert et al., 2008; Bender et al., 2010; Matilainen et al., 2011).

Gjerris et al. (2008) found that gestational age dating in ART pregnancies either by the date of oocyte aspiration (DOA) or by crown-rump length differed significantly by 1.5 days. The gestational age was higher when it was dated according to CRL. The study group speculated that fetuses were larger than expected at the NT scan and their real biological gestational age was lower, therefore, a smaller NT MoM values were observed in assisted reproduction pregnancies (Gjerris et al., 2009). According to a mathematical stimulation method, the use of CRL or DOA for gestational age dating did not significantly influence the detection rate for Down syndrome (Gjerris et al., 2008).

First-trimester screening, which combines maternal age, fetal nuchal translucency thickness, and maternal serum free β-hCG, and PAPP-A, can achieve the detection rate of 90% with the FPR of 5% (Snijders et al., 1998; Nicolaides, 2004; Wojdemann et al., 2005; Spencer, 2007). A further improvement in the screening performance can be achieved by including the assessment of additional, new ultrasound markers. These additional markers are the absence of the nasal bone, and the blood flow in the ductus venosus, and across the tricuspid valve. The absence of the nasal bone, reversed a-wave in the ductus venosus, and tricuspid regurgitation are observed in about 60, 65 and 55% of fetuses with Down syndrome and in 2.6, 3.2 and 0.9%, respectively, of euploid fetuses. The assessment of each of these sonographic markers into first-trimester combined screening, which uses maternal age, NT thickness, and maternal serum free β-hCG, and PAPP-A, can yields a detection rate of 93 - 96% with the false-positive rate of 2.5%. Screening for Down syndrome by maternal age, nuchal translucency thickness and either the ductus venosus, the nasal bone, or the tricuspid flow, at the risk cut-off of 1:100, identified 83, 85, and 85% of cases with false-positive rate of 2.9, 2.7 and 2.7%, respectively (Kagan et al., 2010). Unfortunately, there are no studies concerning these new ultrasound markers in pregnancies conceived after ART.

3. The effect of ART on first-trimester biochemical markers

In pregnancies affected by Down syndrome the maternal serum level of PAPP-A is reduced to about half (Brambati et al., 1993) and the level of free β-hCG is about twice as high when compared with values in chromosomally normal pregnancies (Spencer et al., 1992). Maternal serum PAPP-A and free β-hCG values are affected by many variables, therefore, to estimate accurate patient-specific risks, adjustments in the measured free β-hCG and PAPP-A levels take into account their association with gestational age, maternal weight, ethnicity, and smoking status (Spencer et al., 1999a; Spencer et al., 2003b; Avgidou et al., 2005; Nicolaides et al., 2005). In addition, the mode of conception has an effect on maternal serum screening markers.

Previous studies have shown that serum markers in ART pregnancies differ from natural conception in the second trimester, leading to an increased false-positive rate (Barkai et al., 1996; Ribbert et al., 1996; de Graaf et al., 2000; Niemimaa et al., 2003). Most of the recent studies have reported that first-trimester serum markers are altered in pregnancies conceived after assisted reproduction, when comparing with spontaneous conception. Many studies have shown a reduction, especially in the PAPP-A levels, in ART pregnancies. In our own study (Matilainen et al., 2011), we investigated 282 pregnancies conceived after ART, and in which only one fetus was noted in early ultrasound, and who participated in first trimester combined screening. The control group was comprised of 24.783 spontaneous singleton pregnancies. We found a significant reduction in the PAPP-A concentration level in entire ART group when compared with controls. This is in agreement with most previous studies (Liao et al., 2001; Orlandi et al., 2002; Bersinger et al., 2004; Maymon et al., 2004; Hui et al., 2005; Tul and Novac-Antolic, 2006; Ancaert et al., 2008; Gjerris et al., 2009; Amor et al., 2009).

Some studies have found that PAPP-A levels are decreased in the subgroups of IVF (Liao et al., 2001; Tul and Novac-Antolic, 2006; Amor et al., 2009; Gjerris et al., 2009; Bender et al., 2010; Engels et al. 2010) or ICSI (Ancaert et al., 2008; Amor et al., 2009; Gjerris et al., 2009; Bender et al., 2010; Engels et al., 2010). However, few studies found no differences in the value of maternal serum PAPP-A levels in ART conceptions compared to controls (Ghisoni et al., 2003; Bellver et al., 2005; Lambert-Messerlian et al., 2006). The study by Kagan et al. (2008), which is the largest study so far, reported that PAPP-A levels were reduced 10% in pregnancies conceived after assisted reproduction (n = 2115), when compared to controls (n = 94.688). In our study (Matilainen et al., 2011), we found no statistically significant differences in pregnancies conceived after spontaneous FET or HRT-FET, compared with the control group. There are other studies reported that the median PAPP-A MoM level was not significantly reduced in FET pregnancies (Anckaert et al., 2008; Gjerris et al., 2009). There is also a study in which the median PAPP-A MoM levels were significantly reduced in ICSI pregnancies in the fresh and the frozen-thawed embryo subgroups and in the fresh embryo IVF subgroups as compared to controls (Hui et al., 2005). Amor et al. (2009) studied PAPP-A concentration levels in fresh embryo transfers (n = 773) and frozen embryo transfers (n = 573). PAPP-A levels were reduced in both subgroups when compared with spontaneous pregnancies. However, fresh embryo transfers were associated with significantly lower PAPP-A levels when compared with FET pregnancies.

Studies concerning about the free β-hCG concentration levels in assisted reproduction pregnancies are contradictory. In our study (Matilainen et al. 2011), we found no difference in the median free β-hCG MoM concentrations in between the ART and control groups. This is in agreement with most previous studies (Orlandi et al., 2002; Tul et al. 2006; Bellver et al., 2005; Gjerris et al., 2009; Amor et al., 2009). Yet, there are some studies which have reported the free β-hCG levels to be increased in ART pregnancies (Niemimaa et al., 2001; Liao et al., 2001; Ghisoni et al., 2003; Bersinger et al., 2004; Hui et al., 2005). One study even has reported slightly decreased free β-hCG levels in IVF pregnancies (Engels et al., 2010).

The disintegrin and metalloproteinase domain 12 (ADAM12) is a further first-trimester serum marker for Down syndrome (Laigaar et al., 2003) and other chromocomal aberrations (Spencer & Cowans, 2007). There is only one study concerning the use of ADAM12 as a first-trimester Down syndrome screening marker in ART pregnancies (Laigaard et al., 2009). Study group found no alterations in ADAM12 serum marker levels in ART pregnancies when compared with spontaneous pregnancies.

In our study, the odds ratios for a false-positive rate in the combined first-trimester screening for Down syndrome by maternal age, nuchal translucency, and PAPP-A, and free β-hCG, were not increased in women who conceived following ART, after adjustment for maternal age (Matilainen et al. 2011). This is in agreement with many other studies (Maymon and Shulman, 2001b; Liao et al., 2001; Wojdemann et al., 2001; Orlandi et al., 2002; Bellver et al., 2005). There are also studies which have reported higher FPR in the ART group even after adjustment for maternal age (Orlandi et al., 2002; Amor et al., 2009; Gjerris et al., 2009). Tul and the study group (2006) found a higher FPR in pregnancies after ICSI. Amor et al. (2009) found that PAPP-A levels were reduced and FPR was higher, both in fresh and frozen-thawed embryos, but only in pregnancies in which the mother was administered hormone treatment around the time of embryo transfer. First-trimester Down screening which combines maternal age, NT, and biochemical markers may increase the false-positive result in ART pregnancies, therefore, it increase the likelihood of having amniocentesis or chorionic villus sampling. However, contradictory results from previous published works require larger studies. As more information accumulates on serum marker variations in ART pregnancies, procedure-specific medians for serum markers may need to correct changes in pregnancies conceived after ART. Table 1 summarizes the results of the previous studies.

4. Possible explanations for altered serum marker levels in ART pregnancies

There are many possible confounding factors, which could lead to contradictory results on maternal serum screening markers in pregnancies conceived after assisted reproductive techniques. Multiple corpora lutea and multiple implantation sites have been suggested to be the reason for either increased or decreased marker levels (Weisz et al., 2006). It has been recommended that abnormal marker levels could be due to the underlying subtle metabolic or genetic conditions that can also be the reason for infertility itself (Ribbert et al., 1996). It has also been suggested that lower PAPP-A levels in ART pregnancies might be the result of metabolic impairments related to infertility of the mother (Maymon and Shulman, 2002). However, Amor et al. (2009) found that PAPP-A levels were reduced, both in male-factor infertility, female-factor infertility, and the combination of female and male cause. Anckaert et al. (2008) found that PAPP-A values did not differ between male and female infertility. The same study group found higher median free β-hCG level values in non-male infertility compared with male infertility and spontaneous pregnancies.

Also, a functional delay in fetal and placental development and the higher risk of obstetric complications associated with ART, can lead to changes in serum marker concentrations (Maymon et al., 2004; Helmerhorst et al., 2004; Hui et al., 2005, Williams et al., 2009; Henningsen et al., 2011). Studies have shown that low first-trimester PAPP-A levels indicates placenta-related disorders, such as fetal growth restriction, low birth weight, preeclampsia (Papageorghiou et al., 2007; Gagnon et al., 2008; Pihl et al., 2008; Goetzinger et al., 2010). Studies have also shown that maternal and fetal complications occur more often in assisted reproduction pregnancies (Helmerhorst et al., 2004; Amor et al., 2009; Williams et al., 2009; Henningsen et al., 2011). However, Amor et al. (2009) found that PAPP-A levels were reduced in ART pregnancies with or without pregnancy complications (e.g., preeclampsia or low birth weight). In other study by Zhong et al. (2010), ART pregnancies with low PAPP-A level values were at higher risk for small-for-gestational-age infants or preterm delivery less than 32 weeks of gestation when compared with spontaneous pregnancies with low PAPP-A values.

Recent studies have suggested that vanishing twin might have the impact on serum marker level alterations. Spencer et al. (2010) found that in women with a second empty gestational sac, the median PAPP-A and free β-hCG values were not different from the median values in non-ART pregnancies. Yet, they found that median PAPP-A levels were significantly increased in pregnancies with a vanishing twin and a measurable crown-rump length. Median free β-hCG levels were unchanged in those pregnancies. Amor et al. (2009) found

Study	*Natural pregnancies*	*Assisted reproduction pregnancies*	*Free β-hCG*	*PAPP-A*
Liao et al. (2001)	1233	161 (OI)	←→	←→
		220 (IVF)	↑	↓
		30 (ICSI)	←→	↓
Wojdemann et al. (2001)	3026	63 (OI)	←→	←→
		47 (IVF)	←→	←→
Niemimaa et al. (2001)	4265	49 (IVF)	←→	↑
Orlandi et al. (2002)	370	32 (IVF)	←→	↓
		42 (ICSI)	←→	←→
Maymon and Shulman (2002)	285	71 (IVF)	←→	↓
Ghisoni et al. (2003)	435	145 (ART)	↑	←→
Maymon and Shulman (2004)	1781	99 (IVF)	N/A	↓
Hui et al. (2005)	401	92 (IVF)	↓	↓
		57 (ICSI)	←→	↓
		54 (FET/IVF)	←→	←→
		31 (FET/ICSI)	←→	↓
Bellver et al. (2005)	498	97 (OI)	←→	←→
		47 (IVF)	←→	←→
		222 (ICSI)	←→	←→
		71 (OD/IVF)	←→	←→
		119 (OD/ICSI)	↑	←→
Lambert-Messerlian et al. (2006)	37 070	277 (IVF)	↑	↓
Tul and Novac-Antolic (2006)	914	130 (IVF)	←→	↓
Kagan et al. (2008)	97 294	2115 (IVF)	↓	↑
Gjerris et al. (2009)	2532	992 (ALL ART)	←→	↑
		512 (IVF)	←→	↑
		396 (ICSI)	←→	↑
		84 (FET)	←→	←→
Amor et al. (2009)	50 253	1739 (ALL ART)	←→	↑
		654 (IVF)	←→	↑
		1052 (ICSI)	←→	↑
		773 (Fresh IVF/ICSI)	←→	↑
		573 (FET)	←→	↑
Matilainen et al. (2011)	24 783	176 (IVF/ICSI)	←→	↑
		87 (FET)	←→	←→
		19 (HRT-FET)	←→	←→

OI=ovulationinduction,
↓=decreased,↑=increadec,←→=not different

Table 1. Comparison of first trimester biochemical markers in singleton pregnancies achieved spontaneously and by assisted reproduction.

that in their ART population vanished twins appear to increase the PAPP-A levels rather than decrease them. Gjerris et al. (2009) found no effect on PAPP-A and free β-hCG concentration values in ART pregnancies with an early vanishing twin. It is believed that vanished twins do not decrease the PAPP-A levels, in fact, they might have the opposite effect (Amor et al., 2009).

Maymon and Shulman (2002) suggested that a reduction in PAPP-A levels in pregnancies conceived after assisted reproduction might be an artefact of testing being undertaken at an earlier gestation. Amor et al. (2009) found no difference between ART and non-ART pregnancies in the timing of ultrasound examination or blood sampling. However, they did found a slightly greater crown-grump length for frozen-thawed embryos compared to fresh embryos. They suggested that this difference may reflect a longer in-vitro culture time for frozen-thawed embryos, but the difference would not affect the median PAPP-A MoM levels because these values are adjusted for gestational age.

There are several studies that have suggested that exogenous hormone treatment is the main reason for reduced PAPP-A levels in ART pregnancies (Bersinger et al., 2004; Hui et al., 2005a; Tul and Novak-Antolic, 2006; Amor et al., 2009). Amor et al. (2009) examined the effect of hormone treatment versus no hormone treatment irrespective of FET or fresh embryo transfer and found low PAPP-A levels in transfer cycles with any hormone treatment when compared with cycles without hormone treatment. They also found that PAPP-A levels were reduced regardless of the type of ovarian stimulation. In our study, we also found that PAPP-A concentration levels were reduced in hormonally-stimulated IVF/ICSI pregnancies, but there was no statistically significant difference in spontaneous FET pregnancies (Matilainen et al., 2011). Amor et al. (2009) suggested that administration of exogenous hormones interferes with the normal endocrine changes of early pregnancy, resulting in reduced PAPP-A levels. Tul and Novak-Antolic (2006) found significantly decreased PAPP-A concentration levels with increasing numbers of transferred embryos and also with increasing numbers of retrieved oocytes. The authors hypothesized that the number of oocytes retrieved reflected the number of corpora lutea in pregnancies, supported by their other finding that inhibin A, which is secreted by corpora lutea, was increased with decreasing PAPP-A. They suggested that inhibin A inhibits the secretion of PAPP-A. However, Bender et al. (2010) found no correlation between PAPP-A and free β-hCG values and the transfer of one, two or three embryos in assisted reproduction pregnancies.

5. Down syndrome screening in multiple pregnancies

Twin pregnancies are becoming more frequent in most developed countries due to the increased use of assisted reproductive technologies and advanced maternal age (Spencer 2000). Approximately 25% of pregnancies arising from assisted reproduction are twins or higher order multiples. Despite increasing use of elective single-embryo transfer, double or more embryo transfer was in 2004 occur in more than 80% of all ART procedures (Andersen et al., 2008).

During the last three decades various methods of screening for Down syndrome were introduced in clinical practice, yet, specific problems were encountered when they were applied for twin pregnancies. Screening for Down syndrome in twin pregnancies is considered to be difficult because of the clinical, technical and ethical challenges posed for diagnosis and clinical management of such pregnancies (Cuckle, 1998; Spencer and Nicolaides, 2003).

The value of the prenatal screening for Down syndrome by biochemical test in twins is limited because of the masking effect of normal co-twins and the difficulty of pinpointing the abnormal co-twin (Cuckle, 1998); therefore the ultrasound seems to be the better method for Down syndrome screening both for spontaneous and ART twin pregnancies (Maymon et al., 2002). On the basis of the observation that nuchal translucency thickness measurements were comparable in twins and singleton pregnancies affected by Down syndrome, the application of a combination of maternal age and NT measurement as the tool of assessing the risk of trisomy 21 has been advocated in twins (Pandya et al., 1995; Sebire et al., 1996). The same screening strategy has also been proposed for twins produced from ART pregnancies (Maymon et al. 1999). The detection rates for Down syndrome of 75 - 80% have been reported in twin pregnancies using maternal age and NT for risk calculation (Sebire et al. 1996; Kagan et al., 2007).

Chorionicity has an impact on Down screening measurements and first-trimester evaluation in twins is not completed until an accurate chorionity determination is performed (Sepulveda, 1997). The majority of twin pregnancies conceived after ART are dichorionic, yet, the incidence of monochorionic twin pregnancies after ART has increased (Wenstrom et al., 1993). Chorionicity has an impact on the nuchal translucency thickness. In monochorionic twin pregnancies mean fetal nuchal translucency thickness and inter-twin nuchal translucency thickness were larger when compared with dichorionic twin pregnancies (Cheng et al., 2010). In monochorionic twins the increased nuchal translucency thickness and discordance of NT have been associated with adverse pregnancy outcome, such as perinatal death and twin-twin transfusion syndrome (El Kateb et al., 2007; Kagan et al., 2007). Several studies have reported that the median NT measurements did not differed in twin pregnancies conceived after ART when compared to spontaneous pregnancies (Goence et al., 2005; Hui et al., 2005; Maymon et al., 2005). It is recommended that for dichorionic twins each co-twin fetus is treated as a singleton and its risk is calculated using the published distribution of NT values for singleton pregnancies (Maymon et al. 2005). In monochorionic twins, Down syndrome screening is provided by risk calculation based on the average nuchal translucency thickness measurement of two fetuses (Vandecruys et al., 2005).

Adding the PAPP-A and free β-hCG level measurements to nuchal translucency thickness in twin pregnancies may improve the detection rate about 5 - 6% (Spencer and Nicolaides, 2003), but helped mainly to reduce the higher FPR (Goence et al, 2005, Chasen et al., 2007). In twin pregnancies interpreting all the results of these screening markers is more difficult because the serum marker concentration relates to the pregnancy, while each NT measurement is fetus-specific (Maymon et al., 2005). Chorionity is suggested to have an impact on maternal serum marker levels: one study reported lower PAPP-A levels but indifferent free β-hCG values in monochorionic twin pregnancies when compared with dichorionic pregnancies (Spencer et al., 2008). In other study both markers were decreased in monochoric twin pregnancies (Liskens et al., 2009). In two studies, where no differentiation of chorionicity was made, no differences were found in maternal serum concentrations between assisted twin pregnancies and controls (Orlandi et al., 2002; Gonce et al., 2005). It is recommended that when invasive testing is indicated, NT alone is the screening method women should be counseled to choose, because ultrasound is the best mean of specifically locating the affected co-twin (Spencer and Nicolaides, 2003).

6. Conclusion

Pregnancies conceived after ART represent a group of high-risk pregnancies, which carry a higher psychological and financial burden compared to spontaneous pregnancies (Oddens et al., 1999). ART pregnancies differ from spontaneous pregnancies in many aspects, therefore, Down screening among women pregnant after ART is more complicated. The proportion of women aged 35 years or more is higher in ART pregnancies, therefore, a risk of women having a child affected by Down syndrome is also a higher (Geipel et al., 1999; Pinborg et al., 2004; Weisz and Rodeck, 2006, Gjerris et al., 2008). Risk of chromosomal aberrations is increased in pregnancies conceived after intracytoplasmic sperm injection (Aboulghar et al., 2001; Bonduelle et al., 2002; Jozwiak et al., 2004; Gjerris et al., 2008). The proportion of multi-fetal pregnancies is higher in pregnancies conceived after assisted reproduction (Weisz and Rodeck, 2006, Gjerris et al., 2008). Also fetal and maternal complications occur more often in assisted reproduction pregnancies (Helmerhorst et al., 2004; Amor et al., 2009; Williams and Sutcliffe, 2009; Henningsen et al., 2011). The uptake of amniocentesis and villus biopsy is believed to be lower, because of the higher risk of miscarriage. Women pregnant after ART rather choose non-invasive Down screening before making a decision about invasive testing. (Meschede et al., 1998; Schover et al., 1998; Geipel et al., 1999; Geipel et al., 2004).

A number of different first-trimester ultrasound and biochemical markers have been validated in first-trimester screening for Down syndrome. Method of choice in first-trimester Down screening is combined screening, which measures maternal serum levels of free β-hCG and PAPP-A at 9 - 12 weeks of gestation and nuchal translucency by ultrasound at 11 - 13 weeks gestation. These measurements are combined with maternal age, weight, and gestational age to produce an risk estimate of fetus having a Down syndrome (Wald et al., 2003). For pregnancies with increased risk, an invasive procedure can be offered.

Measurement of fetal nuchal translucency thickness is the most investigated screening method and it is believed to be least affected screening method in ART pregnancies. Some studies have reported a small deviation of NT measurements in pregnancies conceived after assisted reproduction, but these alterations did not influence overall screening performance. The majority of the studies found no difference in NT measurements in ART pregnancies compared with spontaneous conceptions (Liao et al., 2001; Nieminen et al., 2001; Wojdemann et al., 2001; Orlandi et al., 2002; Ghisoni et al., 2003; Lambert-Messerlian et al., 2006 and Matilainen et al. 2011) and no influence on the screening performance and the false-positive rate by combining maternal age and NT for Down syndrome risk assessment (Liao et al., 2001; Ghisoni et al., 2003; Bellver et al., 2005; Lambert-Messerlian et al., 2006; Tul and Novac-Antolic, 2006; Ancaert et al., 2008; Bender et al., 2010; Matilainen et al., 2011). The use of new sonographic markers, such as the absence of the nasal bone, has not been explored in ART pregnancies.

Several studies have reported that first-trimester maternal serum free beta-human chorionic gonadotropin and pregnancy-associated plasma protein-A levels are altered in ART pregnancies and might increase the false-positive rate. The reasons behind these alterations are not unambiguous. It has been suggested that e.g. exogenous hormone treatment, functional delay in fetal, and placental development and the higher risk of obstetric complications associated with ART can lead to changes in serum marker concentrations. Pre- and post-test counseling for women carrying ART-pregnancies is extremely important. Further studies should be determined the viability of altering the risk calculation for pregnancies conceived after ART.

Twin pregnancies are becoming more frequent in most developed countries due to the increased use of assisted reproductive technologies and advanced maternal age (Spencer 2000). Down screening in twin pregnancies is considered to be difficult because of the clinical, technical and ethical challenges posed for diagnosis and clinical management of such pregnancies (Cuckle, 1998; Spencer and Nicolaides, 2003). In twin pregnancies chorionicity is an important confounding variable. It is recommended that for dichorionic twins, each co-twin fetus should be treated as a singleton and its risk should be calculated using the published distribution of NT values for singleton pregnancies (Maymon et al. 2005). In monochorionic twins, Down syndrome screening is provided by risk calculation based on the average nuchal translucency thickness measurement of two fetuses (Vandecruys et al., 2005).

7. References

Aboulghar, H., Aboulghar, M., Mansour, R., Serour, G., Amin, Y., & Al-Inany, H. (2001). A prospective controlled study of karyotyping for 430 consecutive babies conceived through intracytoplasmic sperm injection. *Fertil Steril,* Vol.76, No.2, (August 2001), pp. 249–253.

Amor, DJ., Xu, JX., Halliday, JL., Francis, I., Healy, D., Breheny, S., Baker, HW., & Jaques, AM. (2009). Pregnancies conceived using assisted reproductive technologies (ART) have low levels of pregnancy-associated plasma protein-A (PAPP-A) leading to a high rate of false-positive results in first trimester screening for Down syndrome. *Hum Reprod,* Vol.24, No.6 (June 2009), pp.1330-1338.

Anckaert, E., Schiettecatte, J., Sleurs, E., Devroey, P., & Smitz, J. (2008). First trimester screening for Down's syndrome after assisted reproductive technology: non-male factor infertility is associated with elevated free beta-human chorionic gonadotropin levels at 10-14 weeks of gestation. *Fertil Steril,* Vol.90, No.4, (October 2008), pp.1206–1210.

Andersen, AN., Goossens, V., Ferraretti, AP., Bhattacharya, S., Felberbaum, R., de Mouzon, J., & Nygren, KG,. (2008). Assisted reproductive technology in Europe, 2004: results generated from European registers by ESHRE. *Hum Reprod,*Vol. 23, No.4, (April 2008), pp. 756-771.

Avgidou, K., Papageorghiou, A., Bindra, R., Spencer, K., & Nicolaides, KH. (2005). Prospective first-trimester screening for trisomy 21 in 30 564 pregnancies. *Am J Obstet Gynecol,* Vol.192, No.6, (June 2005), pp.1761–1767.

Barkai, G., Goldman, B., Ries, L., Chaki, R., Dor, J., & Cuckle, H. (1996). Down's syndrome screening marker levels following assisted reproduction. *Prenat Diagn,* Vol.16, No.12, (December 1996), pp. 1111–1114.

Bellver, J., Lara, C., Soares, SR., Ramirez, A., Pellicer, A., Remohi, J., & Serra, V. (2005). First trimester biochemical screening for Down's syndrome in singleton pregnancies conceived by assisted reproduction. *Hum Reprod,* Vol.20, No.9, (September 2005), pp. 2623–2627.

Bender, F., Hecken, J., Reinsberg, J., Reinsberg, J., Berg, C., van der Ven, H., Gembruch, U., & Geipel, A. (2010). Altered first-trimester screening markers after IVF/ICSI: no relationship with small-for-gestational-age and number of embryos transferred. *Reprod Biomed Online.* Vol.20, No.4, (April 2010), pp. 516-22.

Bonduelle, M., Van, AE., Joris, H., Keymolen, K., Devroey, P., Van Steirteghem, A., & Liebaers, I. (2002). Prenatal testing in ICSI pregnancies: incidence of chromosomal anomalies in 1586 karyotypes and relation to sperm parameters. *Hum Reprod,* Vol.17, No.10, (October 2002), pp. 2600–2614.

Brambati, B., Macintosh, MC., Teisner, B., Maguiness, S., Shrimanker, K., Lanzani, A., Bonacchi, I., Tului, L., Chard, T., & Grudzinskas, JG. (1993). Low maternal serum levels of pregnancy associated plasma protein A (PAPP-A) in the first trimester in association with abnormal fetal karyotype. *Br J Obstet Gynaecol,* Vol.100, No.4, (April 1993), pp. 324-326.

Chasen, ST., Pernim SC., Kalish, RB., & Chervenak, FA. (2007). First-trimester risk assessment for trisomies 21 and 18 in twin pregnancy. *Am J Obstet Gynecol,* Vol.197, No.4 (October 2007), pp. 374.e1-3.

Cheng, PJ., Huang, SY., Shaw, SW., Hsiao, CH., Kao, CC., Chueh, HY., & Hsieh, TT. (2010). Difference in nuchal translucency between monozygotic and dizygotic spontaneously conceived twins. *Prenat Diagn,* Vol.30, No. 3 (March 2010), pp. 247-250.

Cuckle, H. (1998). Down's syndrome screening in twins. *J Med Screen.* Vol.5, No. 1, pp. 3-4.

de Graaf, IM., Cuckle, HS., Pajkrt, E., Leschot, NJ., Bleker, OP., & van Lith, JM. (2000). Co-variables in first trimester maternal serum screening. *Prenatal diagnostics,* Vol.20, No. 5, (May 2000), pp. 186-189.

El Kateb, A., Nasr, B., Nassar, M., Bernard, JP., & Ville, Y. (2007). First-trimester ultrasound examination and the outcome of monochorionic twin pregnancies. *Prenat Diagn,* Vol.27, No.10, (October 2007), pp. 922-5.

Engels, MA., Kooij, M., Schats, R., Twisk, JW., Blankenstein, MA., & van Vugt, JM. (2010). First-trimester serum marker distribution in singleton pregnancies conceived with assisted reproduction. *Prenat Diagn,* Vol.30, No.4, (April 2010), pp.372-7.

Frishman, GN., Canick, JA., Hogan, JW., Hackett, RJ., Kellner, LH., & Saller, DN Jr. (1997). Serum triple-marker screening in in-vitro fertilization and naturally conceived pregnancies. *Obstet Gynecol,* Vol.90, No.1, (July 1997), pp. 98–101.

Gagnon, A., Wilson, RD., & Audibert, F. (2008). Obstetrical complications associated with abnormal maternal serum markers analytes. *Journal Obstet Gynaecol Can.* Vol.30, No.10 (October 2008), pp. 918-949.

Geipel, A., Gembruch, U., Ludwig, M., Germer, U., Schwinger, E., Dormeier, A., & Diedrich, K. (1999). Genetic sonography as the preferred option of prenatal diagnosis in patients with pregnancies following intracytoplasmic sperm injection. *Hum Reprod,* Vol.14, No.10, (October 1999), pp. 2629–2634.

Geipel, A., Berg, C., Katalinic, A., Ludwig, M., Germer, U., Diedrich, K., & Gemburch, U. (2004). Different preferences for prenatal diagnosis in pregnancies following assisted reproduction versus spontaneous conception. *Reprod Biomed Online,* Vol.8, No. 1, (January 2004), pp.119-124.

Ghisoni, L., Ferrazzi, E., Castagna, C., Levi Setti, PE., Masini, AC., & Pigni, A. (2003). Prenatal diagnosis after ART success: the role of early combined screening tests in counselling pregnant patients. *Placenta,* Vol.24, No. Suppl B, (October 2003), pp.99-103.

Gjerris, AC., Loft, A., Pinborg, A., Christiansen, M., & Tabor, A. (2008). Prenatal testing among women pregnant after assisted reproductive techniques in Denmark 1995-2000: a national cohort study. *Hum Reprod,* Vol.23, No.7, (July 2008), pp. 1545-1552.

Gjerris, AC., Loft, A., Pinborg, A., Christiansen, M., & Tabor, A. (2009). First trimester screening markers are altered in pregnancies conceived after IVF/ICSI. *Ultrasound Obstet Gynecol,* Vol.33, No.1, (January 2009), pp. 8-17.

Goetzinger, KR., Cahill, AG., Macones, GA., & Odibo, AO. (2010) Association of first trimester low PAPP-A levels with pretesm birth. *Prenatal Diagnosis,* Vol.30, No.4, (April 2010), pp. 309-313.

Goncé, A., Borrell, A., Fortuny, A., Casals, E., Martínez, MA., Mercadé, I., Cararach, V., & Vanrell, JA. (2005). First-trimester screening for trisomy 21 in twin pregnancy: does the addition of biochemistry make an improvement? *Prenat Diagn.* Vol.25, No. 12, (December 2005), pp. 1156-61.

Helmerhorst, FM., Perquin, DA., Donker, D., & Keirse, MJ. (2004). Prenatal outcome of singletond and twins after assisted conception: a systematic review of controlled studies. *BMJ,* Vol. 328, No. 7434, (January 2004), pp. 261-265.

Henningsen, AK., Pinborg, A., Lidegaard, O., Vestergaard, C., Forman, JL., & Andersen, AN. (2011). Perinatal outcome of singleton siblings born after assisted reproductive technology and spontaneous conception: Danish national sibling-cohort study. *Fertil Steril,* Vol.95, No.3, (March 2011), pp. 959-963.

Hui, PW., Lam, YH., Tang, MH., Ng, EH., Yeung, WS., & Ho, PC. (2005). Maternal serum pregnancy-associated plasma protein-A and free beta-human chorionic gonadotrophin in pregnancies conceived with fresh and frozen-thawed embryos from in vitro fertilization and intracytoplasmic sperm injection. *Prenat Diagn,* Vol.25, No.5, (May 2005), pp.390–393.

Hui, PW., Tang, MH., Ng, EH., Yeung, WS., & Ho, PC. (2006). Nuchal translucency in dichorionic twins conceived after assisted reproduction. *Prenatal Diagn,* Vol.26, No.6, (June 2006), pp.510-3.

Kagan, KO., Gazzoni, A., Sepulveda-Gonzalez, G., Sotiriadis, A., & Nicolaides, KH. (2007). Discordance in nuchal translucency thickness in the prediction of severe twin-to-twin transfusion syndrome. *Ultrasound Obstet Gynecol,* Vol.29, No.5, (June 2007), pp.527-32.

Kagan, KO., Wright, D., Spencer, K., Molina, FS., & Nicolaides, KH. (2008). First-trimester screening for trisomy 21 by free beta-human chorionic gonadotropin and pregnancy-associated plasma protein-A: impact of maternal and pregnancy characteristics. *Ultrasound Obstet Gynecol* ,Vol.31, No.6, (June 2008), pp.493-502.

Kagan, KO., Staboulidou, I., Cruz, J., Wright, D., & Nicolaides, KH. (2010). Two-stage first-trimester screening for trisomy 21 by ultrasound assessment and biochemical testing. *Ultrasound Obstet Gynecol,* Vol.36, No.5, (November 2010), pp.542-7.

Jozwiak, EA., Ulug, U., Mesut, A., Erden, HF., & Bahcecim M. (2004). Prenatal karyotypes of fetuses conceived by intracytoplasmic sperm injection. *Fertil Steril,*Vol.82, No.3, (September 2004), pp.628–633.

Laigaard, J., Sørensen, T., Fröhlich, C., Pedersen, BN., Christiansen, M., Schiøtt, K., Uldbjerg, N., Albrechtsen, R., Clausen, HV., Ottesen, B., & Wewer, UM. (2003). ADAM12: a novel first-trimester maternal serum marker for Down syndrome. *Prenat Diagn.* Vol.23, No.13, (December 2003), pp.1086-91.

Laigaard, J., Pedersen, NG., Larsen, SO., Hedley, PL., Wøjdemann, K., Gjerris, AC., Shalmi, AC., Sundberg, K., Tabor, A., & Christiansen, M. (2009). ADAM12 in first trimester maternal serum from pregnancies conceived by assisted reproduction techniques (ART). *Prenat Diagn,* Vol.29, No.6, (June 2009), pp.628-9.

Lambert-Messerlian, G., Dugoff, L., Vidaver, J., Canick, JA., Malone, FD., Ball, RH., Comstock CH., Nyberg, DA., Saade, G., & Eddleman, K., et al. (2006). First- and second-trimester Down syndrome screening markers in pregnancies achieved through assisted reproductive technologies (ART): a FASTER trial study. *Prenat Diagn*,Vol.26, No. 8, (August 2006), pp.672–678.

Liao, AW., Heath, V., Kametas, N., Spencer, K., & Nicolaides, KH. (2001). First-trimester screening for trisomy 21 in singleton pregnancies achieved by assisted reproduction. *Hum Reprod,* Vol.16, No.7, (July 2001), pp. 1501–1504.

Linskens, IH., Spreeuwenberg, MD., Blankenstein, MA., & van Vugt, JM. (2009). Early first-trimester free beta-hCG and PAPP-A serum distributions in monochorionic and dichorionic twins. *Prenat Diagn*,Vol.29, No.1, (January 2009), pp.74-78.

Matilainen, M., Peuhkurinen, S., Laitinen, P., Jarvela, I., Morin-Papunen, L., & Ryynanen, M. (2011). In combined first-trimester Down syndrome screening, the false-positive rate is not higher in pregnancies conceived after assisted reproduction compared with spontaneous pregnancies. Fertil Steril, Vol.95, No. 1, (January 2011), pp.378-81.

Maymon, R., Dreazen, E., Tovbin, Y., Bukovsky, I., Weinraub, Z., & Herman, A. (1999). The feasibility of nuchal translucency measurement in higher order multiple gestations achieved by assisted reproduction. *Hum Reprod* Vol.14, No.8, (August 1999), pp. 2102–2105.

Maymon, R., Jauniaux, E., Holmes, A., Wiener, YM., Dreazen, E., & Herman, A. (2001). Nuchal translucency measurement and pregnancies outcomes after assisted conception versus spontaneously conceived twins. *Hum Reprod,* Vol.16: No.9, (September 2001), pp.1999-2004.

Maymon, R., & Shulman, A. (2002). Serial first- and second trimester Down's syndrome screening tests among IVF-versus naturally -conceived singletons. *Hum Reprod,* Vol.17, No.4, (April 2002), pp. 1081-1085.

Maymon, R., & Shulman, A. (2004). Integrated first- and second-trimester Down syndrome screening test among unaffected IVF pregnancies. *Prenat Diagn,* Vol.24, No.2, (February 2004), pp.125–129.

Maymon, R., Neeman, O., Shulman, A., Rosen, H., & Herman, A. (2005). Current concepts of Down syndrome screening tests in assisted reproduction twin pregnancies: another double trouble. *Prenat Diagn,* Vol.25, No.9, (September 2005), pp.746-50.

Meschede, D., Lemcke, B., Stussel, J., Louwen, F., & Horst, J. (1998). Strong preference for non-invasive prenatal diagnosis in women pregnant through intracytoplasmic sperm injection (ICSI). *Prenat Diagn,* Vol.89, No 7. (July 1998), pp.248-251.

Nicolaides KH. (2004). Nuchal translucency and other first-trimester sonographic markers on chromosomal abnormalities. *Am J Obstet Gynecol,* Vol.191, No.1 (July 2004), pp. 45-67.

Nicolaides, KH., Spencer, K., Avgidou, K., Faiola, S., & Falcon, O. (2005). Multicenter study of first-trimester screening for trisomy 21 in 75 821 pregnancies: results and estimation of the potential impact of individual risk-orientated two-stage first-trimester screening. *Ultrasound Obstet Gynecol, Vol.*25, No. 3, (March 2005), pp. 221–226.

Niemimaa, M., Heinonen, S., Seppala, M., Hippelainen, M., Martikainen, H.,& Ryynanen, M. (2001). First-trimester screening for Down's syndrome in in vitro fertilization pregnancies. *Fertility & Sterility*.Vol.76, No.6, (December 2001), pp.1282-3.

Niemimaa, M., Heinonen, S., Seppala, M., & Ryynanen, M. (2003). The influence of smoking on the pregnancy-associated plasma protein A, free beta human chorionic gonadotropin and nuchal translucency. *BJOG*, Vol.110, No.7, (July 2003), pp.664-667.

Oddens, BJ., den Tonkelaar, I., & Nieuwenhuyse, H. (1999). Psychosocial experiences in women facing fertility problems--a comparative survey. *Hum Reprod.* Vol.14, No.1, (January 1999), pp.225-61.

Orlandi, F., Rossi, C., & Allegra, A. et al. (2002). First trimester screening with free beta-hCG, PAPP-A and nuchal translucency in pregnancies conceived with assisted reproduction. *Prenat Diagn*, Vol.22, No.8, (August 2002), pp.718-721.

Pandya, PP., Hilbert, F., Snijders, RJ., & Nicolaides, KH. (1995). Nuchal translucency thickness and crown-rump length in twin pregnancies with chromosomally abnormal fetuses. *J Ultrasound Med* Vol.14, No.8, (August 1995), pp. 565–568.

Papageorghiou, AT., & Leslie, K. (2007). Uterine artery Doppler in the prediction of adverse pregnancy outcome. *Current Opinion of Obstetrics and Gynaecology.* Vol.19, No.2, (April 2007), pp. 103-109.

Pihl, K., Larsen, T., Krebs, L., & Christiansen, M. (2008). First trimester maternal serum PAPP-A, beta-hCG and ADAM12 in prediction of small-for-gestational-age foetuses. *Prenatal Diagnosis.* Vol.28, No.12, (December 2008), pp.1131-1135.

Pinborg, A., Loft, A., Rasmussen, S., Schmidt, L., Langhoff-Roos, J., Greisen, G., & Andersen, AN. (2004). Neonatal outcome in a Danish national cohort of 3438 IVF/ICSI and 10,362 non-IVF/ICSI twins born between 1995 and 2000. *Hum Reprod* Vol.19, No.2, (February, 2004), pp. 435–441.

Raty, R., Virtanen, A., Koskinen, P., Anttila, L., Forsstrom, J., Laitinen, P., Morsky, P., Tiitinen, A., & Ekblad, U. (2002). Serum free beta-HCG and alphafetoprotein levels in IVF, ICSI and frozen embryo transfer pregnancies in maternal mid-trimester serum screening for Down's syndrome. *Hum Reprod,* Vol.17, No.2, (February 2002), pp.481–484.

Ribbert, LS., Kornman, LH., De Wolf, BT., Simons, AH., Jansen, CA., Beekhuis, JR., & Mantingh, A. (1996). Maternal serum screening for fetal Down syndrome in IVF pregnancies. *Prenat Diagn,* Vol.16, No. 1, (January 1996), pp.35–38.

Schover, LR., Thomas, AJ., Falcone, T., Attaran, M., & Goldberg, J. (1998). Attitudes about genetic risk of couples undergoing in-vitro fertilization. *Hum Reprod*, Vol.13, No.4, (April 1998), pp.862-866.

Sebire, NJ., Snijders, RJ., Hughes, K., Sepulveda, W., & Nicolaides, KH. (1996). Screening for trisomy 21 in twin pregnancies by maternal age and fetal nuchal translucency thickness at 10–14 weeks of gestation. *Br J Obstet Gynaecol* Vol.103, No.10, (October 1996), pp. 999–1003.

Sepulveda, W. (1997). Chorionity determination in twin pregnancies; double trouble. *Ultrasound Obtet Gynecol.* Vol.10, No.2, (August 1997), pp.79-81.

Snijders, RJ., Noble, P., Sebire, N., Souka, A., & Nicolaides, KH. (1998). UK multicentre project on assessment of risk of trisomy 21 by maternal age and fetal nuchal-translucency thickness at 10-14 weeks of gestation. Fetal Medicine Foundation First Trimester Screening Group. *Lancet* Vol.352, No.9125, (August 1998), pp. 343–346.

Spencer, K., Macri, JN., Aitken, DA., & Connor, JM. (1992). Free beta-hCG as first-trimester marker for fetal trisomy. *Lancet,* Vol.339, No.8807, (June 19992), pp.1480.

Spencer, K. (1999). The influence of smoking on maternal serum PAPP-A and free beta-hCG levels in the first trimester of pregnancy. *Prenatal diagnostics,* Vol.19, No.11, (November 1999), pp.1065-1066.

Spencer, K., Souter, V., Tul, N., Snijders, R., & Nicolaides, KH. (1999). A screening program for trisomy 21 at 10–14 weeks using fetal nuchal translucency, maternal serum free beta-human chorionic gonadotropin and pregnancy-associated plasma protein-A. *Ultrasound Obstet Gynecol* Vol.13, No.4, (April 1999), pp. 231-237.

Spencer K. (2000). Screening for trisomy 21 in twin pregnancies in the first trimester using free β-hCG and PAPP-A combined with fetal nuchal translucency thickness. *Prenat Diagn,* Vol.20, No.2, (February 2000), pp.91–95.

Spencer, K., Spencer, CE., Power, M., Dawson, C., & Nicolaides, KH. (2003a). Screening for chromosomal abnormalities in the first trimester using ultrasound and maternal serum biochemistry in a one stop clinic: a review of three years prospective experience. *BJOG,* Vol.110, No.3, (March 2003), pp.281–286.

Spencer, K., Bindra, R., & Nicolaides, KH. (2003b). Maternal weight correction of maternal serum PAPP-A and free beta-hCG MoM when screening for trisomy 21 in the first trimester of pregnancy. *Prenat Diagn, Vol.*23, No. 10, (October 2003), pp. 851–855.

Spencer, K., & Nicolaides, KH. (2003c). Screening fot trisomy 21 in twins using first trimester ultrasound and maternal serum biochemistry in a one-stop clinic: a review of three years experience. Br J Obstet Gynaecol Vol.110, No.3, (March 2003), pp.276-280.

Spencer, K. (2003). Aneuploidy screening in the first trimester. *AmJ med Genet C Semin Med Genet* Vol.145, No.1, (April 2003), pp.18-32.

Spencer, K., & Cowans, NJ. (2007). ADAM12 as a marker of trisomy 18 in the first and second trimester of pregnancy. *J Mater Fetal Neonatal Med* Vol.20, No.9, (April 2007), pp.645-650.

Spencer, K., Kagan, KO., & Nicolaides, KH. (2008). Screening for trisomy 21 in twin pregnancies in the first trimester: an update of the impact of chorionicity on maternal serum markers. *Prenat Diagn.* Vol.28, No.1, (January 2008), pp.49-52.

Spencer, K., Staboulidou, I., & Nicolaides, KH. (2010). First trimester aneuploidy screening in the presence of a vanishing twin: implications for maternal serum markers. *Prenatal Diagnosis.* Vol.30, No.3, (March 2010), pp.235-240.

Tul, N. & Novak-Antolic, Z. (2006). Serum PAPP-A levels at 10-14 weeks of gestation are altered in women after assisted conception. *Prenat Diagn,* Vol.26, No.13, (December 2006), pp.1206-1211.

Vandecruys, H., Faiola, S., Auer, M., Sebire, N., & Nicolaides, KH. (2005). Screening for trisomy 21 in monochorionic twins by measurement of fetal nuchal translucency thickness. *Ultrasound Obstet Gynecol.* Vol.25, No.6, (June 2005), pp.551-3.

Wald, NJ., Cuckle, HS., Densem, JW., Nanchahal, K., Royston, P., Chard, T., Haddow, JE., Knight, GJ., Palomaki, GE., & Canick, JA. (1988). Maternal serum screening for Down's syndrome in early pregnancy. *BMJ* Vol.297, No. 6657, (October 1998), pp. 883-887.

Wald, NJ., White, N., Morris, JK., Huttly, WJ., & Canick, JA. (1999). Serum markers for Down's syndrome in women who have had in vitro fertilisation: implications for antenatal screening. *BJOG* Vol.106, No.12, (December 1999), pp.1304–1306.

Wald, NJ., Rodeck, C., Hackshaw, AK., Walters, J., Chitty, L., & Mackinson, AM. (2003). First and second trimester antenatal screening for Down's syndrome: the results of the

Serum, Urine and Ultrasound Screening Study (SURUSS). *J Med Screen.* Vol.10, No.2, pp.56-104.

Weisz, B.,& Rodeck, CH. (2006). An update on antenatal screening for Down's syndrome and specific implications for assisted reproduction pregnancies. *Hum Reprod Update* Vol.12, No.5, (September-October 2006), pp. 513-518.

Williams, C., & Sutcliffe, A. (2009). Infant outcomes of assisted reproduction assisted repsoduction. *Early Hum Dev.* Vol.85, No.11, (November 2009), pp. 673-677.

Wenstrom, KD., Syrop, CH., Hammitt, DG., & Van Voorhis, BJ., (1993). Increased risk of monochorionic twinning associated with assisted reproduction. *Fertil Steril,* Vol. 60, No.3, (September 1993),pp.510-514.

Wojdemann, KR., Larsen, SO., Shalmi, A., Sundberg, K., Christiansen, M., & Tabor, A. (2001). First trimester screening for Down syndrome and assisted reproduction: no basis for concern. *Prenat Diagn,* Vol.21, No.7, (July 2001), pp. 563-565.

Wojdemann, KR., Shalmi, AC., Christiansen, M., Larsen, SO., Sundberg, K., Brocks, V., Bang, J., Norgaard-Pedersen, B., & Tabor, A. (2005). Improved first-trimester Down syndrome screening performance by lowering the false-positive rate: a prospective study of 9941 low risk women. *Ultrasound Obstet Gynecol* Vol.25, No.3, (March 2005), pp. 227-233.

Zhong, Y., Bradshaw, R., Stanley, AP., & Odibo, AO. (2010). The impact of assisted reproduction technology on the association between first-trimester pregnancy-associated plasma protein-A and human chorionic gonadotropin and adverse pregnancy outcomes. *Am J Perinatol* Vol.28, No.5, (May 2011), pp. 347-354).